Lecture Notes in Computer Science 8315

Commenced Publication in 1973
Founding and Former Series Editors:
Gerhard Goos, Juris Hartmanis, and Jan van Leeuwen

Editorial Board

Jeremy Gibbons   Wendy MacCaull (Eds.)

Foundations of Health Information Engineering and Systems

Third International Symposium, FHIES 2013
Macau, China, August 21-23, 2013
Revised Selected Papers

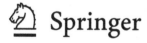 Springer

Volume Editors

Jeremy Gibbons
Oxford University
Department of Computer Science
Wolfson Building, Parks Road
Oxford OX1 3QD, UK
E-mail: jeremy.gibbons@cs.ox.ac.uk

Wendy MacCaull
St. Francis Xavier University
Department of Mathematics
P.O. Box 5000
Antigonish, NS B2G 2W5, Canada
E-mail: wmaccaul@stfx.ca

ISSN 0302-9743   e-ISSN 1611-3349
ISBN 978-3-642-53955-8   e-ISBN 978-3-642-53956-5
DOI 10.1007/978-3-642-53956-5
Springer Heidelberg New York Dordrecht London

Library of Congress Control Number: 2013956644

CR Subject Classification (1998): J.3, D.2.4, H.4.1, H.2.7, D.2.11-12, I.6

LNCS Sublibrary: SL 2 – Programming and Software Engineering

Typesetting: Camera-ready by author, data conversion by Scientific Publishing Services, Chennai, India

Printed on acid-free paper

Springer is part of Springer Science+Business Media (www.springer.com)

Preface

Information and communication technology (ICT) plays an increasingly enabling role in addressing the global challenges of healthcare, in both the developed and the developing world. The use of software in medical devices has caused growing concerns in relation to safety and efficacy. The increasing adoption of health information systems has the potential to provide great benefits but also poses severe risks, both with respect to security and privacy and in regard to patient safety. Hospital and other information systems raise important issues concerning workflow support and interoperability. Regulators, manufacturers and clinical users have pointed out the need for research to develop sound and science-based engineering methods that facilitate the development and certification of quality ICT systems in health care. Such methods may draw from or combine techniques from various disciplines, including but not limited to software engineering, electronic engineering, computing science, information science, mathematics, and industrial engineering.

The purpose of the symposium series on Foundations of Health Information Engineering and Systems (FHIES) is to promote a nascent research area that aims to develop and apply theories and methods from a variety of disciplines, including those listed above, for the purpose of modeling, building and certifying software-intensive ICT systems in healthcare. A particular objective of FHIES is to explicitly include a focus on healthcare ICT applications in the developing world (in addition to systems used in the developed countries), since unique engineering challenges arise in that special setting. Because humans often play a pivotal role in the process of using such systems, theories from the human factors engineering community may need to be integrated with methods from the technology-oriented domains in order to create effective engineering methodologies for socio-technical systems in the healthcare domain. Previous FHIES symposia were held in 2011, in Mabalingwe, South Africa (with post-conference proceedings in Springer LNCS 7151), and in 2012, in Paris, France (with post-conference proceedings in Springer LNCS 7789).

The Third International Symposium on Foundations of Health Information Engineering and Systems (FHIES 2013) took place at the United Nations University International Institute for Software Technology (UNU-IIST) in Macau, between 21st to 23rd August 2013. This volume contains the postproceedings of the symposium.

There were 22 submissions: 14 'full' papers (original research contributions, application experience and case studies, surveys and state-of-the-art reports, position papers describing research projects) and 8 'short' papers (extended abstracts, student papers on work in progress, birds-of-a-feather proposals). Each submission was reviewed by three or four members of the Program Committee, except for 3 short papers that had two reviews each. A week-long online discussion determined the outcome: 19 submissions were accepted and 3 rejected. Two papers were subsequently withdrawn, so in the end there were 13 'full' and 4 'short' contributed papers.

There were also 2 panel sessions and 3 keynote talks on issues central to the mandate of FHIES. The panelists' position statements are included in this volume, as is a full paper co-authored by one of the keynote speakers, Jane Liu, upon which her talk was based. The abstracts of the other two keynote talks were as follows.

Deploying mHealth Technologies in India: Successes, Failures, and Lessons Learned (Bill Thies, Microsoft Research India)
The global spread of mobile phones has ignited broad aspirations regarding the potential role of technology in improving health in impoverished communities. However, researchers and policymakers often meet with surprises when deploying new technologies in resource-poor environment. In this talk, I will describe lessons learned in deploying technologies for health and human development with colleagues in India over the past five years. I will structure the talk around three case studies: a voice portal for citizen reporting, a biometric system for tracking tuberculosis medications, and a mobile data collection tool for childhood malnutrition. I will highlight both successes and failures, and synthesize our experiences into a set of recommendations for future mHealth interventions.

Patient, Heal Thyself: How Technology Can Facilitate Patient Self-Care (Joseph Cafazzo, Centre for Global eHealth Innovation)
Patients have the ability to demonstrate astounding self-care behavior. Who are these patients? What are their identifiable attributes? How can technology elicit this behavior in others for their benefit and the benefit of our strained healthcare delivery system? We know that patients actively seek information for diagnoses, treatment and managing their own care. Our research looks at how access to information and the use of technology affect patient behavior in managing their condition. The aim is to understand how the healthcare system and its providers can support and accommodate these patients for improved, cost-effective, health outcomes.

We thank the members of the Program Committee and the external referees for their care and diligence in reviewing the submitted papers. The review process and compilation of the proceedings were greatly helped by Andrei Voronkov's EasyChair system, which we can highly recommend. We gratefully acknowledge sponsorship from the Macau Foundation and the Macau Science and Technology Development Fund. Finally, we especially thank Wendy Hoi, Alice Pun, Vanessa Madera, and Johannes Faber at UNU, for their organizational efforts, and the participants for making the event a lively success.

November 2013

Jeremy Gibbons
Wendy MacCaull

Organization

Program Committee

Ime Asangansi	University of Oslo, Norway
Tom Broens	Mobihealth, The Netherlands
Lori Clarke	University of Massachusetts, USA
David Clifton	University of Oxford, UK
Gerry Douglas	University of Pittsburgh, USA
Johannes Faber	International Institute for Software Technology, United Nations University, Macau
Jeremy Gibbons	University of Oxford, UK
Jozef Hooman	Embedded Systems Institute and Radboud University Nijmegen, The Netherlands
Michaela Huhn	Technische Universität Clausthal, Germany
Shinsaku Kiyomoto	KDDI R&D Laboratories Inc., Japan
Craig Kuziemsky	University of Ottawa, Canada
Yngve Lamo	Bergen University College, Norway
Insup Lee	University of Pennsylvania, USA
Orlando Loques	Instituto de Computação—Universidade Federal Fluminense, Brazil
Wendy MacCaull	St. Francis Xavier University, Canada
Dominique Mery	Université de Lorraine, LORIA, France
Deshendran Moodley	University of KwaZulu-Natal, South Africa
Jun Pang	University of Luxembourg
Manfred Reichert	University of Ulm, Germany
Ita Richardson	LERO, University of Limerick, Ireland
David Robertson	University of Edinburgh, UK
Christopher Seebregts	Jembi Health Systems, South Africa
Alan Wassyng	McMaster University, Canada

Additional Reviewers

Lu Feng	University of Pennsylvania, USA
Joris Mulder	Tilburg University, The Netherlands

Table of Contents

Patient Safety

Device Safety

Formal Methods

HIV/AIDS and Privacy

Intelligent Tools for Reducing Medication Dispensing and Administration Error

Pei-Hsuan Tsai[1] and Jane W.S. Liu[2]

[1] Inst. of Manufacturing Info. and Sys., National Cheng-Kung University, Tainan, Taiwan
phtsai@mail.ncku.edu.tw
[2] Institute of Information Science, Academia Sinica, Taipei, Taiwan
janeliu@iis.sinica.edu.tw

Abstract. This paper presents an overview of smart medication dispensing and administration devices and software tools designed to minimize dispensing and administration errors. Some of them are for users who take medications on a long term basis without close professional supervision; others are for pharmacy and nursing staffs in hospitals, long term care, and assisted living facilities. These tools should be configurable, customizable, easy to use and effective for diverse users and care-providing institutions. The paper describes approaches taken to meet these objectives.

Keywords: Automated medication management, medication scheduling barcode medication administration, intelligent monitor and alert.

1   Introduction

For years now, professional literature and mass media have been telling us almost everyday of new drugs that can do wonders in curing some previously fatal diseases or help people live with the diseases and chronic conditions better and longer. Unfortunately, they also tell us too often stories (e.g., [1-4]) about medication errors and serious consequences of the errors.

As defined by US FDA (Food and Drug Administration), a medication error is "any preventable event that may cause or lead to inappropriate medication use or patient harm while the medication is in the control of the health care professional, patient, or consumer" [5]. Despite efforts in recent decades to improve medication safety, the rate of medication error remains high even in technologically advanced countries. For example, according to a report published by Institute of Medicine in 2006 [6], a typical (US) hospital patient is subjected to an average of at least one medication error per day. Apparently, this statement is still true today. The Medication Safety Basics webpage of the US CDC (Center for Disease Control and Prevention) [7] states that annually, ADEs (Adverse Drug Events) lead to 700,000 emergency department visits, 120,000 hospitalizations, and $3.5 billion extra medical costs in USA. (Globally, the estimated cost of medication errors is €4.5 – 21.8 billion [8]). CDC expects the numbers of ADEs to grow for reasons including an aging

J. Gibbons and W. MacCaull (Eds.): FHIES 2013, LNCS 8315, pp. 1–21, 2014.
© Springer-Verlag Berlin Heidelberg 2014

population and increasing use of medications for disease prevention. Indeed, according to [9-11], 40 % of people over 65 take 5-9 medications, and 18% of them take 10 or more, on a long term basis without close professional supervision. A consequence is that the rate of ADEs for elderly individuals is many times that of younger people.

These alarming statistics have motivated numerous efforts in development, deployment and assessment of guidelines, methods, systems and tools for prevention of medication errors (e.g., [12-25]). Medication errors can occur throughout the medication use process of ordering, transcribing, dispensing, and administering. Prior to the advent of computerized physician order entry (CPOE) systems [15], errors introduced during ordering and transcribing account for more than half of all errors. CPOE systems are now widely used in hospitals and clinics in developed countries. Data available to date show that together with clinical decision support and electronic patient health record (ePHR) and medication administration record (eMAR) systems, CPOE has been effective [16], [17], [23] [24]. For example, according to Radley, *et al.* [16], data available in 2008 indicate that electronic prescribing through CPOE systems led to 41-55% reduction of prescription errors in US hospitals. Based on the adoption rate of CPOE systems in USA at the time, they estimate a 12.5% reduction in total medication errors, or approximately 17 million fewer errors per year.

Next to prescribing errors, medication administration errors are the most prevalent and contribute 25 – 40% of all preventable medication errors in hospital settings. An *administration error* is a failure to comply with medication directions due to the administration of a wrong drug, with a wrong dosage, at a wrong time, via a wrong route, or to a wrong patient. The chance of making such mistakes can be reduced when medications and patients are identified by their barcode identifiers and when the right medications are given to the right patient is verified at each administration time with the help of barcode medication administration (BCMA) [18] and eMAR systems. Published data (e.g. [20-22]) have shown that institutions using these systems can reduce administration errors significantly (e.g., by 41%) despite challenges in using them in suboptimal settings and potential errors introduced by workarounds [22]. Today, barcode medication administration and dispensing are supported by modern bedside computers, medication carts and medication dispensing systems such as the ones listed at [26] and [27].

This paper presents an overview of two systems of intelligent tools for the reduction of medication dispensing and administration errors: They are *iMAT* (*intelligent medication administration tools*) and *MeMDAS* (*medication management, dispensing and administration system*). iMAT [28-30] is a family of prototype embedded devices, mobile applications and software tools designed to help their users stay compliant to medication directions while providing them with flexibility in scheduling whenever possible and customization in monitoring and alert capabilities. The targeted users are people who take medications outside of health-care institutions, including elderly individuals and people with chronic conditions living independently.

Fig. 1 shows how iMAT fits in the tool chain for medication use process: An iMAT mobile application or embedded device can be used as a point-of-service tool by a hospital to extend its care of a discharged patient who must remain on a rigorous medication regimen for weeks and months. Such tools may also be consumer electronics purchased by the users themselves or by their friends and family members. Indeed, by searching the web and specialty stores, one can find hundreds of pillboxes, medication managers, etc. (e.g., [31-33]) with subsets of iMAT functionalities.

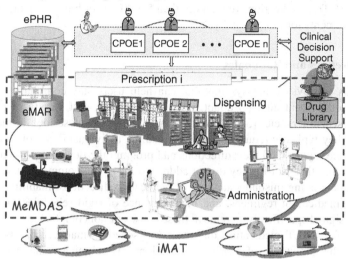

Fig. 1. iMAT and MeMDAS in Tool Chain for Medication Use Process

MeMDAS [34], [35] is a system of intelligent medication dispensing and administration tools for pharmacy and nursing staffs in hospitals, long term care, and assisted living facilities. As Fig. 1 shows, it complements CPOE systems within the tool chain for medication use process. In addition to supporting experimentation with BCMA and barcode medication dispensing (BCMD) by Taiwan University Hospital, the prototype was built to demonstrate several novel concepts and capabilities. They include configurability and customizability of the tools, not only by IT staff of the institutions but also by end-users themselves, and an intelligent monitor, alert and notification (iMAN) tool for detecting user-specified event and action sequences that warrant alerts and notifications be sent to designated person(s) and tools.

The remainder of the paper is organized as follows. Sections 2 and 3 present the motivations, use scenarios and distinguishing capabilities and characteristics of iMAT and MeMDAS, respectively. Section 4 discusses a model-based approach for design, implementation and evaluation of these tools. Section 5 concludes the paper.

2 iMAT - Intelligent Medication Administration Tools

Again, iMAT [28-30] is a system of devices and software tools for reducing the rate and severity of ADEs for people taking medications at home and work, during travels, and so on. Our work on iMAT was a major thrust of the SISARL (Sensor Information Systems for Active Retirees and Assisted Living) Project (2006-2009) [36]. As the project name indicates, its research focus is on technologies for building personal and home automation and assistive devices and systems that can improve the quality of life and self-reliance of their users. Targeted users include the growing population of elderly individuals and people with chronic conditions who are well enough to live active, independent lifestyles. Such a person may take many prescriptions and over the counter (OTC) medications (e.g., more than 5 or 10 according to [9] and [10]) and health supplements for months and years.

2.1   Objectives and Rationales

The benefits of devices and systems that can help users stay compliant and avoid ADEs are self-evident and, no doubt have motivated the vast variety of pillboxes, medication schedulers, etc. [31-33] on the market today. A close look at these tools shows that they typically require the user to load the individual doses of medications into the device, understand their directions and program the device to send reminders accordingly. In other words, they do not address some of the common causes of non-compliance, including misunderstanding of medication directions, inability to adhere to complex medication regimens, and inconvenience of rigid schedules. In contrast, iMAT is designed specifically to remove these causes of noncompliance.

A user of a iMAT medication dispenser and schedule manager has no need to understand the directions of her/his medications. To eliminate the need, iMAT enables the pharmacist of each user to extract a machine-readable *medication schedule specification* (*MSS*) from the user's prescriptions and OTC directions. Once the user's MSS is loaded into his/her iMAT dispenser or schedule manager, the tool automatically generates a medication schedule that meets all the constraints specified by the specification. Based on the schedule, the tool reminds the user each time a dose of some medication should be taken and provides instructions on how the dose should be taken (e.g., with 8 oz of water, no food within 30 minutes, etc.). In this way, iMAT helps to make complex regimens easy to follow.

For users on medications for months and years, tardiness in response to reminders is unavoidable. Directions of modern medications typically provide some flexibility in choices of dose size and time and instructions on what to do in case of late or missed doses. The iMAT scheduler uses scheduling models and algorithms [37-39] that can take advantage of this leeway to make the user's medication schedule easy to adhere. To tolerate user's tardiness, the tool monitors the user's response to reminders, adjusts the medication schedule as instructed by the MSS when the user is tardy, and when a non-compliance event becomes unavoidable, sends alert and notification in ways specified by MSS (e.g., notify the user's physician) and the user (e.g., record the miss). Thus, the tool helps to reduce the rate and ill effects of non-compliance.

Dispensing can be a weak link in medication safety for people taking medications outside care-providing institutions. A typical user targeted by iMAT may be under the care of multiple physicians and given prescriptions ordered via multiple CPOE systems. While each of the user's prescriptions is error free, it may fail to account for interactions between medications ordered by other prescriptions. The user may also take OTC and herbal medicines that may interact with her/his prescription drugs. To reduce the chance for errors due to drug interactions, iMAT imposes on the user two usage restrictions: First, the user lets his/her iMAT manage all his/her prescription and OTC medications since no tool can be effective otherwise. Although the tool does not manage food, it must take into account of user's preferences and habits in meals and snacks when they interfere with some of the user's medications. Second, the user's MSS is generated from the directions of all his/her medications by the user's pharmacist using an authoring tool [30], [40]. A function of the tool is to merge all the human-readable directions and translate them to a standard machine-readable format to enable automatic scheduling as stated above. The other critical function is to check all the directions for possible conflicts (i.e., drug interactions that have not been properly taken into account by the user's prescriptions and directions). When the tool detects possible conflict(s), it alerts the pharmacist to have the conflict resolved. For this purpose, as well as for the generation of MSS, iMAT also has a database containing medication directions in XML format, the format used by the iMAT prototype. We will return shortly to provide specifics. Fig. 2 shows where this tool, called the MSS Authoring tool in the figure, is used in a scenario assumed by iMAT.

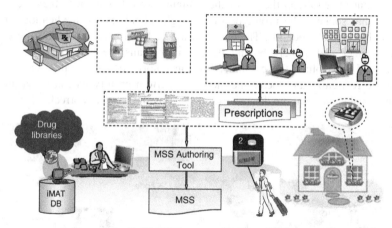

Fig. 2. iMAT Use scenario (From [30])

2.2   Structures and Key Components

Specifically, Fig. 2 assumes that the user has a medication dispenser. It holds his/her medications and helps him/her take them at home: The tool makes sure that the user retrieves the right dose of each medication from the right container when he/she responds to reminder at each dose time. The medication scheduler component of the dispenser can serve as a schedule manager. When the user is away from home and carries the medications with him/her on the road, the schedule manager provides reminders to the user by sending text and voice messages, with or without pictures of the medications, to his/her smart phone, as the lower right part of the figure illustrates. When the dispenser is connected to the Internet, the user can acknowledge the receipt of each reminder and report his/her action taken as response to the reminder.

The scenario assumes that the user's pharmacy supports the dispenser and has access to the user's medication record. When the user goes to fill a new prescription or purchase some OTC drug, the pharmacist uses the MSS authoring tool to process the new direction(s) together with the directions of medications currently taken by the user according to the user's record and after making sure all conflicts have been resolved, generate a new MSS for the user's dispenser. The pharmacist gives the user the MSS in a memory card (or loads the MSS to the user's dispenser via the Internet) and new supplies of medications in containers. Each container holds a medication marked by the universal identifier of the medication.

Fig. 3 shows two dispenser prototypes. They are similar in general: Each dispenser has a base. Medication containers are plugged in the base. An interlock mechanism in the base makes sure that the containers, once plugged in, are locked in place. A container can be removed, or its lid can be opened, only when a dose of the medication in it is due to be taken and the user responds in time to the dispenser's reminder by pressing the PTD (Push-To-Dispend) button. The prototype on the left tags each container by the radio frequency identifier (RFID) of the medication. When the user plugs a container into an empty socket in the base, the action triggers the dispenser controller to read the tag of the container and thus identify the medication located at that socket. The prototype on the right identifies the medications in the containers by their barcode ids. The one shown here has a window in the front with a barcode scanner and camera behind it. The user scans the barcode of each new container and then plugs the container into an empty socket and thus enables the dispenser to recognize and locate the medication. Both prototypes can use a built-in webcam to make sure that the dose sizes retrieved by the user are correct.

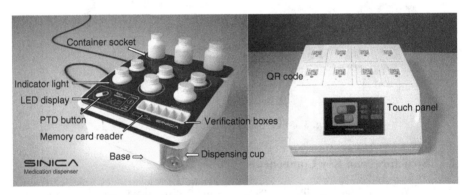

Fig. 3. Physical appearance of two prototype dispensers

Fig. 4 shows alternative configurations of iMAT: The dotted box encircles the software components and data that are essential for all configurations. A user who does not want a stand-alone dispenser can have these components run on a smart-phone platform, as a self-contained schedule manager and monitor such as the one described in [41]. The mobile application offers most of the schedule management and compliance monitoring functions of an iMAT dispenser. This configuration is depicted in the right part of the figure.

The flexible configuration shown in the left half of the figure may be chosen by a user who has multiple computers and mobile devices at home and work: The software components run on a PC and uses one or more laptop computers and mobile devices for its interaction with the user. A user may start with only these parts and incur no expense of special-purpose hardware. As he/she starts to take more and more medications, the user can get one or more dispensers, less the software components, and connect them to the computer as peripheral devices. As an example, Fig. 4 shows a dispenser connected locally to the PC and a dispenser connected remotely for a user who has a dispenser at home and another at work.

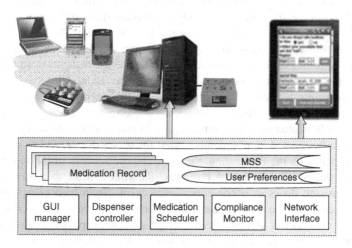

Fig. 4. Alternative configurations (From [30])

2.3   Medication Schedule Specification

As stated earlier, the prototype iMAT intends to demonstrate the feasibility and safety of flexible medication schedules. Today even low-cost computing devices can store gigabytes of data and carry out mega-instructions per second. A medication schedule manager can take advantage of such resources to exploit fully timing and dosage flexibilities provided by directions of most medications and thus make the medication schedules less rigid, more considerate of user preferences, and more tolerant to user tardiness. The scheduling models and several heuristic algorithms for scheduling multiple medications for this purpose can be found in [28] and [37-39].

Firm and Hard Constraints. The iMAT medication scheduling model incorporates the concept of firm and hard constraints that has been developed and used to build safety critical real-time systems [42]. The remainder of this section describes how these constraints are defined within the medication schedule specifications.

We use the terms firm and hard constraints in the same sense as they are used in real-time systems literature. *Firm constraints* are typically more stringent. The scheduler tries to meet all the firm constraints whenever possible. Violations of firm constraints can occur, often due to user's tardiness or forgetfulness. The scheduler allows such violations when it cannot find a schedule to meet all firm constraints.

When the user is so late that a firm timing constraint is violated, the schedule manager recomputed the time for the late dose and possibly a new dose size as specified by the MSS. Such adjustments in the schedule may degrade the rigor of compliance (i.e., increase the change of ADE) and quality of the schedule (e.g., be less convenient for the user) but are nevertheless acceptable. Take Fosamax as an example. According to PDRHealth [17], Fosamax in tablet form is used to prevent or treat oosteoporosis. Suppose that the user is directed to take a 5 mg tablet every morning at least 30 minutes before taking any other medication or food. The direction also says that in case of a miss dose, skip the missed dose and resume the regular schedule the next day. So, a tablet each day is a firm constraint. The MSS may simply say to cancel the current dose and inform the user of the cancellation if he/she responds to the reminder for taking Fosamax too late: Here, being too late means after eating breakfast or when some other medication must be taken without delay.

Hard constraints are less stringent; they limit the degree to which medication directions are allowed to be relaxed and schedule quality to degrade. A violation of a hard constraint is treated as a non-compliant event and warrants an action (e.g., warn the user, call a designated family member, alert the user's doctor, and so on.) Clearly, the action depends on the medication, the user, and the severity of the violation; it is specified by the MSS. In case of Fosamax, the user's MSS may say to treat 7 consecutive missed doses as a non-compliance event. So, a hard constraint is time between consecutive dose is no greater than 7 days. When the event occurs, the user (or a family member) is alerted. He/she may ask his/her physician to change the prescription to "one 35mg tablet once a week". By switching to a less frequent schedule, he/she risks a higher chance of side effects such as painful acid reflux.

In general, for each medication M managed by the user's iMAT, the MSS contains a section extracted by the authoring tool from an XML file of directions stored in the iMAT database. Table 1 lists the parameters contained in the section for M.

Specifically, the section of M in MSS provides general information (e.g., name(s), granularity and picture(s) of the medication and the duration the user is supposed to be on it). The tool needs this information to manage and schedule the medication. The section has a dosage parameters (DP) part: DP defines the size and timing constraints for doses of M when the medication does not interact with other medications of the user. If some of the user's medications interact with M, the section also contains a special instructions (SI) part. SI specifies changes in dosage parameters and additional timing constraints to account for the interactions.

Dosage Parameters. The parameters in lines 1 and 2 in the DP part of the table define firm constraints of the medication. Specifically, line 1 gives the *nominal dose size range*; it bounds the sizes, in term of multiples of granularity of M, of individual doses of M. Line 2 gives the *nominal separation range* in terms of the minimum length and maximum length of time between two consecutive doses of the medication. The medication scheduler computes the normal schedule of the medication based on these parameters.

Table 1. Parameters of medication schedule specification (From [30])

- *M*: Name of the medication
- *g*: Granularity of dose size
- [T_{min}, T_{max}]: Minimum and maximum durations
- Other relevant attributes
- Dosage Parameters (DP)
  1. [d_{min}, d_{max}]: Nominal dose size range
  2. [s_{min}, s_{max}]: Nominal separation range
  3. [D_{min}, D_{max}]: Absolute dose size range
  4. [S_{min}, S_{max}]: Absolute separation range
  5. (*B, R*): Maximum intake rate defined by an upper bound *B* of total size of doses in a specified time interval *R*
  6. (*L, P*): Minimum intake rate defined by a lower bound L of total size of doses in a specified time interval P
  7. Non-compliance event types and corresponding actions.
- Special Instructions (SI)
  1. *N*: Name of an interferer
     a. Change list
     b. $\sigma_{min}(M, N)$: Minimum separation from *M* to *N*
     c. $\sigma_{min}(N, M)$: Minimum separation from *N* to *M*
  2. L: Name of another interferer
     ...

In contrast, the *absolute dose size* range and *absolute separation range* in lines 3 and 4, respectively, define hard constraints. The medication scheduler never uses dose size and separations outside these ranges. The constraints in lines 5 and 6 are called *maximum intake rate* (*B, R*) and *minimum intake rate* (*L, P*), respectively. The former specifies the total size of all doses within any time interval of length *R* to be no more than *B*. The latter requires that total size of all doses within any interval of length *P* to be at least equal to *L*. The scheduler treats these constraints (or the less stringent rates $(B+\beta, R)$ and $(L-\lambda, P)$ for some small β and λ no less than zero) as hard constraints.

As an example, the direction of Tylenol reads "Take one tablet every 4 to 6 hours. If pain does not respond to one tablet, two tablets may be used. Do not exceed 8 tablets in 24 hours." The DP part of this medication has [d_{min}, d_{max}] = [1, 2], [s_{min}, s_{max}] = [4, 6], (*B, R*) = (8, 24); granularity of time is one hour. The values of these parameters follow literally from the direction. Since the drug is to be taken as needed, [D_{min}, D_{max}] = [0, 2] and [S_{min}, S_{max}] = [4, ∞]. Moreover, there is no required minimum total dose size for this drug; hence (*L, P*) = (0, 24).

While the maximum intake rate is imposed to prevent overdose, the minimum intake rate constraints the number of missed doses. As an example, suppose that the physician of a user taking Propranolol for hypertension ordered for him/her one low dose tablet 3 times a day and wants to make sure that he/she does not skip any dose, or at most a dose occasionally. This constraint is specified as (*L, P*) = (3, 24), or more relaxed (*L, P*) = (2, 24) or (20, 168) (i.e., skip one dose per day or one per week).

Finally, we note that the "if you miss a dose" instruction within directions typically leads to an absolute separation range [S_{min}, S_{max}] containing the nominal range. As an example, the nominal and absolute separation ranges of a once a day medication are [24, 24] and [12, 48] or [8, 48], respectively, when its missed dose instruction reads "If you miss a dose, take it is when you remember. If it is close to the time for the next dose, skip the one you miss and go back to regular schedule."

Special Instructions (SI). In Table 1, the term an *interferer* of a medication M refers to a medication (or food) that interacts with M so much that some changes in the directions of M are warranted. The SI part in the section of MSS for M has an entry for each interferer N of M. The dose size and separation ranges of M may need to be changed to take account of their interactions. Such changes are specified by the change list in the entry. The dosage parameters in the change list are in effect as long as the user is on both M and N.

The entry for an interferer N may also define additional separation constraints: The time separation between each dose of M and any dose of the interferer N must be within the specified range: The minimum separation σ_{min} (M, N) from M to N specifies a lower bound to the length of time from each dose M to any later dose of N, and σ_{min} (N, M) from N to M is a lower bound to the time from each dose to N to any later dose of M. For example, the constraint that Fosamax must be taken before any food and at least 30 minutes before breakfast is specified by σ_{min} (Fosamax, Food) = 30 minutes and σ_{min} (Food, Fosamax) = 4 hours. The technical report [39] discusses additional constraints, such as maximum inter-medication separation constraints.

3   Medication Management, Dispensing, and Administration

Again, the acronym MeMDAS stands for Medication Management, Dispensing and Administration System [34], [35]. It is a distributed system of tools that supports medication dispensing and administration stages of medication use process as shown in Fig. 1. Its primary users are nursing and pharmacy staffs in hospitals, long term care, and assisted living facilities.

3.1   Capabilities

The system provides the users with tools similar to the ones in state-of-the-art mobile carts and medications stations (e.g., [26] [27]), as well some distinct capabilities:

- Medication (and medical supply) delivery and inventory monitoring;
- Barcode medication dispensing and administration (BCMD and BCMA);
- Work and time management (WTM);
- Configuration and customization tools and user interface functions;
- Information access and labor-saving capabilities, such as generating shift report from data and notes collected during the user's shift, tracking medication and medical supply usages and automating requests for replenishments; and
- Intelligent monitor, alert and notification (iMAN) [42].

A user can use the modern WTM tool as a personal digital assistant and have it maintain not only medication schedules and appointments of patients under the user's care, but also track the user's daily work plans and personal schedule (e.g., meetings and tasks). For example, it enables the user to schedule times for various tasks (e.g., prepare a patient three days ahead of the patient's colonoscopy appointment and warm up a patient before a physical therapy session) and gets reminders from the tool at those times. Adjustment in patient schedules is unavoidable. The WTM tool is capable of enforcing rules governing patient schedules. A change of the schedule time of a patient event requested by the user can take effect only after the tool has confirmed that the changed schedule satisfies all rules.

Just like iMAT described in the previous section, flexibility is a distinct characteristic of MeMDAS. By being *flexible*, we mean easily configurable and customizable. Medication administration processes vary from hospital to hospital, department to department, and even patient to patient. Protocols and rules governing ideal administration processes for a patient in an ICU (Intensive Care Unit) and a patient in a general ward are typically different. For this reason, MeMDAS tools and component systems are built to be easily configurable and customizable, in most cases by end users themselves: Nursing and pharmacy staffs with proper authorization can customize for themselves majority of the MeMDAS tools and user interface functions to follow the protocols and enforce the policies and rules of their respective institutions, departments and patient wards.

The intelligent monitoring and notification tool [42] complements interlock and control mechanisms to enhance error prevention. Like similar tools for safety critical systems, iMAN also enables the user to analyze and determine the causes of errors after they occur. iMAN is unique in its capability to detect events and action sequences deemed by the user as having a high likelihood to cause errors and when such an event is detected, notify designated persons to take preventive actions. An easy to use and reliable iMAN is particularly important for monitoring and tracking common workarounds and protocol violations such as the ones reported in [22].

3.2   Component Systems

A MeMDAS has three types of component systems. They are MUMS (multiple-user medication station), iNuC (intelligent nursing carts), and BaMU (basic mobile unit) as depicted in part (a) of Fig. 5.

The term *medication station* refers to a system of smart cabinets with barcode controlled containers monitored and operated by a small server. Medication stations such as the ones listed in [26] and [27] typically operate in fully automated mode: When a user comes to retrieve medications for a patient, the station opens automatically all the containers holding the medications due to be administered to the patient at the time. Operating in this mode, a station can serve only one user at a time. In a ward with many nurses (e.g., 5-10) caring for patients on frequent medications, the added burden on the nurses to stand in line for retrieval of medications or to adjust their work plans in order to minimize queuing time often more than offsets the advantages of using the station. MeMDAS medication stations are configurable so that they can also operate in a semi-automatic mode. When operating semi-automatically, the station server collaborates with the users and their mobile carts to ensure correct dispensing of medications to multiple users concurrently.

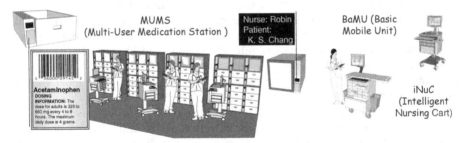

(a) Component systems (above) (b) Workflow-based structures of iNuC and MUMS (below)

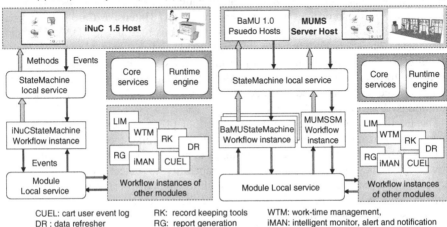

CUEL: cart user event log   RK: record keeping tools   WTM: work-time management,
DR : data refresher   RG: report generation   iMAN: intelligent monitor, alert and notification

Fig. 5. Component Systems of MeMDAS

Both iNuC and BaMU are mobile nursing carts. iNuC [35] is a self-contained system. Each cart serves a user (usually a nurse). The drawers in it carry the daily doses of medications for each of the patients cared for by the user. The block diagram in the left half of part (b) of the figure shows the structure of a workflow-based version of iNuC. Except for dispensing, an iNuC offers its user all the capabilities listed above without help from MUMS, and, in events of network and hospital information system outages, can function stand-alone.

A BaMU is a light-weight system of mobile tools for use during barcode dispensing of medications from MUMS and for transporting the currents doses retrieved for each patient from MUMS to the patient's bedside. It relies on a MUMS server to provide work planning, scheduling and monitoring and alert functions. Some BaMU do not have the medication administration and patient record keeping tools. Some of such BaMU's are used in wards that have computers at patients' bedsides for these purposes. Such a BaMU can also function as an intelligent medication supply cart for use by pharmacy staff.

3.3   Alternative Configurations

The MeMDAS prototype was partially funded by National Taiwan University Hospital (NTUH) and designed and developed by the SISARL project [36] in close collaboration with the hospital's nursing and pharmacy departments. At the time (2008-2010), the hospital used computers on mobile carts to provide nursing staff with a web-based interface via which they can access the hospital information system and read and update their patients' records. The hospital was in the process of introducing barcode ids of medications and patients. An objective of MeMDAS was to support the hospital's experimentation with BCMA.

The hospital was also planning to experiment with alternative dispensing workflow processes. As with most hospitals in Asian-Pacific region, a centralized dispensing process was used throughout the hospital at the time: According to this process, the pharmacy prepares and delivers daily to each ward a supply cart with drawers. Daily doses of medications for each patient in the ward are in one or more drawers. To support this process, one or more MUMS can be used in the pharmacy, and BaMU's can be used as intelligent supply carts. Together, they support barcode medication dispensing and make the process of preparing supply carts less error prone.

The hospital was planning to adopt distributed dispensing in departments where patients' prescriptions change frequently, including ICU and OR. MUMS and BaMU were intended for such departments: The pharmacy monitors and stocks the cabinets in the station with all or most medications needed for patients in each ward. At times when some medications are due to be administrated to one or more of her/his patients, each nurse retrieves individual doses of the medications for each patient from the cabinets under the control of the station server and his/her BaMU. We will return in Section 4 to describe this collaborative process.

Distributed dispensing tends to increase workload for nurses. Hybrid workflow process is a compromise: In this case, some medications are dispensed and delivered via supply carts by the pharmacy. The ward also has a medication station and uses it to hold controlled drugs and frequently used medications, making it possible for nurses to get newly ordered medications on a timely basis.

In wards where dispensing is centralized or hybrid, nurses uses iNuC for BCMA: To put a medication drawer of a patient under the control of an iNuC, the nurse removes the drawer from the supply cart, scans the barcode patient id in the drawer to capture the id and then puts the drawer in any empty drawer slot of his/her iNuC. Sensing that a drawer is placed in the slot, the RFID reader of the cart reads the tags on the drawers and acquires the association between the id of the new drawer, its location in the cart and patient's barcode id. From this information, it creates the mapping between the drawer location and the patient id. Later, when the patient is due to take some medication(s), the nurse can have the cart open the patient's drawer at bedside by scanning the patient's barcode id in the wristband worn by the patient.

As stated earlier, a distinguishing characteristic of MeMDAS is flexibility: MUMS can be easily configured to run in automatic or semiautomatic mode. The software system controlling operations, GUI and user interactions of the mobile carts can be configured to make an iNuC work as a BaMU and vice versus. This is accomplished by building the component systems on workflow-based structures depicted in part (b) of Fig. 5. Section 4 will elaborate this design choice.

3.4   User-Centric Design and Development

MeMDAS was prototyped in a user-centric manner collaboratively by researchers from the SISARL project and representative users from NTUH. The approach was motivated by studies such as [24] that recommend close involvement of the targeted users throughout the development process as a way to eliminate sources of errors known to occur when new automation systems are deployed.

Following this approach, the requirement capture process for each component system started with presentations of the concepts and functions of the system to representatives of NTUH nursing staffs from many departments and pharmacy staffs. Discussions during these meetings provided the design team with clearer understanding of users' needs, wishes and views. After the meetings, likely early adopters were identified. The development team met with them regularly until concrete use scenarios were developed and requirements were defined and prioritized. Later, when the alpha version of the prototype became available, they used it on a trial basis and their assessments helped to improve the system.

Requirement specifications in textual and diagrammatic forms, even when augmented by formal specifications, are ineffective communication channels between users and developers. For this reason, we used mockups for requirement solicitation, definition and documentation purposes. Take iNuC as an example. Except for the absence of the physical medication drawers with the interlock mechanism and real patient data and nurse ids, the mockup gives the evaluators the look and feel of a real iNuC. We used it to collect information on what the users want the system to do, how the tools interact with them, what and how the display shows, what their preferences in input/output devices and mode of operations are, and so on.

Mockups proved to be as effective as we had hoped them to be. Through them, we indeed obtained valuable feedback and suggestions. They also enabled us to identify design defects and potential bugs that were likely to remain unnoticed until the prototypes are deployed. As an example, during the administration of a medication, iNuC GUI provides a table entry in which the user is required to record the actual quantity of the medication consumed at the time if the quantity differs from the prescribed quantity. This information is used by the tool to track the supplies more accurately. The label and placement of the entry displayed by the iNuC mockup misled some evaluators to think that the user can change the dose size of the medication. Changing dose size by the nurse is, of course, not allowed for most medications. As another example, a sign-in/login feature provided by the mockup for sake of user convenience may leave some of patients unattended during shift changes. To fix this design error, a new role-based access control policy was developed to take into account delays and other anomalies during shift changes.

4   Model-Based Design, Implementation and Evaluation

Flexibility (i.e., configurability and customizability) of MeMDAS prototypes was achieved by building them on a workflow-based architecture. The basic building blocks of a workflow-based application/system are called *activities*. An activity may be the execution of a program, scan of a barcode, transmission of a message, etc. Activities are composed into module-level components called *workflows*. The order and conditions under which activities in a workflow are executed and the resources needed for their execution are defined by the developer of the workflow. The workflow approach [45-49] has been widely used in enterprise computing systems for automation of business processes.

We use the workflow paradigm in two ways: for flexible integration of reusable components and for modeling the system, users and their interactions. Specifically, workflow-based MeMDAS component systems run on Windows Embedded Standard and .NET Workflow Framework [49]. Part (b) of Fig. 5 shows the workflow-based structures of iNuC and MUMS server. The block diagrams intend to highlight the commonalities between iNuC and MUMS Server. (To save space, we omitted the diagram for BaMU, which is essentially the same as that of iNuC.) Only boxes representing the host and state machine workflow are labeled by the names of the systems; the systems differ primarily in these parts. In particular, the state machine local service interface and module local service interface in all systems are the same. Similarly, the workflows provided by other modules are identical. By replacing iNuC state machine workflow with a BaMU state machine workflow, we can make the GUI and the cart behave like a BaMU.

We also use workflows as models of the systems and tools throughout the development process. According to the workflow-based model [50], jobs and tasks done by the system are modeled as activities and workflows. They are called *device activities and workflows*. Many operations of MeMDAS are semi-automatic. Actions taken and tasks done by human user(s) are modeled by *user activities* and *workflows*. Interactions between the user and the system are modeled by local services for workflow to workflow communication. The model also incorporates workflow definitions of GOMS (Goals, Objectives, Methods and Selections) and MHP (Model Human Processor) [51] [52] model elements commonly used in user-interface design to characterize human users with different attributes and skills.

Throughout the development process, the behavior of the new system or tool is defined by its *operational specification*. The specification consists of a model of the system defined in terms of device workflows and a model of the user(s) defined in terms of user workflows. The definitions also specify the resources (e.g., barcode scanner, interlocks, executables, and human users) required by each activity. In the design phase before the actual resources are available, the workflow definitions call for virtual resources (i.e., device simulators, dummy code, user models, etc.) as resource components. As the development process progresses, the virtual resources are replaced by physical devices and programs. Device workflows modeling module-level components become implementations of the components. User workflows provide use scenarios and scripts for testing purposes.

An advantage of specifying operations of the system and modeling user(s) and user-device interactions in terms of workflows is that such specifications and models are executable. By executing the models, the developer can assess the design, usability and performance of the system at each stage of the development process. The simulation environment described in [50] was developed for this purpose.

As a case study, we used workflow models of MUMS, BaMU, and users in a series of simulation experiments to determine whether the MUMS server, multiple users and their BaMUs work correctly in semi-automatic medications dispensing. By being correct, we mean that every user gets correct medications from MUMS and puts the medications in the correct patient drawer for every patient.

Fig. 6 shows a scenario to illustrate the process. The scenario takes place in a ward where a MUMS is used to support distributed dispensing. At the start of each shift, the MUMS server plans for each nurse in service an administration schedule for all of his/her patients. At the time when one or more of his/her patients is due to take some medications, the server sends a reminder to the nurse. In response to the reminder, the nurse (called Robin in Fig. 6) logs on a BaMU (BaMU-4 in the figure) and thus acquires exclusive use of the cart and informs the MUMS server that she is using the cart. She then selects RetrieveMedications command via the GUI of BaMU-4. Upon receiving the command, MUMU server sends the list of Robin's patients due to take medications at the time to the cart.

The part of the scenario illustrated by Fig. 6 starts from the solid arrow in the upper left corner of the figure. The arrow represents the transmission of patient list. (Other solid arrows also indicate transmission of data while dashed lines or arrows represent elapse time.) Upon receiving Robin's patient list, BaMU-4 displays the list, unlocks the empty drawers in the cart and then waits for Robin's selection of a patient from the list. At the MUMS with the cart, Robin selects a patient from the list displayed by the cart and opens an unlocked drawer. Sensing a drawer is opened, BaMU-4 stores the mappings of drawer-location-patient-id and drawer-id-patient-id and sends the mappings to the MUMS server. The server will need them later to ensure that the nurse takes the right drawer to the right patient.

In response to Robin's patient selection, BaMU-4 sends (BaMU-4, Robin, Patient Id) to the server, informing the server that Robin is retrieving medications for the specified patient. The server responds by having the displays on the containers holding medications to be retrieved for the patient to show Robin's name and the patient's name. To retrieve a dose from one of these containers, Robin uses the barcode scanner on BaMU-4 to read the barcode on the label of the container. The captured reading is sent to the MUMS server. After verification, the server unlocks the container, allowing Robin to retrieve a dose from it. Once Robin finishes retrieving all the medications of the selected patient, she closes the open cart drawer.

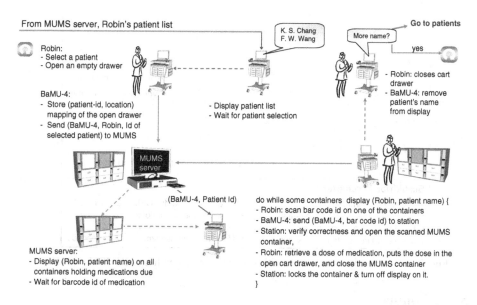

From MUMS server, Robin's patient list

K. S. Chang
F. W. Wang

More name?

Go to patients
yes

Robin:
- Select a patient
- Open an empty drawer

BaMU-4:
- Store (patient-id, location) mapping of the open drawer
- Send (BaMU-4, Robin, Id of selected patient) to MUMS

- Display patient list
- Wait for patient selection

- Robin: closes cart drawer
- BaMU-4: remove patient's name from display

MUMS
server

(BaMU-4, Patient Id)

MUMS server:
- Display (Robin, patient name) on all containers holding medications due
- Wait for barcode id of medication

do while some containers display (Robin, patient name) {
- Robin: scan bar code id on one of the containers
- BaMU-4: send (BaMU-4, bar code id) to station
- Station: verify correctness and open the scanned MUMS container,
- Robin: retrieve a dose of medication, puts the dose in the open cart drawer, and close the MUMS container
- Station: locks the container & turn off display on it.
}

Fig. 6. Semi-automatic dispensing from MUMS

The drawer is locked in place in the cart. Robin can have the drawer opened and removed only by scanning the barcode id of the patient.

In all the simulation runs carried out in our attempt to detect errors and malfunctions caused by user-system interactions, we observed none. Examination of event logs generated during simulation shows that the complicated process illustrated by Fig. 6 in fact is not error prone: While the MUMS server allows multiple users to access the cabinets at the same time, it correctly permits only one user at a time to open any container. The fact that each user has exclusive use of his/her own cart and barcode scanner is the main reason.

We also simulated different numbers of users retrieving medications from a MUMS to determine the responsiveness the system as a function of concurrent users. The estimated times taken by a user to operate the BaMU GUI were obtained using the CPM variant of the GOMS model [51]. The amounts of time for other user actions, (e.g., open a drawer, walk a distance, etc.) were obtained by measuring the amounts of time taken by several test subjects to carry out the actions. Fig. 7 shows the result of such a simulation experiment. In this case, the MUMS has only one cabinet with 138 containers. The result show that the average time spent by a user waiting to access containers remains small compared to the average amount of time required to retrieve medications from containers when the number of nurses using the MUMS concurrently is no more than three.

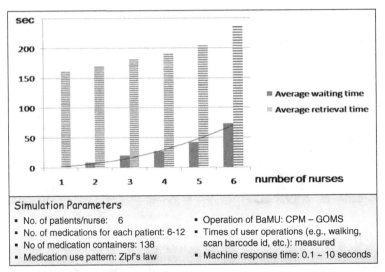

Fig. 7. Average retrieval time and waiting time of dispensing from MUMS (From [50])

5   Summary

Previous sections described two systems of tools for reduction of medication administration and dispensing errors. iMAT is for people who take medications on their own, i.e., outside care-providing institutions. MeMDAS provides mobile carts and smart cabinets similar to the ones listed in [26] and [27].

A distinguishing characteristic of both systems is flexibility. iMAT exploits flexibilities provided by directions of typical medications to make the user's medication schedule easy to adhere to and tolerant of user's tardiness whenever scheduling flexibility does not jeopardize compliance. MeMDAS allows users with authorization to tailor the tools for their own institutions, departments and patient wards. Both systems try to prevent errors by providing their users with reminders and instructions on when and how medications are administrated. Both systems enable user actions and anomalous events to be monitored and alerts and notifications to be sent as specified, in case of iMAT, by the user's MSS, and in case of MeMDAS, by users with proper authorization.

Several prototype iMAT dispensers and schedule managers, as well as a MSS authoring tool, were built to prove concepts ranging from medication scheduling, user-centric design, device models and architectures and adaptability. To assess usability and effectiveness of mobile schedule managers, we conducted a small field trial on ten test subjects with ages ranging from 25 to 60 and different education background [28]. Their occupations include student, engineer, housewife, retiree, and businessman. Their medications were for diabetes, hypertension, heart disease, asthma, and other chronic diseases. Before the subjects started to use a version of the iMAT schedule manager running on smart phones, we logged their medication compliance using questionnaires on paper. According to the logs, they missed 1/3 of the doses of their prescription medications and were late in dose time by one to three hours on the average. The results show that the tool was effective (and easy to use) for subjects who are busy and who are often not sure when and what medications should be taken. It was particularly effective in improving compliance for three subjects: They are (1) a 30-year-old software engineer who is a diabetic and takes 11 types of medications at least four times a day; (2) a 24-year-old graduate student who has two medications that must be taken every 12 hours for controlling her asthma; and (3) a 60-year-old businessman who takes eight types of medications at least three times a day for treatment of hypertension and diabetes. Commonalities among them are their complex medication regimens, long work days and irregular hours, and the inconvenience of taking medications during work and at night. As expected, for subjects who do not want to take medications because of other factors, the tool did not work well. Some subjects live at relatively slow pace. They can manage their schedules without the tool and hence were not motivated to use the tool.

A missing piece in the iMAT tool set is a sufficiently complete database of medication directions in the XML format. Currently, the iMAT database contains directions for a few hundred commonly used medications. They were obtained by manual translation of directions in PDRHealth [17] to XML format. We are developing a translator to automate the translation process.

MeMDAS component system prototypes are in different stages of maturity. Their code can be found at the open source software repository http://openfoundry.org and are released under GPL license. A commercial version of the medication station based on the MeMDAS prototype is currently being used on trial basis in a hospital in Taipei, Taiwan.

Acknowledgments This work was partially supported by the Taiwan Academia Sinica thematic project SISARL, a grant from National Taiwan University Hospital, the Flexible Medication Management Systems Project supported by the Taiwan Ministry of Economic Affairs, and by the Center of IET, National Taiwan University under MOE Grant AE-00-00-06.

References

1. Strategies to reduce medication errors: working to improve medication safety, http://www.fda.gov/Drugs/ResourcesForYou/Consumers/ucm143553.htm
2. Medication errors led to severe harm or death in 36 Ontario cases. Canadian Press (August 2013), http://www.cbc.ca/news/health/story/2013/08/21/medication-errors-ontario-hospitals.html
3. Emily's Story, http://emilyjerryfoundation.org/emilys-story/
4. Kowalczyk, L.: Brigham and Women's airing medical mistakes – hospital reports errors to staff in drive for improvement. Boston Globe (April 2013)
5. Medication Errors, Food and Drug Administration, http://www.fda.gov/drugs/drugsafety/medicationerrors/default.htm
6. Preventing medication errors, Institute of Medicine Report. National Academies Press, Washington, DC (2006)
7. US CDC Medication Safety Program, Medication Safety Basics, http://www.cdc.gov/medicationsafety/basics.html#Key
8. Medication errors, European Medicine Agency, http://www.ema.europa.eu/ema/index.jsp?curl=pages/special_topics/general/general_content_000570.jsp

9. Koper, D., et al.: Frequency of medication errors in primary care patients with polypharmacy. Family Practice (June 2013)
10. Budnitz, D.S., et al.: Emergency hospitalizations for adverse drug events in older Americans. New England Journal Medicine (November 2011)
11. Hall, H.: Reducing the risk of adverse drug events. posted in January 2012 at, http://www.sciencebasedmedicine.org/reducing-the-risk-of-adverse-drug-events/
12. Health information technology in the United States: better information systems for better care (2013) Published by Harvard School of Public Health, Mathematica Policy Research and Robert Wood Johnson Foundation, http://www.rwjf.org/content/dam/farm/reports/reports/2013/rwjf406758
13. Addressing medication errors in hospitals: a practical toolkit, California Health Foundation, http://www.chcf.org/publications/2001/07/addressing-medication-errors-in-hospitals-a-practical-toolkit
14. Prevention of medication error, American Academy of Orthopaedic Surgery (2008), http://www.aaos.org/about/papers/advistmt/1026.asp
15. Computerized Physician Order Entry, http://en.wikipedia.org/wiki/Computerized_physician_order_entry
16. Radley, D.C., et al.: Reduction in medication errors in hospitals due to adoption of computerized provider order entry systems. J. Am. Med. Inform. Assoc. (February 2013)
17. PDRHealth, Physicians' Desk References, http://www.pdrhealth.com/drug_info/
18. Bar-coded medication administration, http://healthit.ahrq.gov/ahrq-funded-projects/emerging-lessons/bar-coded-medication-administration
19. Poon, E.G., et al.: Effect of Barcode technology on the safety of medication administration. New Engl. Journal Medicine (May 2010)
20. Montesi, G., Lechi, A.: Prevention of medication errors: detection and audit. J. Clin. Pharmacol. (June 2009)
21. Schneider, R., et al.: Bar-Code Medication Administration: A Systems Perspective. Am. J. Health Syst. Pharm. (2008)
22. Koppel, R., et al.: Workarounds to barcode medication administration systems: their occurrences, causes, and threats to patient safety. J. Am. Med. Inform. Association 15(4) (July-August 2008)
23. Kuperman, G.J., et al.: Medication related clinical decision support in computerized provider order entry systems: A Review. J. Am. Med. Inform. Assoc. (2007)
24. Koppel, B., et al.: Role of Computerized Physician Order Entry Systems in Facilitating Medication Errors. Journal of AMA 293(10) (2005)
25. Kawamoto, K., et al.: Improving clinical practice using clinical decision support systems: a systematic review of trials to identify features critical to success. BMJ (April 2005)
26. Rx Showcase, http://www.rxinsider.com/prescription_dispensing_automation.htm
27. Pyxis point-of-care verification, http://www.carefusion.com/medical-products/medication-management/point-of-care-verification/, and Pyxis Medication Station http://www.carefusion.com/medical-products/medication-management/medication-technologies/pyxis-medstation-system.aspx
28. Tsai, P.-H., Shih, C.-S., Liu, J.W.-S.: Mobile reminder for flexible and safe medication schedule for home users. In: Jacko, J.A. (ed.) Human-Computer Interaction, Part III, HCII 2011. LNCS, vol. 6763, pp. 107–116. Springer, Heidelberg (2011)

29. Tsai, P.H., Yu, C.Y., Shih, C.S., Liu, J.W.S.: Smart medication dispensers; design, architecture and implementation. IEEE Systems Journal (March 2011)

30. Tsai, P.H., Yu, C.Y., Wang, W.Y., Zao, J.K., Yeh, H.C., Shih, C.S., Liu, J.W.S.: iMAT: intelligent medication administration tools. In: Proceedings of IEEE International Conference on E-Health (July 2010)

31. e-pill, Pill Dispensers for Home and Institutional Use, http://www.epill.com/pillstation.html

32. Automatic Pill Dispensers with Alarms, http:// www.dynamic-living.com/automated_medication_dispenser.htm

33. My Pill Box, http://www.mypillbox.org/mypillbox.php

34. Liu, J.W.S., Shih, C.S., Tan, C.T., Wu, V.J.S.: MeMDAS: medication management, dispensing and administration System. Presented at Mobile Health Workshop (July 2010)

35. Tsai, P.H., Chuang, Y.T., Chou, T.S., Shih, C.S., Liu, J.W.S.: iNuC: an intelligent mobile medication cart. In: Proceedings of the 2nd International Conference on Biomedical Engineering and Informatics (October 2009)

36. SISARL (Sensor Information Systems for Active Retirees and Assisted Living), http://sisarl.org

37. Tsai, P.H., Shih, C.S., Liu, J.W.S.: Algorithms for scheduling interactive medications. Foundations of Computing and Decision Sciences 34(4) (2009)

38. Tsai, P.H., Yeh, H.C., Yu, C.Y., Hsiu, P.C., Shih, C.S., Liu, J.W.S.: Compliance Enforcement of Temporal and Dosage Constraints. In: Proceedings of IEEE Real-Time Systems Symposium (December 2006)

39. Hsiu, P.C., Yeh, H.C., Tsai, P.H., Shih, C.S., Burkhardt, D.H., Kuo, T.W., Liu, J.W.S., Huang, T.Y.: A general model for medication scheduling. Institute of Information Science, Academia Sinica, Taiwan. Technical Report TR-IIS-05-008 (July 2005)

40. Yeh, H.C., Hsiu, P.C., Shih, C.S., Tsai, P.H., Liu, J.W.S.: APAMAT: A prescription algebra for medication authoring tool. In: Proceedings of IEEE International Conference on Systems (October 2006)

41. Wang, W.Y., Zao, J.K., Tsai, P.H., Liu, J.W.S.: Wedjat: A mobile phone based medication reminder and monitor. In: Proceedings of the 9th IEEE International Conference on Bioinformatics and Bioengineering (June 2009)

42. Liu, J.W.S.: Real-Time Systems. Pearson (2000)

43. Lin, H.C.: Intelligent monitoring, alert and notification tool. MS thesis, Department of Computer Science. National Tsing University, Taiwan (2011)

44. iNuC code, MeMDAS code, http://www.openfoundry.org/of/projects/1530

45. Pandey, S., et al.: Workflow engine for clouds. In: Cloud Computing, Principles and Paradigms. Wiley Series on Parallel and Distributed Computing (2011)

46. WfMC: Workflow Management Coalition, http://www.wfmc.org/

47. XPDL (XML Process Definition Language) Document (October 2005), http:// www.wfmc.org/standards/docs/TC-1025_xpdl.2.2005-10-03.pdf

48. Pajunen, L., Chande, S.: Developing workflow engine for mobile devices. In: Proc. of IEEE International Enterprise Distributed Object Computing Conference (2007)

49. Bukovics, B.: Pro WF: Windows Workflow Foundation in.Net 4.0. Apress (2009)

50. Chen, T.-Y., et al.: Model-Based Development of User-Centric Automation and Assistive Devices/Systems. IEEE Systems Journal 6(3) (2012)

51. John, B.E., Kieras, D.E.: The GOMS family of user interface analysis techniques: comparison and contrast. ACM Trans. Computer-Human Interaction (1996)

52. Card, S.K., et al.: The Psychology of Human-Computer Interaction. Lawrence Erlbaum Associates (1983)

Panel Position Statements

Kudakwashe Dube[1], Deshendran Moodley[2], Bill Thies[3],
Jane W.S. Liu[4], Joseph Cafazzo[5], and Oleg Sokolsky[6]

[1] School of Engineering and Advanced Technology, Massey University, New Zealand
K.Dube@Massey.ac.nz

[2] UKZN/CSIR Meraka Centre for Artificial Intelligence Research and Health
Architecture Laboratory, School of Mathematics, Statistics and Computer Science,
University of KwaZulu-Natal, Durban, South Africa

[3] Microsoft Research India
thies@microsoft.com
http://research.microsoft.com/~thies/

[4] Institute of Information Science, Academia Sinica, Taipei, Taiwan
janeliu@iis.sinica.edu.tw

[5] Centre for Global eHealth Innovation
Joe.Cafazzo@uhn.ca
http://www.ehealthinnovation.org/

[6] Department of Computer & Information Science, University of Pennsylvania
sokolsky@cis.upenn.edu

1 Health Informatics in the Developing World: Is This Our Problem?

The western world enjoys a far greater degree of sophistication in computer technology than the developing world; challenges include the fact that infrastructure and resources in the developing world lag far behind; education to use and maintain the technology is often lacking; and cultural and societal issues prohibit its use. Questions include: What is the role of the first world in promoting more widespread use of technology for health informatics? What are the advantages to the first world in promoting more widespread use? What is the role of scientists in the first world in developing technology suitable for less technologically savvy regions? Should we interfere in cultures that do not use technology as we do? What can we practically expect to positively influence by engaging with developing world? How do we engage with the developing world in a sustainable way? Finally, modern vaccines have made huge differences in health the world over; can we expect similar positive transformation from increased computer/information technology in the developing world?

Moderated by Zhiming Liu

1.1 Kudakwashe Dube

Introduction. *The western world enjoys a far greater degree of sophistication in computer technology than the developing world.* This lack of sophistication in

J. Gibbons and W. MacCaull (Eds.): FHIES 2013, LNCS 8315, pp. 22–31, 2014.

Information and Communication Technology (ICT) can be an opportunity for health informaticians to introduce new technologies without some of the adoption barriers that are associated with the ICT sophistication found in the developed world. The major challenges in developing countries are chronic, numerous and are in addition to well-known challenges encountered in *Health Informatics* (HI) in the developed world [Adjorlolo2013][Dare2005].

First, *infrastructure and resources in the developing world lag far behind* [Foster2012]. However, introduction of new ICT has been observed to attain high levels of speedy adoption that are unparalleled by any in the developed world. This is usually accompanied by new and innovative uses that solve problems that are unique and endemic to the developing countries. A typical example is the adoption of wireless cellular telephony [Juma2012] and the mobile web-based technologies, which led to the new form of payment system based on transfer of mobile phone top-up balances from one phone number to another. Thus, health informaticians, with the benefit of experiences gained in the developed world, should participate in shaping the adoption of HI technologies in new ways that may not have been foreseen in the developed world.

Second, *education to use and maintain the technology is often lacking* [Braa1995]. This is mainly due to the non-availability of the technology. With some developing countries, like Zimbabwe, that are attaining above 90% literacy rates even in the midst of political and economic problems, educating the population to use and maintain the technology will take very short periods of time.

Third, *cultural and societal issues prohibit the use of Computer Technology.* Although this may be largely true, there are regions of the developing world where these issues make it easier to introduce ICTs than in developed world [Bell2006]. For instance, in some cultures in Africa, access to personal information may be tolerated within the context of the large extended family and friends. Privacy is associated more strongly with the physical body than with information about the physical body. Concepts like *ubuntu* that permeates the fabric of culture and society, make individuals become more prone towards emphasising the attainment of the common good, even at the expense of individual privacy, preferences and freedoms. Thus, through persuasion and education, it may be much easier to introduce ICT and HI technologies in some developing regions than in developed regions of the world. This could be viewed as an opportunity for HI researchers to engage with the aim of developing solutions that will have far-reaching impact in developing countries.

The Role of Health Informatics Researchers in Developing Countries.
There is now a critical mass of a wide range of advanced HI technologies, experience and hindsight from several decades of research outputs in developed countries. The adoption of these advances usually takes a long time despite technological sophistication. Developing countries are still in their infancy in the adoptions of ICTs, not only in healthcare, but in many other domains. Even the first generation *Health Information Systems* (HIS) have not yet been adopted. There is a unique opportunity for HI researchers to define their critical roles and

to provide leadership and expertise as well as to further enhance research works for use in the introduction and adoption of both first and second generation HIS.

Advantages to the First World of Promoting Adoption of Health Informatics Technologies in the Third World. There are a number of advantages to the first world in promoting more widespread use of HI technologies in developing regions of the world. Most of these advantages could be realised if HI researchers in developed countries initiate collaborative environments with researchers and practitioners in developing countries.

First, developing countries make up the *novel context that offers a unique, flexible and malleable environment for new ways, paradigms and approaches to many aspects of HI* that focus on achieving the desired outcomes in the context of severely limited resources. The malleability of this environment arises from the fact that ICTs are not yet in widespread use in many countries, which lag many years behind. This makes it easy to introduce new technologies together with new paradigms and new ways of thinking that may be harder to introduce in developed regions that are subject to technological inertia and other challenges that result from introducing technological changes.

Second, the developing country environment offers researchers *the unique push to rethink their theories, methods and techniques and modify them for high efficiency, impact and outcomes within the context of severely limited resources.* The result will benefit both worlds. Third, theory, techniques and technological advancement within the area of HI will be enhanced and strengthened by subjecting the outcomes of HI research works to diverse environments and contexts. The developing countries offer new environments and, possibly, novel contexts and challenges that may provide opportunities for making HI theory and technologies more robust or even extended in ways that may not have been conceivable in the developed world.

A typical example of the above two advantages was the announcement of efforts to create the $100-laptop for children in the developing countries. This attracted a lot of efforts that had significant impact on the engineering and development of low-power consumption computing devices (laptops, tablets and smart phones) that are currently benefiting both developed and developing countries. The original drive was to develop low-cost, low-power consuming and yet functioning computing devices that are suitable for resource- and power-limited environments in developing countries. Research outputs that are optimised for developed countries will also work for developed countries. Thus, the result of research work that optimises solutions for the environment that is the *lowest common denominator* benefits both worlds.

Fourth, every individual has a vested interest in the *availability of efficient and effective healthcare systems with effective disease monitoring and reporting capabilities everywhere on earth.* Globalisation trends that are characterised by rapid movements of people from one region of the world to another have led to diseases spreading quickly between developed and developing regions of the world. The widespread use of HI technologies from developed countries in developing countries is a major contribution towards the achievement of efficient healthcare systems, including disease surveillance and monitoring systems, and, hence, a safe world for everyone.

The Role of Scientists in the First World. Scientists in the first world have a invaluable role to play in developing technology suitable for less technologically savvy regions of the world. From a more general point of view, the less technologically savvy regions of the world constitute the *lowest common denominator* for a world whose resources are limited and diminishing. It is, therefore, the universally moral and ethical as well as a duty of first world scientists (in fact, all scientists) to develop technological solutions that work first within the context of the *lowest common denominator* in order for the management of the world's limited resources to be sustainable. Such technologies would be optimised for limited resources as a key requirement. Such technologies need not be backward solutions that amounts to the return to antiquated and inefficient ways of solving problems in both the developing and the developed world. The developed world scientists have the resources to lead the challenge of searching for the simplest solution that require the fewest resources. In doing so, their central focus and major priority would be to develop technologies that work for less technological savvy regions of the world. Such technologies are expected to be resource-efficient, modern and effective appropriate functional solutions to problems in both developing and developed regions of the world. Health Informaticians in the developed world would be expected to take up the challenge of creating new technologies or foundations of new technological innovations that would be available for use everywhere in the world. It is not inconceivable, that such technologies will also become adopted later for use in developed regions of the world. For example, although mobile phone-based payment systems arose as a result of the introduction of mobile phone technologies in remote villages in Africa where there is lack of cash and no banks, there are discussions of introducing this novel developing world technology into developed regions of the world in European countries and Japan.

Interference in Cultures that Do Not Use Technology. The process of interfering with other cultures to introduce new technologies that were not used before has been one of the the driving forces behind human technological development, enrichment and advancement since time immemorial. It has worked positively over centuries. The modern developed world cannot claim to be originators of all modern technologies being used in their cultures as there is evidence that the technological foundations, theories and principles originate from other cultures around the world.

An important point to note here is the fact that there is no culture in the world that does not use technology and that does not change with changing technology. Technological changes can originate internally or externally to a culture. The impact on culture and society of technological changes that originate internally is not different from that of technological changes that originate externally. Furthermore, it could be argued that there is no such thing as interference when introducing new technology into a another culture even though the technology may have a positive or negative impact on the the culture. This is so because cultures are dynamic and as technologies are introduced and substituted, the cultures adapt and change with either positive or negative impact to members of the society.

Given that HI researchers are not oblivious to codes of ethics nor are they immune to ethical, social and professional scrutiny and audit processes, there is the expectation that any interference required to introduce new HI technologies into any culture around the world would be well-intended and would not bring deliberate or foreseeable harm to the target culture while at the same time passing the various forms of ethical and professional scrutiny from all stakeholders and agents of international development.

Practical Expectations of What to Positively Influence by Engaging the Developing World. There are many areas in which HI researchers and practitioners in the developed world could have practical expectations of exerting positive influence through engagement with the developing world researchers. These include the following:

1. The development of policies that encourage the adoption of new locally customised HI technologies in public and private healthcare organisations.
2. The empowerment of local experts to participate and carry out the local customisation work on the HI technologies to be transferred as well as the knowledge and information contents of these technologies.
3. The stimulation of collaborative research works/projects and work groups at universities in developing countries and development of local centres of excellence and engagement with the developed world.
4. The encouragement of local researchers and experts to participate in efforts that seek to introduce the technologies targeted at the developing world.
5. The facilitation of discussions and exchanges of innovative research problems, ideas, methods and outcomes of technology adoption efforts through joint conferences and similar forums.

Sustainable Engagement with the Developing World. To be sustainable, any form of engagement with the developing world must incorporate the following key elements:

1. The contribution towards empowering local researchers, practitioners and policy makers to build their own capacity for engaging in international collaborations for facilitating bi-directional technology transfer.
2. The involvement of local institutions that are agents of sustainable human capital replenishment, focusing on young people, in particular, at universities, research centres and technical institutes in projects that seek to develop technologies that are suitable for the developing world.
3. The involvement of local practitioners and policy makers, e.g., Ministries of Health and of Higher Education as well as clinicians' professional associations. This should be coupled with a contribution towards an environment that brings practitioners and policy makers to work together with researchers at universities.

4. The recognition that the role and use of the HI technologies to be "transferred" will need to be redefined in the terms of the language, culture and general social and economic contexts of the developing world and then learned [Braa1995]. Only then sustainable maintenance and innovations that extend and develop further the "transferred" HI technologies can be realised in a way that may also benefit the developing world.

Expectations of Positive Transformation from Increased Use of ICT in the Developing World. Clearly, modern vaccines have made huge differences in health the world over. Such direct positive transformation may be hard to expect from increased computer/information technology use in the developing world, especially in the short- to medium-term. This is due to the fact that the developing world is still struggling with the basic necessities of their Healthcare Systems. However, if the introduction of the new technologies is harmonised with and targeted towards the major problem areas of these Healthcare Systems, it could be reasonable to expect the same positive transformation as that being seen from modern vaccines.

Conclusion: *Challenges in Health Informatics in the Developing World.* The major challenges for HI in the developing world are dictated by key trends that will shape health concerns in these regions of the world as well as create novel opportunities for Health Informatics to address major challenges that the area will be facing. These trends have been identified in many government reports across the developing world as well as through studies conducted by private bodies [Robertson2009] and international organisations [WHO-HMN2011]. The trends may be summarised as follows:

1. Increasing the private sector role in regions where health monitoring and reporting is generally handled by the public sector, which may lead to under-reporting at the national level. The HI challenge is supporting interoperability and monitoring across the public and private sectors;
2. Changing profiles of disease challenges due to escalating economic developments. The HI challenge is to provide decision-support systems that accommodate the old and emerging disease profiles;
3. The threat of pandemic risk will span both the developed and developing world. The HI challenge is to support monitoring and control of pandemics in ways that are beneficial to both the developing and developed world;
4. Treatments enhancements will result from advances in medical technology but their distribution will be hampered by lack of infrastructural improvements;
5. The brain-drain from health systems of the developing world to the developed world will escalate as a result of globalisation. The HI challenge is the development of knowledge-rich decision-support systems that can be used by clinicians with low-levels of qualification and training and that should be run on low-cost and wirelessly networked mobile computing devices.

It will be necessary for HI in developing countries to address the problems that arise from these trends in order to have any positive impact. The developing world defines our technological lowest common denominator that should be our target for sustainable technological advancements in a world that is tending towards diminished resources.

Thus, HI in the developing world is our problem if the technologies that we are developing are to be robust, sustainable and continuously innovative. Even if our target is the developed world, the solutions that we develop must be relevant to the technological lowest common denominator in order to be sustainable everywhere.

References

Adjorlolo2013. Adjorlolo, S., Ellingsen, G.: Readiness Assessment for Implementation of Electronic Patient Record in Ghana: A Case of University of Ghana Hospital. Journal of Health Informatics in Developing Countries (JHIDC) 7(2), 2013, http://www.jhidc.org/index.php/jhidc/article/view/104/144 (accessed: October 31, 2013)

Bell2006. Bell, G.: The Age of the Thumb: A Cultural Reading of Mobile Technologies from Asia. Knowledge, Technology and Policy 19(2), 41–57 (2006)

Braa1995. Braa, J., Monteiro, E., Reinert, E.S.: Technology Transfer vs. Technological Learning: IT Infrastructure and Health Care in Developing Countries. Information Technology for Development 6(1) (1995)

Dare2005. Dare, L., Buch, E.: The Future of Health Care in Africa Depends on Making Commitments Work in and Outside Africa. British Medical Journal (BMJ) 331, 1–2 (2005)

Foster2012. Foster, R.: Health Information Systems: A High-Level Review to Identify Health Enterprise Architecture Assets in Ten African Countries. Report of the Jembi Health Systems - Health Enterprise Architecture Project (2012), http://www.hiwiki.org/PHTF/images/e/e2/R_Foster_HEA_Review.pdf (accessed: October 31, 2013)

Juma2012. Juma, K., Nahason, M., Apollo, W., Gregory, W., Patrick, O.: Current Status of e-Health in Kenya and Emerging Global Research Trends. International Journal of Information and Communication Technology Research 2(1(2), 50–54 (2012)

Robertson2009. Robertson, J., DeHart, D., Tolle, K.M.: Healthcare Delivery in Developing Countries: Challenges and Potential Solutions. In: Hey, T., Tansley, S., Tolle, K.M. (eds.) The Fourth Paradigm, pp. 65–73. Microsoft Research (2009) ISBN: 978-0982544204

WHO-HMN2011. WHO-HMN. Country Health Information Systems: A Review of the Current Situation and Trends; Report of the Health Metrics Network (HMN) under the World Health Organization (WHO), (2011), http://www.who.int/occupational_health/healthy_workplace_framework.pdf (accessed: October 31, 2013)

1.2 Deshendran Moodley

Globally, it is apparent that much still needs to be done in terms of health ICT. There are fundamental challenges with existing health ICT solutions which seems to indicate that a quantum leap in research and innovation is required. Despite the fact that there are challenges in terms of e.g. privacy and confidentiality, we should be further along in health ICT than we currently are. One can draw money from ATM machines and pay with a VISA card in Kigali but cannot access a shared health record. It is clear that health lags behind other industries in the application of ICT. We believe that ICT has the potential to have a higher impact in health care delivery in developing countries than the developed world. Discussion points, issues, challenges and future directions:

1. A deeper understanding of the social, cultural and political environment is required to create and deploy effective technologies. Systems must cater for the local situation which can be highly dynamic. While lessons can be learnt from experiences in high income countries, innovation is required to tailor solutions for local settings.
2. There is a need to develop local ICT innovators, to strengthen Computer Science departments at local universities, and improve capacity for technology creation rather than just technology use.
3. Is ICT for Health (ICT4H) a Computer Science research area? Is this "applied" Computer Science or purely a software development exercise?
4. Open architectures and frameworks are required to facilitate interoperability between fragmented health applications and systems, from aggregated reporting systems that operate at the population level to EMR systems at the individual level.
5. Other areas where advanced technologies are required include: capturing of sharable clinical knowledge and process models, real-time clinical decision support, public health simulation to support policy making and revision of health priorities.

1.3   Bill Thies

Designing for Technology Transfer. One of the most under-appreciated design challenges for health informatics in the developing world is that of technology transfer. If you look at vaccines, there are often decades of high-tech research and development that is delivered in a single shot—an exemplar of good technology transfer. Some areas of computing offer similar benefits. For example, a randomized algorithm may be very difficult to design or prove efficient, but it is often very easy to use. Unfortunately, the situation is often reversed for health informatics. Many information systems that we attempt to transfer to the developing world are easier to produce than they are to maintain! When this is true, we do a disservice by developing them as outsiders, as it only exacerbates the challenges of localization and maintenance. I will explore the implications of this observation, including an intentional focus on designing for technology transfer as well as an openness to prioritizing education and training over the development of new technology artifacts.

2 Human Factors in Health Informatics: Something We Should Be Bothered with?

The potential of computer technology in modern medicine and health services is vast, but in many instances is hampered by low uptake on the part of the users. Challenges include inability to use existing technology, refusal on the part of both individuals and organizations to invest in the time to change to new methodologies, refusal to share via electronic media, and suitability of technology across the age, cultural and other spectra. Questions include: How much of these problems can we expect to just "fade away" as people grow up a computerized world? Whose job is it to address these problems—i.e., is this simply a marketing problem or what kind of ownership should each of us take for each of these issues? How can we address these problems both as individuals and as a group? How much are we willing to allow and/or encourage funding agencies to support this somewhat "soft" science? How can we convince vendors to be more sensitive to the needs of the customer? Finally, can we, in fact, really make technology more user-friendly or should we expect people to just "deal with it"?

Moderated by Alan Wassyng

2.1 Jane Liu

Many devices and applications for wellness management and health care (including intelligent medication schedulers and dispensers; mobile heart-beat, blood pressure and pulse rate monitors; and individual personal health electronic records) are user-centric: They are used on a discretionary basis by people with diverse needs, personal preferences and skills and run on platforms owned and maintained by the users. In addition to being able to adapt to changes in user's needs while in use, a user-centric device must be easily configurable and customizable by the user. Some user-centric devices and applications require little or no training of their users but may rely on the users to perform some mission-critical functions. Such a device or application must be able to monitor and respond to user actions in order to ensure that the user and device together never do any harm and all unavoidable errors are either recoverable or tolerable. These challenges must be overcome for the devices and applications to be widely used and indispensable tools.

2.2 Joseph Cafazzo

To ignore this aspect of the design of healthcare IT systems, is to deny its full utility. Far too many systems exist in practice that do not fully realize the promise of creating a safer more efficient healthcare system, largely due arbitrary design that does not consider the complexity of human cognition and performance, and the environment in which they work. Moving beyond the provision of healthcare services in the traditional sense, we cannot create the next generation of patient self-care tools without creating a user-experience that will elicit positive health behaviours, that ultimately will lead to improved health outcomes and reduced dependency on traditional care.

2.3   Oleg Sokolsky

Human factors in health informatics are one of the most important factors in patient safety. It is critical that engineers developing new information technologies for health care be aware of the following two aspects of human factors. On the one hand, developers of information technology have to be aware of workflows and clinical guidelines that caregivers follow in their daily routine. A tool that does not fit into these workflows either remains unused, wasting its potential, or—worse—creates new safety hazards for patients through workarounds and shortcuts that caregivers are forced to apply in order to use the tool. On the other hand, behavior of tools have to match mental models that caregivers have. That is, caregivers have to have unambiguous understanding of what the tool is telling them and what it expects as input. Mode confusion, that is, a mismatch between the tool actual state and the state perceived by a caregiver, creates further safety hazards for patients. A necessary but not sufficient condition for avoiding mode confusion is to provide intuitive and unambiguous user interfaces.

Modelling Care Pathways
in a Connected Health Setting

Padraig O'Leary[1,2], Patrick Buckley[1,3], and Ita Richardson[1,2]

[1] ARCH – Applied Research for Connected Health
University of Limerick
[2] Lero – the Irish Software Engineering Research Centre
University of Limerick, Ireland
[3] Kemmy Business School,
University of Limerick, Ireland
{padraig.oleary,patrick.buckley,ita.richardson}@ul.ie

Abstract. Connected Health involves the use of ICT to improve healthcare quality and outcomes. In a connected heath environment, stakeholders can struggle to make best use of this information coming from a variety of sources. Given this, we are investigating the challenge of how to use available information to make informed decisions about the care pathway which the patient should follow to ensure that prevention and treatment services are efficient and effective. In this paper, we outline our research into care pathway and information modelling in a Connected Health setting. The research is currently underway, and follows a series of stages using sources in industry and academia. In this paper, we present an overview of the project work packages including an explanation on how the different stages of the research form a continuum in which the developed models will be continually adjusted. We describe how empirical evidence will be used in the development of the models through following an evolutionary multi-method research approach.

1 The Challenge

The design, development and implementation of effective Healthcare Information Systems (HIS) is the pre-eminent concern of the Health Informatics discipline. In a report entitled *Crossing the Quality Chasm: A New Health System for the 21st Century,* the American Institute of Medicine recognises that "IT has enormous potential to improve the quality of healthcare" [1]. However, the same report recognized that the fulfilment of this potential represented an enormous, multifaceted challenge that tests both practitioners and the academic community.

An innovative approach to healthcare provision which has gained considerable interest in recent years is Connected Health. Connected Health encompasses terms such as wireless, digital, electronic, mobile, and tele-health and refers to a conceptual model for health management where devices, services or interventions are designed around the patient's needs, and health related data is shared, in such a way that the patient can receive care in the most proactive and efficient manner possible [2].

J. Gibbons and W. MacCaull (Eds.): FHIES 2013, LNCS 8315, pp. 32–40, 2014.

The incentive behind Connected Health is to develop and deliver healthcare solutions that can increase quality of life and reduce the risk to patients while lowering the overall cost of care.

These Connected Health solutions require new clinical pathways and care delivery mechanisms. Clinical pathways, traditionally focused in primary and secondary care, are extending into the community. This repositioning of care provision will dramatically affect the volume and character of data that healthcare professional will have available to them. Care homes, hospices, hospitals and pharmacists will be interacting in a loosely connected, patient defined network. Patients will use mobile technology to record, store and transmit medical data. The difficulty healthcare professionals are faced with is how to use this data to make informed decisions about the care pathway which the patient should follow. Effective use of this data will require the creation of new and advanced health information systems that ensure that preventions and treatments are efficient and effective.

These health information systems "... *formally model guidelines, workflow or care pathways and provide support for clinical decisions that extend over time*" [3]. Health information systems are active, dynamic. And contain a large number of interacting components and subsystems. Artefacts in such a system include hardware components; actors such as healthcare professionals, IT experts and patients; and data that represents the state of the system at any moment in time.

The development of health information systems is supported by the use of models of both systems and processes [4]. These models support requirements capture and analysis. They are used to design, control and monitor system development and often serve a role in post-development validation and implementation.

The model of an information system is different and distinct from an instance of that information system. Similarly, the model of a health information system will be different and distinct from an instance of a health information system. A model will always be simpler and more abstract than an instantiated health information system. Crucially, models of workflows and care pathways must be understood by many different stakeholders, who may have different experiences, backgrounds and knowledge [5]. In the healthcare context, modelling is recognized as providing a unique challenge caused by factors such as the unpredictable and dynamic nature of workflows [6].

The research presented in this paper aims to model care pathways and information flow based on Connected Health solutions. Initially, we will focus on understanding and modelling the clinical preventions, treatments and control of dementia in the elderly. To do this, we will establish the information which comes from different healthcare professionals, systems and medical devices, how that information should be managed to provide effective and efficient care and the clinical pathways within which this information will be used. This will be carried out in conjunction with those healthcare professionals who are managing elderly patients, and will result in models and a software prototype for presenting these models which we will evaluate during the project. Therefore, the two aims of the research are as follows:

1. To unambiguously model the care pathways and information required by the variety of stakeholders in a health network.
2. To use software prototyping to develop an understanding how best these models can be presented to healthcare professionals.

In this paper we outline our planned programme of research for meeting these aims. The paper is organized as follows: Section 2 provides an overview of the research plan. Section 3 describes the work to date. Section 4 describes the planned work and key work packages to be delivered. Finally section 5 concludes our paper with a summary of the project.

2   Research Plan

Based on international best practice and input from local healthcare professionals, we will develop care pathways and information models that can be used by healthcare professionals in a Connected Health network, which will include home-care and hospitalization. We will develop models and software for the distribution and presentation of care pathways and information models throughout this Connected Health Network.

This research will be delivered across five work-packages:

- WP1 – Requirements Capture
- WP2 – Development and Modelling of Care pathways
- WP3 – Development and Modelling of Information Requirements
- WP4 – Prototype of Care pathways and Information Requirements
- WP5 - Evaluation of Information Utilization

The goal of our research is to present an evidence based care pathway for dementia which is disseminated to Connected Health stakeholders in a manner that informs and expedites effective decision making. With this in mind, we will describe each of the proposed work packages. As we have commenced WP1 we present how we are eliciting the requirements for a care pathway support system and our initial decisions on our modelling approach. Our future work discusses WP2, 3, 4 and 5 - how we will develop and evaluate a care pathway support system that will use the care pathway models.

3   Research to Date

3.1   WP1 - Requirements Capture

The purpose of this work-package is to identify the key requirements for the modelling of care pathways and information flow in the Connected Health network. We are answering the following question - "What are key requirements for representing care pathways and information flow?" These include the information, knowledge, clinical and medical device requirements that are required. Defining the data that must be collected regarding individual patients, the aggregated sets of data which are required by healthcare professionals and other Connected Health partners, the use of medical devices in the care and support of the dementia patients and the pathway which is followed by health professionals as they carry out their jobs. In addition it is important to understand the requirements for out of bounds data which indicates the occurrence of exceptional events thus requiring immediate interventions.

To date, we have considered both the state-of-the-art in workflow modelling and expert knowledge from practitioners and academics. We are systematically identifying and analysing requirements from the literature. We are commencing a qualitative meta-synthesis which will be performed on studies published in English that addressed the modelling process and reported the exposition of a new methodology, model, system implementation, or system architecture. Thematic analysis will be used to capture the underlying 'requirement' themes.

We have developed an initial definition of the requirements based on which we conducted surveys among experts to assess the relevancy, completeness, and relative importance of our initial requirements. We prioritized and refined the requirements based on experts' opinion. We merged some requirements based on the experts' suggestions and rephrased some requirements to address misunderstandings and ambiguities found. Furthermore, when refining the requirements we took into account additional requirements suggested by the experts.

Using the identified requirements, we performed an evaluation of current modelling languages. A modelling language is any artificial language that can be used to express information or knowledge or systems in a structure that is defined by a consistent set of rules [7]. There is an enormous variety of modelling languages in existence.

Modelling languages can be graphical (e.g. UML [8]), textual (e.g. PML [9, 10]), mathematically based formal languages or a combination of these (e.g. Petri-Nets [11] or Little-Jil [12]). Modelling languages are designed in such a way as to balance a large number of competing attributes including, but not limited to, how easy they are to understand, how well they support the representation of a process and what kinds of different syntactic structures such as loops and conditional branching they support.

Different modelling languages balance these competing requirements in different ways, and the syntax of a modelling language will have a major impact on the models that are created with it Therefore, since the efficiency of any Connected Health solution is determined in part by the utility of the model, which is in turn partly determined by the choice of modelling language, it stands to reason that the choice of modelling language used is an important determinant of the eventual success or failure of a Connected Health solution.

Based on our evaluations, we have identified a 'best-fit' language that advocates the value of low-fidelity models for documenting and analysing knowledge-intensive work in health care setting [13]. A low fidelity model does not seek to capture every detail and nuance of a knowledge-intensive process; rather, it documents the major activities of a process, and the primary sequence in which they are performed.

Coordination among concurrent activities performed by different actors is modelled as resource flow: dependencies among coordinated activities are represented by the resources shared by concurrent activities.

4   Further Research Being Undertaken

4.1   WP2 – Development and Modelling of Care Pathways

We used previous experience in the development of a process reference model [14] to design a research method which will result in an empirically-grounded model of care pathways in dementia. An initial review of the relevant literature indicated that while high level descriptions of dementia care pathways are available there are few low-level pathway descriptions. Furthermore, no guidance is provided on how the pathway descriptions could be applied or tailored to specific setting. Documented pathways require customisation where the defined process needs to be specialised and a lower level frequently needs to be constructed in order to create a working model.

We will use a multi-method research design as advised in [15]. This is "the conduct of two or more research methods, each conducted rigorously and complete in itself, in one project" [16]. By using triangulation between methods and data, our research will allow more plausible interpretations to emerge.

According to [17] multi-method research may be conducted from a complementary or evolutionary perspective. In the development of our models, we will follow an evolutionary approach. We will undertake an initial exploratory study. We will gather qualitative data, exploring a wide range of topics. We will analyse the results, and use it to develop an initial pathway model. Using a variety of research methods, we will collect and analyse data, and update the model over three cycles. Our approach will be influenced by [18] and is focused on empirically grounded and valid process model construction. In an analogy with systems engineering, the overall construction process is based on a cyclic structure to allow for corrections to the model from preceding construction stages via feedback-loops. Although the stages are dealt with sequentially, they contain cyclic sub-stages. The research approach will be compatible with common suggestions for qualitative research designs in process models [18] and is presented in Figure 1.

Version one of the model will be developed through available literature and clinical guidelines. Version two will be based on ethnographically informed practitioner evidence. Key stakeholder activities will be observed and observations extracted. These observations will be used to design an interview protocol to be used during a series of semi-structured interviews. From these interviews, key concepts will be extracted combined to form a pathway model. Version three of the model will be based on process mining techniques as proposed by van der Aalst [19]. The goal of process mining is to use event data to extract process related information, e.g., to automatically discover a process model by observing events recorded by systems used throughout the Connected Health network. There have been several documented case studies [19] of the use of process mining techniques in clinical settings.

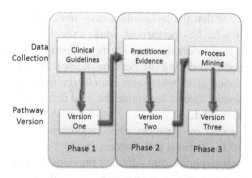

Fig. 1. Modelling phases

When developing the model, we will be identifying the key process indicators required to measure patient care and subsequent improvements, and will use these to develop data dashboards. These will be based on the dashboards which we are currently using within a local hospital. We will establish the key inputs, process and outputs required to ensure that medical devices and data from medical devices are used efficiently and effectively in these pathways.

From our past experience in developing and implementing H-QAP in a local hospital, we recognize that there is a need to "reverse engineer" the clinical process from a systems perspective. This gives us the opportunity to analyse where the efficiency points are, where the system fails, where system intervention is needed and where human contact from healthcare professionals is required. Using H-QAP will guide us in the identification of policies, procedures, protocols, and guidelines, key process indicators (KPI) and patient satisfaction ratings. These research stages will form a continuum in which the focus of the research, the model, is continually adjusted based on the results of the previous stage.

4.2   WP3 – Development and Modelling of Information Requirements

Using the information collected in WP1, a data dictionary will be developed which models the information requirements of the various stakeholders in the Connected Health network. Where required, techniques and algorithms to collate, compress and aggregate the data captured by the various Connected Health solutions will also be identified and defined. Models will be created which explicitly includes the information requirements of the various Connected Health stakeholders.

4.3   WP4 – Prototype

We will develop a system which will meet the requirements for a care pathway support system and which is more explanatory in nature than enforcing. Rather than prescribing a list of actions to be performed at each and every stage of the pathway, we will adopt a reactive approach, whereby a Connected Health stakeholder is provided with guidance only when they explicitly ask for it. The pathway support system is 'descriptive', in the sense that the stakeholder does not even need to inform the system about the activities he has performed while executing a pathway. Rather, the pathway enactment engine infers the state of the pathway by examining the state of products created or modified during the performance of the process's tasks. Then, if an actor requires guidance as to what tasks should (or may) be performed next, the system can use the inferred state to determine the next action to be taken, according to the underlying pathway model.

The prototype will gather information, where appropriate aggregate it, and provide targeted information to the various stakeholders in the Connected Health network in line with their information requirements defined previously. It will provide a support system for the care pathways that have been identified. We expect that it will support the decisions that a healthcare professional will make about a patient such as what clinical care is required, where this should be carried out (in the community or hospital), what medical devices can support this care and what data is required for this care to be carried out effectively. Healthcare professionals will be provided with dashboards which will aggregate data to measure their defined KPI, highlighting where problems and potential problems exist. It will also take into account software quality regulations commensurate with a research project [20]. We will develop this prototype to ensure that the information can be accessed on a wide variety of device's including, but not limited to desktop PC's, laptops, tablets and mobile phones.

4.4   WP5 - Evaluation of Information Utilization.

This task will focus on evaluating the impact of the optimized information and care pathways delivery to healthcare professionals. Using relevant evaluation frameworks, the overall effectiveness and efficiency of the software prototype will be evaluated. This work package will evaluate the utilization of the information collected and its effectiveness on the decisions which are being made in the prevention and treatment during the dementia care pathway. This task will focus particularly on ensuring that the information being captured and collated is valid, and that decisions being made are supporting the efficiency and effectiveness of the clinician. It will also examine the utilization of the information provided by the software system on clinical decision making, and look for changes in patient outcomes and care in terms of previously identified KPI.

Second, this task will focus on evaluating the effectiveness of the methods by which the data is presented to healthcare Professionals. In this task, experimental research will compare a variety of ways of presenting information to healthcare professionals, with a view to empirically identifying best practice for delivering information to healthcare professionals in a manner that aids decision making.

5   Conclusion

In response to a need for pathway support in Connected Health, the authors identified the following research objectives: First, to unambiguously model the care pathways and information required by the variety of stakeholders in a health network. Second, to use software prototyping to develop an understanding how best this information can be presented to healthcare professionals.

By meeting these objectives, we hope to assist stakeholders in dementia care networks as to how to use available data to make informed decisions about the care pathway which the patient should follow to ensure that preventions and treatments are efficient and effective.

In this paper, we have documented our approach for the support of care pathways in Connected Health and the research design decisions made. For Connected Health to reach its potential there is a need to define and present evidence-based pathways and this research is a step in this direction. The plan we present is high level. Further research is needed to support the definition of what, when and how tasks are used for specific contexts, domains or organization in the Connected Health setting. It would also be interesting to consider a more rigorous information systems development approach which considers the interplay between various system stakeholders.

Acknowledgements. This work was partially supported by ARCH – Applied Research for Connected Health funded by Enterprise Ireland, IDA Ireland and by Science Foundation Ireland grant 10/CE/I1855. Many thanks to Sinead O'Mahony for proof reading and suggested improvements.

References

1. AIOM: Crossing the Quality Chasm: A New Health System for the 21st Century, http://www.nap.edu/openbook.php?record_id=10027&page=170
2. Caulfield, B.M., Donnelly, S.C.: What is Connected Health and why will it change your practice? Qjm Mon. J. Assoc. Physicians (2013)
3. Gooch, P., Roudsari, A.: Computerization of workflows, guidelines, and care pathways: a review of implementation challenges for process-oriented health in-formation systems. J. Am. Med. Inform. Assoc. (2011)
4. Bennett, S., McRobb, S., Farmer, R.: Object-oriented Systems Analysis and Design Using UML 2/e. McGraw-Hill Education (2001)
5. Shelly, G.B., Rosenblatt, H.J.: Systems Analysis and Design. Cengage Learning (2011)
6. Hicheur, A., Ben Dhieb, A., Barkaoui, K.: Modelling and Analysis of Flexible Healthcare Processes Based on Algebraic and Recursive Petri Nets. In: Weber, J., Perseil, I. (eds.) FHIES 2012. LNCS, vol. 7789, pp. 1–18. Springer, Heidelberg (2013)
7. Modeling language (2013), http://en.wikipedia.org/w/index.php?title=Modeling_language&oldid=547030508
8. OMG Unified Modeling LanguageTM (OMG UML), http://www.omg.org/spec/UML/2.4.1/
9. Noll, J., Scacchi, W.: Specifying process-oriented hypertext for organizational computing. J. Netw. Comput. Appl. 24, 39–61 (2001)
10. Atkinson, D.C., Noll, J.: Automated validation and verification of process models. In: Proceedings of the 7th IASTED International Conference on Software Engineering and Applications (2003)

11. Kurt, J.: Coloured Petri Nets: Basic Concepts, Analysis Methods and Practical Use. Springer (1996)
12. Wise, A.: Little-JIL 1.5 Language Report. Department of Computer Science. University of Massachusetts (2006)
13. O'Leary, P., Buckley, P., Richardson, I.: Modelling Care Pathways in a Con-nected Health Setting. Presented at the Third International Symposium on Foundations of Health Information Engineering and Systems, Macau (August 21, 2013)
14. O'Leary, P., de Almeida, E.S., Richardson, I.: The Pro-PD Process Model for Product Derivation within software product lines. Inf. Softw. Technol. 54, 1014–1028 (2012)
15. O'Leary, P., Richardson, I.: Process reference model construction: implementing an evolutionary multi-method research approach. Iet Softw. 6, 423–430 (2012)
16. Morse, J.M., Niehaus, L.: Mixed method design: principles and procedures. Left Coast Press (2009)
17. Wood, M., Daly, J., Miller, J., Roper, M.: Multi-method research: An empirical investigation of object-oriented technology. J. Syst. Softw. 48, 13–26 (1999)
18. Fettke, P., Loos, P.: Reference modeling for business systems analysis. Idea Group Inc., IGI (2007)
19. Van der Aalst, W.M.P.: Process Mining: Discovery, Conformance and Enhancement of Business Processes. Springer Publishing Company (2011) (incorporated)
20. Richardson, I., Shroff, V.: Software Quality Plan for TRANSFoRm (2011), http://www.transformproject.eu/

A Resource Flow Approach to Modelling Care Pathways

Padraig O'Leary[1,2], John Noll[2], and Ita Richardson[1,2]

[1] ARCH – Applied Research for Connected Health
University of Limerick, Ireland
[2] Lero – the Irish Software Engineering Research Centre
University of Limerick, Ireland
{padraig.oleary,john.noll,ita.richardson}@ul.ie

Abstract. Attempts to extend process management to support pathways in the health domain have not been as successful as workflow management for routine business processes. In part this is due to the dynamic nature of knowledge-intensive work such as care pathways: the actions performed change continuously in response to the knowledge developed by those actions. Also, care pathways involve significant informal communications between those involved in caring for the patient and between these carers and the patient / patient family which are difficult to capture. We propose using an approach to supporting care pathways that embraces these difficulties. Rather than attempting to capture every nuance of individual activities, we seek to facilitate communication and coordination among knowledge workers to disseminate knowledge and pathway expertise throughout the organization.

1   Introduction

Connected Health encompasses terms such as wireless, digital, electronic, mobile, and tele-health and refers to a conceptual model for health management where devices, services or interventions are designed around the patient's needs, and health related data is shared, in such a way that the patient can receive care in the most proactive and efficient manner possible [1]. All stakeholders in the pathway are 'connected' by means of timely sharing and presentation of accurate and pertinent information regarding patient status through smarter use of data. Essentially "Connected Health" is the utilization of "connecting" technologies (i.e. communication systems – broadband, wireless, mobile phone, fixed phone lines), medical devices for healthcare applications and healthcare information systems. In addition, technologies relating to sensors, alert systems, vital sign monitoring devices, health informatics and data management systems are also fundamental to the development of Connected Health solutions.

These Connected Health solutions provide an opportunity to establish new care pathways and care delivery mechanisms. Care pathways, traditionally focused in primary and secondary care, are extending into the community. Standards of care, conventionally maintained and reinforced in a hospital/clinic setting, must now be supported in a community setting and encompass the new information flows from

J. Gibbons and W. MacCaull (Eds.): FHIES 2013, LNCS 8315, pp. 41–58, 2014.
© Springer-Verlag Berlin Heidelberg 2014

Connected Health solutions. This affords a significant opportunity to improve care pathways and develop best practices around Connected Health solutions.

As a model for healthcare provision, Connected Health offers many potential benefits. It is anticipated that these solutions will increase quality of life and reduce the risk to patients while lowering the overall cost of care. However, the conceptual shift from a model of healthcare where patient care is provided by an individual doctor to a model where care is provided by a team of heath care professionals also poses many challenges. It comes from teams of healthcare professionals who can have access to a lot of, often, too much, information. These healthcare professionals work together to understand prevention and treatments, and often use individual patient data, aggregated data and information from multiple sources. Patients may be using medical devices from mobile phone applications to regulated monitors, which are also data collection points. The difficulty healthcare professionals are faced with is how to use this data to make informed decisions about the care pathway which the patient should follow to ensure that preventions and treatments are efficient and effective.

In this paper, we report on applying a modelling approach to define care pathways and information flow in a Connected Health environment. The model specification can then be parsed and interpreted by a pathway support system. The modelling approach enables pathways to be modelled as independent "pathway fragments" representing activities performed by a single actor. Each fragment is a specification of the control flow from one action to the next that leads to the completion of an action. Coordination among concurrent activities performed by different actors is modelled as resource flow while dependencies among coordinated activities are represented by the resources shared by concurrent activities. This work contributes to a larger project which seeks to model workflow and information flow in connected health settings [2].

In Section 2 we provide a background to applying this approach. In Section 3 we show the rational and application of the approach using a simple example. In Section 4, we describe an implementation of process modelling using an idealized evidence-based pathway for a dementia patient. Finally, in Section 6 we describe our conclusion.

2   Workflow in Healthcare

The healthcare domain relies on knowledge intensive work. Knowledge intensive work is different from routine work in that actors may perform knowledge intensive actions in different ways, depending on their intuition, preferences, and expertise. For example, novice actors who are performing the work for the first time may not have any knowledge about how to do the work. More experienced actors who have done the work before have some insight about how things should be done. Finally, there are experts, who know the process thoroughly and can readily improvise new solutions to problems. Due to this difference in their respective knowledge levels, different actors may do the same work in different ways. Consequently, the amount and nature of guidance required while doing the work is different. Thus, a modelling language for supporting knowledge intensive work must be flexible.

Continuous change is also a key issue in the health domain. Changes may result from the introduction of new devices, new software applications, new personnel, or new guidelines, regulatory requirements or standards. Still other changes come as reactions to errors that have recently occurred locally. In part, this is due to the dynamic nature of such activities: actors in knowledge-intensive environments continually adapt their activities to reflect increasing understanding of the problem at hand, which understanding results from performing the knowledge intensive activities. Thus, the performance or enactment of knowledge-intensive work processes involves a continuous cycle of planning, action, review, and refinement. Any representation of workflow in healthcare must be able to handle this continuous change.

A workflow modelling language is any artificial language that can be used to express information or knowledge or systems in a structure that is defined by a consistent set of rules [3]. There is an enormous variety of modelling languages in existence. Modelling languages can be graphical (e.g. UML [4]), formal (e.g. Petri-Nets [5] or Little-Jil [6]), or control flow (e.g. PML [7, 8]).

2.1   Formal Modelling

Formal modelling processes is one paradigm for describing processes [9, 10]. This approach relies on rules or logical descriptions to describe the actions and then generates a model from the dependencies specified in the actions. The main advantage of this approach is that the modeller need only specify individual actions, and the associated tools will automatically generate a model with consistent dependencies. Two of the most popular formal modelling approaches in healthcare are Petri-Nets and Little-Jil.

Petri-Nets [5, 11] is an example of a formal modelling language and uses constructs underpinned by a mathematical model [12] to describe workflow. The advantages of Petri-Nets are the explicit synchronisation and concurrency, plus mechanisms for sequencing and routing of tasks in workflows. However Petri-Nets has a number of disadvantages [13] not least of which is the difficulty in representing data-flow. It is also difficult to model conditions that relate to attributes and information objects. These are required for modelling collaborative workflows that are typical for integrated health information systems for the effective sharing of health information and care resources.

Little-Jil [6] is formal modelling language based on co-ordination of agents. Little-JIL is based on a graphical representation of processes. This graphical representation is used to describe the order and communication between actions. A compiler is developed to translate a Little-JIL model into a finite-state machine. Properties of a workflow are specified as a property of the state machine. Finite state machine model checkers are used for verification of the model.

Through both Petri-Nets and Little-Jil are formal approaches they have a graphical representation. The advantage of this approach is that the process is displayed as a graph or flowchart that can be easily followed. However, the advantage of a graphical display erodes as the detail of the model increases.

The complexity of the language should not prevent a person without strong technical background from using the language. A non-technical person should be able to model the process without being encumbered by the syntactic requirements of the language. However, both Little-Jil and Petri-Nets assume some level of technical familiarity using syntax such as 'interface', 'agent' and 'exception'.

For the modeller, formal modelling approaches can make it difficult to control the order of actions in the process. If two steps are independent, but the modellers wants them to be performed in a sequence, then a false dependency must be introduced in order to achieve the desired results, which adds an unnecessary layer of complexity. This can produce undesirable results especially at high levels of abstraction. The semantics to provide control to a process are too low-level to adequately control an abstract model. If no rules are specified, then it is difficult to generate a model that accurately depicts the process at a high-level.

Common formal modelling approaches to adding flexibility is enabling exception handling capabilities. The focus is on changing the running instances of the process model to handle exceptional situations which may or may not be anticipated and which require the actor to deviate from the normal flow of work. The idea is that once systems have such capability, they will be able to handle dynamic work processes. Little-Jil uses exceptions to increase flexibility. Petri-Nets have been adapted to allow for exceptions [14]. Recursive Workflow Nets (RecWF-Nets) [15] are another formalism for the modelling and analysis of flexible clinical pathways. They allow users to deviate from the pre-modelled process plan during run-time by offering other alternatives (creating, deleting or reordering some sub-processes).

However these approaches are counterintuitive to how people think about processes. The order in which actions are performed is a primary concern when defining a process and the modeller should be able to control it. Therefore, rather than implementing the care pathway with a formal modelling language, the language we advocate is control-based with a resource flow focus, an approach called PML [7, 8].

2.2   Process Modelling Language

PML (Process Modelling Language) enables control to be specified by the modeller, which allows her to describe the flow of control in the pathway. This method can be used to model abstract pathways, detailed pathways, and every layer of abstraction between the two [16]. At a high level of abstraction, the control is sequential, which allows the modeller to imply the dependencies without actually having to specify them. If it is later decided that the model should be more specific, the actual dependencies can be introduced. This method is more intuitive and reflects the steps that healthcare professionals normally take.

Previous work has demonstrated the value of resource flow models for documenting and analysing knowledge-intensive work [7, 17]. A resource flow model does not seek to capture every detail and nuance of a knowledge-intensive process; rather, it documents the major activities of a process, and the primary sequence in which they are performed through the production and consuming of artefacts. Using a resource flow specification of the pathway, the current state of the pathway can be inferred by observing the current state of the artefacts in the environment. Then, when the actor asks for advice, the pathway support system uses this inferred state and the process specification to provide guidance on what to do next. Since there is no enforcement of the nominal flow of actions specified in the process model, deviations can be easily supported. The only requirement for these deviations is the availability of required resources.

Modelling pathway using resource flow models yields several benefits [16]:

- Resource flow models are low-fidelity, easy to specify, and can be generated rapidly.
- A resource flow model still captures the essential facets of a process, especially the resources consumed and artefacts produced by a given set of activities.
- Because they seek to represent only high-level detail, resource flow models are relatively stable; that is, they continue to be accurate descriptions of the high-level process, even as the details of process activities evolve in response to knowledge and experience gained with the problem.

Ultimately, we will use resource–flow care pathways to develop a support system that will guide stakeholders through pathway execution. For example, when a doctor requests assistance on the next steps for a suspected dementia case our model should provide them support in doing this. It is currently difficult for medical professionals to stay up-to-date on the latest recommended protocols without such assistance. Providing updated process models that can provide on-line guidance would help address this problem.

Our proposed approach targets the facilitation of communication and collaboration among knowledge workers to disseminate process expertise as widely as possible. In this approach, actors are given high-level guidance about what activities to perform, and how to perform them, through the use of low-fidelity process models. These specify a nominal order of actions, but leave actors free to carry out their activities as their expertise and the situation dictates.

In the following section, we will demonstrate the potential for this type of low-fidelity control flow modelling for care pathway representation.

3   Resource Flow Pathway Modelling

An example of a low-fidelity model depicting a pathway is shown in Figure 1. This model shows the nominal sequence of activities involved in the treatment of a set of symptoms: the patient presents himself to a specialist clinician, an examination is undertaken and after which a diagnosis is made followed by a course of treatment.

This model captures both the important activities in a clinical treatment, and the main sequence, and is thus useful for discussing the pathway. But it does not capture all of the possible transitions between activities. Many experienced healthcare professions may delay diagnosis, may refer the patient to another clinician, or may attempt to treat patient symptoms if diagnosis is not possible. Occasionally, it is necessary to iterate over the examine and diagnose cycle – as a clinician attempts to diagnose from the generic to the specific. Figure 2 shows these additional transitions, represented by dashed edges.

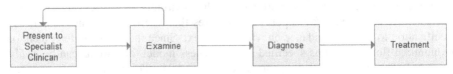

Fig. 1. Specialist assessment pathway

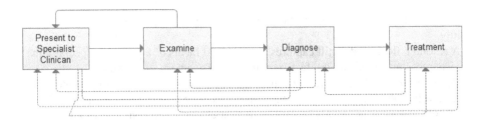

Fig. 2. Specialist assessment pathway, augmented

While this depiction is more complete, in that it represents all of the plausible transitions between actions, it is not completely accurate. For example, although the graph shows a transition from "Present to Specialist Clinician" to "Diagnose", it is not possible to take this transition until the "Examine" step has been successfully completed at least once: "Diagnose" requires examination artefacts, which is the output of the "Examine" step. Further, it's not clear that Figure 2 is more useful than Figure 1. As a guidance tool, a novice clinician might find the numerous transitions confusing, while an expert would already know that these additional transitions are possible.

The modelling approach we have adopted is based on the notion of low-fidelity process models. A low-fidelity model seeks to capture the essence of a process, while abstracting away as many details as possible. The modelling language allows the modeler to capture both the nominal control flow (the solid edges in Figure 2), and the conditions that constrain transitions outside the nominal flow (the dashed lines in Figure 2).

A PML specification of the model in Figure 1 is shown in the following page. The nominal control flow is represented explicitly by the iteration constructs and the ordering of actions in the specifications. The constraints on other transitions are expressed by `provides` and `requires` statements. These are predicates that express the inputs and outputs of each step (action) in the pathway, and thus the pre and postconditions that exist at each step in the pathway. Note that this simple specification captures the constraint that `Diagnose` cannot proceed until `Examine` is successful: the `Diagnose` action require a resource called `examinationArtefacts`, which is produced (provided) by the "Examine" action. Thus, until this action succeeds, `Diagnose` is not possible.

PML representation of Clinical Assessment Pathway

```
process ClinicalAssessment {
  iteration {
    iteration {
      action PresentToSpecailistClinician{
        requires { reportedSymptoms }
        provides { scheduleExamination}
      }
      action Examine {
        requires { scheduleExamination }
        provides { examinationArtefacts }
      }
    }
    action Diagnose {
      requires { examinationArtefacts }
      provides { diagnosis }
    }
    action Treatment{
      requires { diagnosis}
    }
  }
}
```

3.1 Modelling Parallel Pathways

A further complication in modelling the care pathway is that the clinical assessment pathway shown in Figures 1 and 2 does not exist in isolation. Other pathways produce and consume resources from this pathway, as depicted in Figure 4. This figure shows two cooperating pathways: the clinical assessment pathway of Figure 1 and Figure 2, and a parallel lab test pathway.

These pathways cooperate to result in an assessment for the patient: both start with some symptoms to develop their respective artefacts. In addition, the laboratory assessment pathway needs the output of the clinical assessment pathway (the examination artifact and the diagnosis artifact) to run laboratory tests. This dependency between the two pathways could be represented by an explicit link between the "Treat" and "Run Tests" actions (represented by the solid edge in Figure 3). But this approach has several difficulties.

First, it creates an explicit connection between the two pathways that does not always exist: healthcare professions could employ any of a number of different treatment pathways.

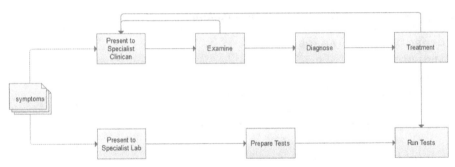

Fig. 3. Coordinated Pathways

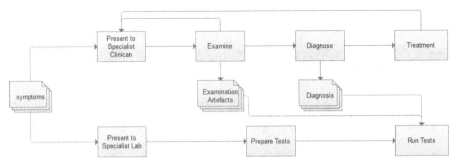

Fig. 4. Resource flow between pathways

Second, it requires both pathways to be maintained as a single model, which is often not the case. Different organizations are responsible for different pathways that they develop independently. Finally, it doesn't capture the true relationship between the pathways. Typically the laboratory assessment pathway requires a "Diagnosis" and "Examination Artefacts", which could, for example, include blood samples to run test so that the actual relationship is between "Diagnose" and "Run Tests" as opposed to "Treat" and "Run Tests." But the patient must have been examined before it can be accepted for testing so there is also a relationship between "Examine" and "Run Tests". From the test pathway point of view there is an "and" style relationship between "Diagnose" and "Examine", and "Run Tests".

The essential relationship between the two pathways is that the clinical assessment pathway produces examination and diagnosis artefacts for the lab pathway to test (Figure 4). It is not important to the laboratory pathway how the clinical assessment pathway diagnoses the patient or how they produce the examination artefacts. What is important is that they exist in a state suitable for the "Run Tests" action.

This relationship is represented in PML as the *PML representation of Laboratory Assessment Pathway*. This specification shows that the beginning of the laboratory assessment pathway depends on the availability of "symptoms". More importantly, the "Run Tests" action cannot begin until the "Present to Specialist Lab" and the "Prepare Tests" actions are completed.

Because the pathways are indirectly coupled, it is not necessary for all actions to be modelled, or enacted. Through a shared resource, enacted pathways can be coordinated with ad-hoc work or activities in another organization. Thus, the "RunTests" action can begin as soon as the "examinationArtefacts" and "diagnosis" resources are available, but these resources can be produced by any pathway, including a completely spontaneous ad-hoc pathway.

PML representation of Laboratory Assessment Pathway

```
process LabAssessment{
  action PresentToSpecialistLab{
    requires { symptoms }
    provides { testPlan }
  }
  action PrepareTests{
    requires { testPlan }
    provides { testSuite }
  }
  action RunTests{
    requires { testSuite && examinationArtefacts
      && diagnosis }
    provides { diagnosis.status == "tested" }
  }
}
```

4   Modelling Clinical Guidelines

In the initial year of the research we are focusing on the understanding and modelling of the clinical preventions, treatments and control of dementia in the elderly. Recently, the National Health Service in the United Kingdom has made the Map of Medicine (MoM) available to healthcare professionals.

The Map of Medicine [18] is a visualization of the ideal, evidence-based patient journey for common and important conditions that can be shared across all care settings. The decentralized nature of care pathways relies on the guidance of a defined pathway to provide cohesion between various stakeholders. The MoM is a web-based tool that can help drive clinical consensus to improve quality and safety in any health-care organization. In the MoM the key interventions are described and references to the guidelines and the overall available literature are made available. The pathways can be one of the tools to organize daily clinical practice, based on the evidence-based content of the MoM.

The MoM care pathway for dementia has two components: assessment of dementia and management of dementia. The first entails detailing how dementia should be assessed and diagnosed. The second is based on managing dementia until end of life. Each stage is comprised of a series of actions related to fulfilling the next stage in development. The management of dementia pathway is given in Figure 5 and provides a summary of the actions involved. In the following section, we discuss our experiences in modelling this pathway using PML.

4.1 Modelling Map of Medicine Dementia Management

On first inspection of the map it is clear that the model is in a basic state in that it includes control and resources, but no attributes or expressions. Inconsistencies are typically introduced into a model because of a failure to specify requirements for an action. In PML, this translates to the failure to require or provide a resource in an action. Each graphical activity contains a detailed description of the underlying pathway. Interpreting a natural language pathway descriptions, such as that used by the MoM, is based on user interpretation.

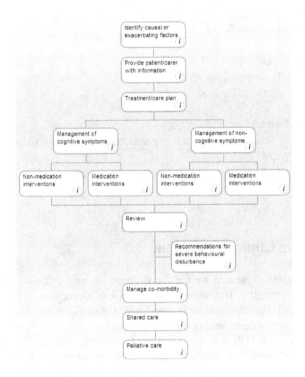

Fig. 5. Action flow in Map of Medicine

Since the top level map is described graphically, we first captured the control flow as a PML model with empty actions. Abstraction and hierarchical decomposition facilitates developing the model incrementally. We had to continually make choices about the number of levels into which an action should be decomposed and about the level of abstraction that was required. A first pass was made to understand and represent the pathway only involving step decomposition and control flow.

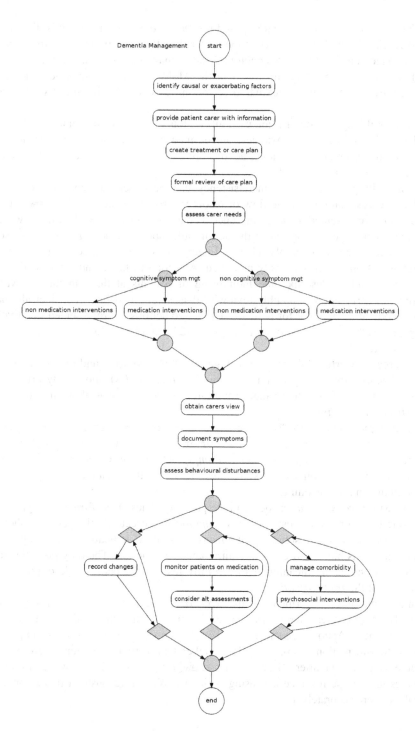

Fig. 6. Resource flow representation of Dementia Management

When examining provided and required resources, the MoM pathway is discussed at two levels of detail. High level actions refer directly to activities (Treatment/care plan, Management of cognitive symptoms, and Management of non-cognitive symptoms) which are graphically illustrated in the MoM. The lower level activities are extracted from the pathway textual descriptions associated with the higher level activities.

The natural language description used allows lots of room for user interpretation in the description of activities. Artefacts are defined but never used, artefacts are required but never created, high level actions are explicitly documented but low level activities are implicitly defined.

By modelling the MoM an inconsistency can be observed between the MoM graphical representation and the flow of resources. For instance, the `Review` action in the map is represented as occurring once as part of a linear control flow. However the natural language description of the action talks about the action being "assessed and recorded at regular intervals" [18]. In Figure 6 this is represented as the `Record Changes` action and is iteratively modelled. A second instance and a sub section of the `Review` action describes the monitoring of patients at three month intervals: "continue to carry out 3-6 monthly review of disease progression", "consider alternative methods of assessment for patient". These two actions are represented iteratively in Figure 6 as "`monitor patients on medication`" and "`consider alt assessments`".

Resource flow errors fall into four categories: those requiring and providing no resources (*empty*), those only requiring resources (*black holes*), those only providing resources (*miracles*), and those that provide resources other than those that they require (*transformations*).

For example, the actions "`Management of non-cognitive symptoms`" and "`Management of cognitive symptoms`" do not require or produce any resources therefore we can class them as *empty* actions. However, both actions are filtering patients based on a set of symptoms. However the resource that is providing symptom information is omitted.

In the MoM *transformations* occur in the pathway. These *transformations* typically occur due to two possibilities: the *transformation* is correct and the pathway should not consider the created resource, or the *transformation* is indicative of a change to a resource that was not specified as a requirement to the action. The only possible way to determine the actual meaning is to carefully inspect the pathway description and the context of the *transformation*.

An example of a transformation is the "`create_treatment_or_care_plan`" action. The required resource is "`patient_history`" and the produced resource is "`care_plan`". Action "`formal_review_of_care_plan`" is an example of where a transformation is improper. Here rather than a transformation where a new resource is produced after "`formal_review_of_care_plan`" we consolidate resources to a single resource and using attributes. We can reconstruct the action and describe it more accurately as:

PML description of formal review action

```
action formal_review_of_care_plan {
    agent {person && carer}
    requires {care_plan}
    provides {care_plan.reviewed == "true"}
}
```

Though a report of an unprovided resource can mean a misrepresentation of process, it can also be indicative of a resource that should pre-exist the process. "Iden-tify_causal_or_exacerbating_factors" requires the resource "Guide-lines_For_Treatment_Of_Patients" but this is the first action in the MoM pathway which means the resource cannot be specified prior to its use. Therefore identifying resources that should be considered inputs to the pathway is a key pre-determinant for pathway execution. Outputs to the process should also be specified.

Resources that are provided by an action but are not later used in the pathway could be the result of a misspecified resource or an action does not note that it requires a certain resource. "care_plan" in action "monitor_patients_on_medication" is produced but not consumed in the pathway.

Correcting the mistakes found in the previous revision results in a model that produces no errors when checked, which ensures that the model is satisfied with the way dependencies are built. Though this does not indicate that there are no problems in the pathway, the model errors have been effectively removed. The final model is shown in Figure 6.

Our experience suggests that these sorts of detailed and complex pathway models should be developed incrementally. This would allow high level, more-abstract views of the pathway to be validated before more-detailed models are developed. The scope and granularity of the model should be determined by the questions the model is intended to address. There is no doubt that detailed models require more effort to develop and maintain, but provide more definitive, in-depth feedback.

PML representation of Map of Medicine Dementia Management pathway

```
process Dementia_Management {
  action identify_causal_or_exacerbating_factors {
    requires { Guidelines_For_Treatment_Of_Patients }
  }
  action provide_patient_carer_with_information {
    agent {GP && patient && carer}
    requires {patient_record.Confirmed_Dementia  }
    requires {patient_record.requests_privacy == "false"
}
    provides { information_to_carer }
  }
```

```
action create_treatment_or_care_plan {
   agent {memory_assessment_service}
   agent {GP && clinical_psychologiest && nurses && oc-
cupational_therapists && phsiotherapists &&
speech_and_language_therapists && social_workers && vol-
untary_organisation}
   requires { patient_history }
   provides { care_plan }
}
action formal_review_of_care_plan {
   agent {person && carer}
   requires {care_plan}
   provides {care_plan.review}  /* XXX Maybe,
care_plan.reviewed == "true" */
}
action assess_carer_needs {
   agent { carer}
   provides {care_plan.respite_care}
}
branch  {
   branch cognitive_symptom_mgt {
      action non_medication_interventions {
provides {support_for_carer}
provides {info_about_servicesAndInterventions}
provides {(optional) cognitive_simulation}
      }
      action medication_interventions {
agent {specialist}
agent {carer}
requires {(intangible)carer_view_on_patient_condition }
provides {prescription}
      }
   } /* end of management_of_cognitive_symptoms  */
   branch non_cognitive_symptom_mgt {
      action non_medication_interventions {
agent {carer && patient}
requires {(nontangible)non_cognitive_symptoms || (non-
tangible) challenging_behaviour}
provides {early_assessment}
      }
      action medication_interventions {
requires {(intangible) risk_of_harm_or_distress}
provides {medication}
      }
   } /* end of management_of_non_cognitive_symptoms */
```

```
  } /* end cognitive/non-cognitive symptoms branch */
  action obtain_carers_view {
    agent {carer}
    provides {(intangible) view_on_condition}
  }
  action document_symptoms {
    agent {patient}
    provides {patient_record.symptoms}
  }
  /* optional, if required */
  action assess_behavioural_disturbances {
    agent {patient}
    requires {(intangible)
risk_of_behavioural_disturbance}
    provides {care_plan.appropriate_setting}
  }
  branch {
    iteration {
      action record_changes {
  agent {patient}
  provides {patient_record.symptoms}
  provides {(optional) medication}
      }
    }
    iteration  {
      action monitor_patients_on_medication{
  agent {patient }
  provides {(optional)care_plan.medication}
      }
      action consider_alt_assessments {
  requires {patient_record.disability || pa-
tient_record.sensory_impairment || pa-
tient_record.lingustic_problems || pa-
tient_record.speech_problems}
  provides {care_plan.alternative_assessment_method}
      }
    }
    iteration {
      action manage_comorbidity {
  /*requires { }*/
  provides {comorbidity.depression}
  provides {comorbidity.psychosis}
  provides {comorbidity.delirium}
  provides {comorbidity.parkinsons_disease}
  provides {comorbidity.stroke}
```

```
      }
      action psychosocial_interventions {
  requires {comorbidity.depression || comorbid-
ity.anxiety}
  agent {carer}
      }
    }
  } /* branch */
} /* process */
```

5   Conclusion

The application of a low fidelity model does not seek to capture every detail and nuance of a knowledge-intensive process. Rather, it documents the major activities of a process, and the primary sequence in which they are performed. Our preliminary work offers considerable promise that low fidelity resource modelling approaches are very suited to modelling medical processes.

One of the benefits of a resource-flow approach is that you can ensure that each action's required resources are produced by some earlier action; otherwise, either there is a flaw in the model, or an input to the pathway. In the MoM we can assess were there cases where the natural-language description overlooked an action or failed to mention a resource that was required later in the pathway? This is one of the biggest benefits of creating formal models: they force a certain level of rigor and therefore examination that could otherwise cause flaws to be overlooked.

5.1   Future Work

By adopting a process modelling approach developed for the software development domain, we have described an approach for care pathway modelling. This approach to pathway modelling needs further evaluation with some optimisation for the health domain. Currently we are involved in modelling dementia pathways, initially looking at clinical guideline based pathways by NICE [19] and Map of Medicine [18].

One of the concerns of the approach is its ability to scale to a large care pathway. Further investigation is required into possible issues when organising pathway fragments via required and provided resources. One possible solution that we will investigate is the use of resource scope, where a resource is only viable within the context of a specific pathway. Alternatively pathway resources could mimic the characteristics of class variables from object oriented languages such as Java. As part of this investigation, we will apply resource flow models to a large scale critical process from the medical domain.

Other interesting issues include how to maintain coherence between the actual pathway and the pathway model. Medical guidelines change frequently, however, so at least the generic versions of these models would need to be updated regularly and then re-customized. Related questions revolve around the customization of the care pathways and the degree to which each local setting has to create custom pathways. In theory, for well-designed pathway models, the customization of a general pathway to a particular hospital setting should mostly involve changes to the low-level pathway steps.

Acknowledgements. This work was partially supported by ARCH – Applied Research in Connected Health funded by Enterprise Ireland, IDA Ireland and by Science Foundation Ireland grant 10/CE/I1855. Many thanks to Sinead O'Mahony for proof reading and suggested improvements.

References

1. Caulfield, B.M., Donnelly, S.C.: What is Connected Health and why will it change your practice? Qjm Mon. J. Assoc. Physicians (2013)
2. O'Leary, P., Buckley, P., Richardson, I.: Modelling Care Pathways in a Con-nected Health Setting. Presented at the Third International Symposium on Foundations of Health Information Engineering and Systems, Macau (August 21, 2013)
3. Modeling language (2013), http://en.wikipedia.org/w/index.php?title=Modeling_language&oldid=547030508
4. OMG Unified Modeling LanguageTM (OMG UML), http://www.omg.org/spec/UML/2.4.1/
5. Kurt, J.: Coloured Petri Nets: Basic Concepts, Analysis Methods and Practical Use. Springer (1996)
6. Wise, A.: Little-JIL 1.5 Language Report. Department of Computer Science. University of Massachusetts (2006)
7. Noll, J., Scacchi, W.: Specifying process-oriented hypertext for organizational computing. J. Netw. Comput. Appl. 24, 39–61 (2001)
8. Atkinson, D.C., Noll, J.: Automated validation and verification of process models. In: Proceedings of the 7th IASTED International Conference on Software Engineering and Applications (2003)
9. Klingler, C.D., Nevaiser, M., Marmor-Squires, A., Lott, C.M., Rombach, H.D.: A case study in process representation using MVP-L. In: Proceedings of the Sev-enth Annual Conference on Computer Assurance, COMPASS 1992. Systems Integrity, Software Safety and Process Security: Building the System Right. pp. 137–146 (1992)
10. Junkermann, G., Peuschel, B., Schäfer, W., Wolf, S.: Merlin: Supporting Cooperation in Software Development through a Knowledge-based Environment. Software Process Modelling and Technology. pp. 103–129. John Wiley & Sons Inc. (1994)
11. Aalst, W.V.D., van Hee, K.M.: Workflow Management: Models, Methods, and Systems. MIT Press (2004)
12. Gooch, P., Roudsari, A.: Computerization of workflows, guidelines, and care pathways: a review of implementation challenges for process-oriented health information systems. J. Am. Med. Inform. Assoc. 18, 738–748 (2011)
13. Bertolini, C., Schäf, M., Stolz, V.: Towards a Formal Integrated Model of Collaborative Healthcare Workflows. In: Liu, Z., Wassyng, A. (eds.) FHIES 2011. LNCS, vol. 7151, pp. 57–74. Springer, Heidelberg (2012)

14. Huang, W., Shi, Y.: Research on Exception Monitoring and Handling Based on Petri Nets. In: International Conference on Information Management, Innovation Management and Industrial Engineering, ICIII 2008, pp. 335–338 (2008)
15. Hicheur, A., Ben Dhieb, A., Barkaoui, K.: Modelling and Analysis of Flexible Healthcare Processes Based on Algebraic and Recursive Petri Nets. In: Weber, J., Perseil, I. (eds.) FHIES 2012. LNCS, vol. 7789, pp. 1–18. Springer, Heidelberg (2013)
16. Noll, J.: Flexible Process Enactment Using Low-Fidelity Models. In: Proceedings of the International Conference on Software Engineering and Applications, Marina del Rey, USA (2003)
17. Scacchi, W., Noll, J.: Process-driven intranets: life-cycle support for process reengineering. IEEE Internet Comput 1, 42–49 (1997)
18. Medicine, M. of: Dementia - management, http://healthguides.mapofmedicine.com/choices/map-open/dementia2.html
19. NHS NICE Guidelines - Dementia Overview (2013), http://pathways.nice.org.uk/pathways/dementia/dementia-overview

ICT-powered Health Care Processes
(Position Paper)

Marco Carbone[1], Anders Skovbo Christensen[3], Flemming Nielson[2],
Hanne R. Nielson[2], Thomas Hildebrandt[1], and Martin Sølvkjær[3],*

[1] IT University of Copenhagen, Rued Langgaardsvej 7, 2300 Copenhagen, Denmark
{hilde,mcarbone}@itu.dk
http://www.itu.dk
[2] DTU Compute, Matematiktorvet 303B, 2800 Kgs. Lyngby, Denmark
{fnie,hrni}@dtu.dk
http://www.dtu.dk
[3] IMT Region H, Innovation & Configuration Borgervænget 3, 2., 2100 Copenhagen, Denmark
{martin.soelvkjaer,anders.christensen}@regionh.dk
http://www.regionh.dk

Abstract. The efficient use of health care ressources requires the use of Information and Communication Technology (ICT). During a treatment process, patients have often been tested and partially treated with different diagnoses in mind before the precise diagnosis is identified. To use ressources well it becomes necessary to adapt the prescribed treatments to make use of the tests and partial treatments already performed, rather than always starting from square one. We propose to facilitate this through the design of *declarative process models* accounting for the involvement of distributed groups of medical specialists and the adaptation of treatments, and through the evaluation of the *trustworthiness of models* taking account of test results and actual treatments compared to the clinical guidelines.

Keywords: Clinical guidelines, declarative and stochastic process models, adaptability, trustworthiness.

1 Challenges and Project Hypothesis

Health care is a fundamental service offered by the society, and as a consequence of the demographic development and the discovery of new medical treatments there is an increasing pressure on getting more and better health care from a fixed budget. A key trend is the use of better work flow in order to reduce errors [47] and make more efficient use of health care resources, and this increasingly dictates the use of Information and Communication Technology (ICT) powered Health Care Processes.

A particular challenge in the health care sector is that the needs of patients are individual and do not directly fit standard work flows (or pathways) as seen in e.g. originally developed for mass production of consumer goods. The patient may have a number of general or specific symptoms, some of which may be variations over normality, whereas others could point to different diagnoses requiring different treatments or tests.

---

* Authors listed alphabetically.

J. Gibbons and W. MacCaull (Eds.): FHIES 2013, LNCS 8315, pp. 59–68, 2014.

Seen from the point of view of the traditional organization of health care, the general practitioner performs an initial screening of the symptoms before patients are referred to more specialized treatment; each group of specialists will focus on one particular type of diagnosis, making further tests and examinations, and carry out treatment only if the hypothesized diagnosis is confirmed.

Seen from the point of view of the patient, this may lead to a sequence of partial treatments and re-referrals before end of treatment. Even more challenging are the needs of patients with co-morbidities — patients suffering from several illnesses at the same time and where symptoms may overlap and there may even be conflicts between the treatments offered by different groups of specialists.

We therefore see the Electronic Health Record (EHR) as giving a record of both tests and partial treatments, representing (multiple) diagnosis, that change with executed experiments and tests and, therapies given to reflect these (multiple) diagnoses. As new tests are made, and as the recovery of the patient is evaluated, the treatment plan may be adjusted to focus on alternative or more specialized diagnoses. There is a need to be able to exploit previous tests and treatments, and to match them to the new prescribed treatment as well as possible, rather than starting out all over again.

The processes of diagnosis and treatment of these multimorbid conditions are, seen in their entirety, thus generally spread between GPs, hospitals, specialty doctors and maybe combined with social service or nursing by the local municipal health units. This makes control, coordination, communication and compliance a special challenge.

Also, a very intensive trend in the e- and mHealth agendas, is the active involvement of the patient via cooperation active roles within the processes or direct patient control. The patient, with the rights of a citizen, takes an active role as an extra provider of own healthcare services and executes (sub)segments of the clinical procedure, reports data directly to the EHR or enters them via telemonitoring equipment or a telemedicine communication channel [8].

This project will study these challenges in the area of cancer treatment, in collaboration with Region Hovedstaden (one of the key Danish health care providers and responsible for the treatment of all Danes living around Copenhagen). In the words of the Danish National Board of Health 2008 (translated by Naja Holten Møller):

> A significant number of patients may not follow the course of a pathway from start to finish. These are, for instance, patients with other diseases or conditions that will affect the diagnosing and treatment. These also include patients where the picture of suspected or [later on] confirmed cancer is unclear. Or it may be patients with relapse after end of treatment.

As described here, it is necessary for the formulation and ICT support of such distributed health care processes to not only reflect the clinical content and data, but also to represent coordination, initiation and assignment of roles to the different steps in a procedure. Examples are

- elective, booked procedures and/or services, incl. self-booked,
- time-slot procedures and/or services (come when you like),
- self service, self initiated or self managed procedures and/or services.

This nature of cross-sectorial cooperation, handover of control, patient empowerment and online medicine makes it necessary to widen the scope of procedure definition beyond traditional flow models.

The main hypothesis of the project is that ICT powered *process models*, as studied in embedded, workflow management and service oriented systems, can be adapted to fit these challenges better than techniques based on procedural workflows and pathways. This involves the difficult question of how to design *declarative process models* to account for the involvement of distributed groups of specialists that need to collaborate in a virtual manner in confirming the diagnosis (or diagnoses) of the patient, adapting and carrying out treatments that are both cost-effective and of high quality. It also involves the difficult question of how to evaluate the *trustworthiness of models* of both the data representing test results, of the diagnoses that may fit the symptoms in varying degrees, and of the conformance of the actual treatment to the one prescribed in clinical guidelines.

The results of this project are likely to benefit the future organization of health care and to lead to new ICT systems that may be developed by software companies. As part of the project we will prepare researchers to take part in working with both health care providers and software companies in achieving these goals.

2 Theoretical Foundations

Process calculi and algebras [30] have been developed to describe the higher-level functioning of modern IT systems, which are to a large extent distributed and operating concurrently. More recent process algebras focus on *coordination* mechanisms between distributed agents, on the *orchestration* of a number of distributed services offered by various agents, and on the *choreography* of a number of distributed and independent services performed by agents that are not under central control; many of these development have been funded by European Union projects, mentioning just Software Engineering for Service-Oriented Overlay Computers (SENSORIA) [45] in which we participated.

Declarative specifications expressed using adaptations of mathematical logic, such as Linear Temporal Logic and Computation Tree Logic [1], provide the basis for model checking hardware components and software systems against specifications and are used extensively by major companies like Intel and Microsoft. During the last five years declarative process notations with implicit control flow, including our own work on Dynamic Condition Response Graphs [33], have been researched as a means to provide support for *flexibility in execution* [51] and *dynamic adaptability* of business process and workflow management systems in general [32–34, 40, 41], and health care processes in particular [27, 35, 36]. Currently, a working group under the Object Management Group (OMG) is preparing a proposal of a declarative case management modeling notation [54] to extend the Business Processing Model and Notation (BPMN 2.0) [39], the current industrial standard for business process modeling defined by the OMG. In the proposed project, we aim to research to which degree declarative models allow to adapt the prescribed operation by adding and removing new activities and constraints, as may result from initiating a new concurrent diagnosis or treatment subprocess within a treatment process.

Trustworthiness is a problem well known from ICT systems where security challenges include both confidentiality (or privacy) and integrity (or trust) of the data. In particular, the notion of trust seems relevant for tagging data bases and EPRs with information about the extent to which test results, diagnoses and treatments can be trusted. During the last two decades there has been numerous work on type systems for the confidentiality of data, and type systems for integrity of data are often dual to these (in a precise formal sense); examples include the Decentralized Label Model [37] developed for the programming language Java. The challenge will be to formulate type systems for *process models* that can accurately propagate trustworthiness information throughout the processes so as to make qualified decisions about the quality of treatment. A recent addition is our own Quality Calculus [16] addressing the problems of how to prescribe actions when insufficient guidance has been received and how to determine the quality of the actions performed under such circumstances. In particular, we aim to research the extent to which a given sequence of partial treatments live up to the expectations as may be prescribed in clinical guidelines. For the latter we anticipate that important insights may be obtained from constraint solving (of both hard and soft constraints [2]) as well as stochastic model checking [1] (using reward and cost structures). In short, given a process model one may construct the set of acceptable traces and consider whether the process model is consistent with a given specification.

Supplementary Methods and Techniques. Along the primary project dimensions of *Declarative Process Models* and *Trustworthiness of Models* we anticipate incorporating a number of cross-cutting methods and techniques, in particular *Type and Effect Systems* [38], *Session Types* [20], *Stochastic Model Checking* [1] and *Constraint Solving* [2].

Type and Effect Systems is a method for annotating software programs with high-level information about their behavior, which can be verified by performing *type checking* before the program is executed. Type systems traditionally just focus on making sure that data types are used consistently like not trying to add integers to character strings. They have been extended also with considerations from security like confidentiality and integrity levels. Effect systems go one step further and provide summaries of the communications performed by the software programs (see e.g. [38]). *Session Types*, also referred to as *behavioral types*, is a refinement of type and effect systems for annotating distributed process models with the behavioral patterns of interaction between the individual actors and ICT systems (see e.g. [20]). That is, in addition to ensuring that the interchanged data has the correct format, the behavioral types also guarantee that each participant follows the same protocol. In this way, session type checking can sometimes guarantee that actors will never end in a deadlock situation, waiting for each other and not being able to progress. *Stochastic Model Checking* is a set of fully automatic techniques for determining whether process models live up to expectations as expressed using mathematical logic (see e.g [1]). The consideration of stochastic models and logics makes it possible to deal with probabilities (including probabilities of events that are not stochastically independent) as well as expectations of waiting times. Recent work has extended models and logics with reward (or cost) structures that make it possible to obtain information about the expected quality of behavior (like waiting times exceeding the recommendations from the clinical guidelines). *Constraint Solving* traditionally focuses on *hard* constraints that must be met [2]. More recent work also incorporates *soft* constraints that express preferences and where the objective is to obtain as high a score as possible while adhering to the hard constraints. This is made more challenging in the presence of multiple optimization criteria in which case the identification of Pareto frontiers (as studied in Economics) may be the best one can hope for. Solvers are often developed using the framework of Satisfaction Modulo Theories [9].

3   Work Packages and Milestones

WP1: Processes and Practice Cases. This work package is mainly to be conducted by a postdoc hired for one year and should start as soon as possible after the project has been granted. The purpose of WP1 (Processes and Practice Cases) is to identify a set of representative and critical healthcare processes within cancer treatment, and to study the challenges in the current workflows for handling these processes. Focus will be on previously identified challenges related to ad-hoc initiated pre-diagnosis processes, co-morbidities, and distributed collaboration [31]. This will likely involve some amount of interviewing health care professionals in order to describe workflows, the challenges in existing workflows, and the challenges in interactions between existing cancer treatment packages. In addition to a description of the study itself, an important delivery of the work package is a number of representative cases of healthcare processes and current medical practice in the primary and/or secondary health care sector. These need to be described in such a way that they can be approached by the PhD students; they will mainly have a background in Information and Communication Technology, and will approach the cases with the more technically oriented techniques of declarative process models (the topic of WP2) and trustworthiness of models (the topic of WP3). This work should start well before the other work packages and should terminate during the first year of work packages WP2 and WP3.

Milestones of WP1:   1) Survey of previously identified challenges related to ad-hoc initiated pre-diagnosis pro- cesses, co-morbidities, and distributed collaboration 2) A set of representative and critical healthcare processes within cancer treatment.

WP2: Declarative Process Models. This work package is mainly to be conducted by a PhD student who should be hired within six months of commencing the project and should work for three years. Based on the cases of processes and practice from work package WP1, a PhD student will in this work package be guided towards a background in declarative process models. The initial focus of WP2 (Declarative Process Models) will be on extending and modifying existing technologies for declarative process models [7,18,21,44,48,51,52] to be able to deal with the challenges offered by the cases. The subsequent focus will be on extending and modifying existing methods and techniques for distribution [11,17,19,24,43,50,53], adaptation [10,25,40,49] and analysis [13,29] of declarative process models in order to provide qualitative (and perhaps quantitative) information about the quality of service. Especially in the initial phase we foresee considerable interaction with work package WP3; in the later phase we foresee interaction with work packages WP4 and WP5.

Milestones of WP2: 1) PhD student trained in declarative process models. 2) Existing technologies for declarative process models extended to be able to deal with the challenges offered by the cases identified in WP1. 3) Existing methods and techniques for distribution, adaptation, and analysis of declarative process models extended to provide qualitative (and perhaps quantitative) information about the quality of service.

WP3: Trustworthiness of Models. This work package is mainly to be conducted by a PhD student who should be hired within six months of commencing the project and should work for three years. Based on the cases of processes and practice from work package WP1, a PhD student will in this work package be guided towards a background in trust models and their formalisation [6]. The initial focus of WP3 (Trustworthiness of Models) will be on extending and modifying existing formalisms for trust models [6] to be able to deal with the challenges offered by the cases. The subsequent focus will be on extending and modifying existing methods and techniques for the analysis of trust process models in order to provide qualitative (and perhaps quantitative) information about the quality of service. Especially in the initial phase we foresee considerable interaction with work package WP2; in the later phase we foresee interaction with work packages WP4 and WP5.

Milestones of WP3: 1) PhD student trained in trust models and their formalisation. 2) Existing technologies for trust models extended to be able to deal with the challenges offered by the cases identified in WP1. 3) Existing methods and techniques for analysis of trust process models extended to provide qualitative (and perhaps quantitative) information about the quality of service.

WP4: Stochastic Analysis or Constraint Solving. This work package is mainly to be conducted by a postdoc hired for one year during the second half of the project; the exact time will depend on the needs of the project and the availability of the right person (likely a PhD graduate or postdoc from the MT-LAB research centre). The focus of WP4 (Stochastic Analysis or Constraint Solving) is to apply techniques for stochastic analysis and constraint solving to the models resulting from WP2-WP3 We anticipate that our consideration of probabilistic and stochastic phenomena may present new challenges beyond those normally studied in embedded and service oriented systems. We also anticipate that our consideration of hard and soft constraints may require solution techniques beyond our current repertoire of techniques. We therefore intend to hire a PhD graduate or postdoc with expertise in one of these areas. This work should interact with work packages WP2 and WP3.

Milestones of WP4: Demonstration of Stochastic Analysis or Constraint Solving for process models identified in WP 2-3.

WP5: Prototype Development. This work package is mainly to be conducted by a postdoc hired for one year during the second half of the project; the exact time will depend on the needs of the project and the availability of the right person (likely a PhD graduate from an industrial PhD programme). Towards the end of the project we would like to assess the feasibility of the results coming out of primarily work packages WP2 and

WP3. To facilitate assessing the feasibility of the results coming out of in particular WP2 and WP3 we have created a special work package (WP5) for prototype development, and decided to allocate a postdoc with experience in the field, to make sure that there is enough focus and man power on this important part of the project. This work should interact strongly with our end users as well as work packages WP2 and WP3.

Milestones of WP5: Prototype(s) demonstrating ICT-powered Health Care services based on WP2 and WP3.

4   Conclusion

We have described a research project proposal focussed on the design of *declarative process models* and *formal models of trustworthiness* for healthcare treatment processes, accounting for the involvement of distributed groups of medical specialists, dynamic adaptation of partially completed treatment processes, and evaluation of the *trustworthiness of models* by applying techniques for stochastic analyasis and/or constraint solving, taking account of test results and actual treatments compared to the clinical guidelines.

We have so far established a collaboration with the *SOAMED* graduate school in Berlin. In addition to the IT, Medico and Telephony (IMT) section in the capital region of Denmark, we have identified an industrial partner who has experience in collaborating with universities and is specialized in developing case and knowledge management systems base on declarative process models. We are currently applying for funding for the research project and we are continuously looking for potential collaborators and related projects.

References

1. Baier, C., Katoen, J.-P.: Principles of Model Checking. MIT Press (2008)
2. Bartak, R.: Modelling soft constraints: A survey. Neural Network World 12, 421–431 (2002)
3. Bates, D.W., Cohen, M., Leape, L.L., Overhage, J.M., Shabot, M.M., Sheridan, T.: White paper - reducing the frequency of errors in medicine using information technology. Journal of the American Medical Informatics Association 8(4), 299–308 (2001)
4. Berg, M.: The search for synergy: interrelating medical work and patient care information systems. Methods of Information in Medicine 42, 337–344 (2003)
5. Bernstein, K., Bruun-Rasmussen, M., Vingtoft, S., Andersen, S.K., Nohr, C.: Modelling and implementing electronic health records in denmark. Stud. Health Technol. Inform. 95, 245–250 (2003)
6. Bhatti, R., Bertino, E., Ghafoor, A.: A trust-based context-aware access control model for web-services. Distrib. Parallel Databases 18(1), 83–105 (2005)
7. Chesani, F., Mello, P., Montali, M., Storari, S.: Testing careflow process execution conformance by translating a graphical language to computational logic. In: Bellazzi, R., Abu-Hanna, A., Hunter, J. (eds.) AIME 2007. LNCS (LNAI), vol. 4594, pp. 479–488. Springer, Heidelberg (2007)
8. European Commission. ehealth action plan 2012-2020 - innovative healthcare for the 21st century. Webpage (December 2012),
https://ec.europa.eu/digital-agenda/en/news/ehealth-action-plan-2012-2020-innovative-healthcare-21st-century

9. de Moura, L.M., Bjørner, N.: Satisfiability modulo theories: introduction and applications. Commun. ACM 54(9), 69–77 (2011)
10. Divitini, M., Simone, C.: Supporting different dimensions of adaptability in workflow modeling. Computer Supported Cooperative Work 9(3-4), 365–397 (2000)
11. Dong, G., Hull, R., Kumar, B., Su, J., Zhou, G.: A framework for optimizing distributed workflow executions. In: Connor, R.C.H., Mendelzon, A.O. (eds.) DBPL 1999. LNCS, vol. 1949, pp. 152–167. Springer, Heidelberg (2000)
12. Dumas, M., van der Aalst, W.M., ter Hofstede, A.H.: Process Aware Information Systems: Bridging People and Software Through Process Technology. Wiley-Interscience (2005)
13. Fahland, D.: Towards analyzing declarative workflows. In: Koehler, J., Pistore, M., Sheth, A.P., Traverso, P., Wirsing, M. (eds.) Autonomous and Adaptive Web Services. Dagstuhl Seminar Proceedings, vol. 07061, p. 6. Internationales Begegnungs- und Forschungszentrum fuer Informatik (IBFI), Schloss Dagstuhl (2007)
14. Grimshaw, J., Eccles, M., Thomas, R., Mac Lennan, G., Ramsay, C., Fraser, C., Vale, L.: Toward evidence-based quality improvement. evidence (and its limitations) of the effectiveness of guideline dissemination and implementation strategies 1966-1998. J. Gen. Intern. Med. 21, 14–20 (2006)
15. Grol, R., Grimshaw, J.: From best evidence to best practice: effective implementation of change in patients' care. The Lancet 362(9391), 1225–1230 (2003)
16. Nielson, H.R., Nielson, F., Vigo, R.: A calculus for quality. In: Păsăreanu, C.S., Salaün, G. (eds.) FACS 2012. LNCS, vol. 7684, pp. 188–204. Springer, Heidelberg (2013)
17. Hildebrandt, T., Mukkamala, R.R., Slaats, T.: Designing a cross-organizational case management system using dynamic condition response graphs. In: 2011 15th IEEE International on Enterprise Distributed Object Computing Conference (EDOC), August 29-September 2, pp. 161–170 (2011)
18. Hildebrandt, T., Mukkamala, R.R.: Declarative event-based workflow as distributed dynamic condition response graphs. In: Post-proceedings of PLACES 2010 (2010)
19. Hildebrandt, T., Mukkamala, R.R., Slaats, T.: Declarative modelling and safe distribution of healthcare workflows. In: International Symposium on Foundations of Health Information Engineering and Systems, Johannesburg, South Africa (August 2011)
20. Honda, K., Yoshida, N., Carbone, M.: Multiparty asynchronous session types. In: POPL, pp. 273–284 (2008)
21. Hull, R.: Formal study of business entities with lifecycles: Use cases, abstract models, and results. In: Proceedings of 7th International Workshop on Web Services and Formal Methods. LNCS, vol. 6551 (2010)
22. Rahmanzadeh, A., Fox, J., Johns, N.: Disseminating medical knowledge: the proforma approach. Artificial Intelligence in Medicine 14, 157–182 (1998)
23. Kawamoto, K., Houlihan, C.A., Andrew Balas, E., Lobach, D.F.: Improving clinical practice using clinical decision support systems: a systematic review of trials to identify features critical to success. BMJ 330(7494), 765 (2005)
24. Kindler, E., Martens, A., Reisig, W.: Inter-operability of workflow applications: Local criteria for global soundness. In: van der Aalst, W.M.P., Desel, J., Oberweis, A. (eds.) Business Process Management. LNCS, vol. 1806, pp. 235–253. Springer, Heidelberg (2000)
25. Klein, M., Dellarocas, C., Bernstein, A.: Introduction to the special issue on adaptive workflow systems. Computer Supported Cooperative Work 9(3-4), 265–267 (2000)
26. Lenz, R., Blaser, R., Beyer, M., Heger, O., Biber, C., Baumlein, M., Schnabel, M.: It support for clinical pathways–lessons learned. International Journal of Medical Informatics 76(suppl. 3), S397–S402 (2007); Ubiquity: Technologies for Better Health in Aging Societies - MIE 2006

27. Lyng, K.M., Hildebrandt, T., Mukkamala, R.R.: From paper based clinical practice guidelines to declarative workflow management. In: Proceedings of 2nd International Workshop on Process-oriented information systems in healthcare (ProHealth 2008), Milan, Italy, pp. 36–43. BPM 2008 Workshops (2008)

28. Lyng, K.M.: Clinical guidelines in everyday praxis, implications for computerization. Journal of Systems and Information Technology (2009)

29. Maggi, F.M., Montali, M., Westergaard, M., van der Aalst, W.M.P.: Monitoring business constraints with linear temporal logic: An approach based on colored automata. In: Rinderle-Ma, S., Toumani, F., Wolf, K. (eds.) BPM 2011. LNCS, vol. 6896, pp. 132–147. Springer, Heidelberg (2011)

30. Milner, R.: Communicating and Mobile Systems: the Pi-Calculus. Cambridge University Press (1999)

31. Møller, N.H., Bjørn, P.: Layers in sorting practices: Sorting out patients with potential cancer. Computer Supported Cooperative Work 20, 123–153 (2011)

32. Montali, M.: Specification and Verification of Declarative Open Interaction Models: A Logic-Based Approach. LNBIP, vol. 56. Springer (2010)

33. Mukkamala, R.R.: A Formal Model For Declarative Workflows - Dynamic Condition Response Graphs. PhD thesis, IT University of Copenhagen (March 2012) (forthcomming)

34. Mukkamala, R.R., Hildebrandt, T., Tøth, J.B.: The resultmaker online consultant: From declarative workflow management in practice to ltl. In: Proceedings of the 2008 12th Enterprise Distributed Object Computing Conference Workshops, EDOCW 2008, pp. 135–142. IEEE Computer Society, Washington, DC (2008)

35. Mulyar, N., Pesic, M., van der Aalst, W.M., Peleg, M.: Towards the flexibility in clinical guideline modelling languages. BPM Center Report (Ext. rep. BPM-07-04) 8 (2007)

36. Mulyar, N., Pesic, M., van der Aalst, W.M.P., Peleg, M.: Declarative and procedural approaches for modelling clinical guidelines: Addressing flexibility issues. In: ter Hofstede, A.H.M., Benatallah, B., Paik, H.-Y. (eds.) BPM Workshops 2007. LNCS, vol. 4928, pp. 335–346. Springer, Heidelberg (2008)

37. Myers, A.C., Liskov, B.: A decentralized model for information flow control. In: SOSP, pp. 129–142 (1997)

38. Nielson, F., Nielson, H.R., Hankin, C.: Principles of program analysis (2. corr. print). Springer (2005)

39. Object Management Group BPMN Technical Committee. Business Process Model and Notation, version 2.0. Webpage (January 2011),
http://www.omg.org/spec/BPMN/2.0/PDF

40. Pesic, M., Schonenberg, M.H., Sidorova, N., van der Aalst, W.M.P.: Constraint-based workflow models: Change made easy. In: Meersman, R., Tari, Z. (eds.) OTM 2007, Part I. LNCS, vol. 4803, pp. 77–94. Springer, Heidelberg (2007)

41. Pesic, M.: Constraint-Based Workflow Management Systems: Shifting Control to Users. PhD thesis, Eindhoven University of Technology, Netherlands (2008)

42. Quaglini, S., Stefanelli, M., Lanzola, G., Caporusso, V., Panzarasa, S.: Flexible guideline-based patient careflow systems. Artificial Intelligence in Medicine 22(1), 65–80 (2001); Workflow Management and Clinical Guidelines

43. Reichert, M.U., Bauer, T., Dadam, P.: Flexibility for distributed workflows. In: Handbook of Research on Complex Dynamic Process Management: Techniques for Adaptability in Turbulent Environments, pp. 32–171. IGI Global, Hershey (2009)

44. Robertson, D.: A lightweight coordination calculus for agent systems. In: Leite, J., Omicini, A., Torroni, P., Yolum, p. (eds.) DALT 2004. LNCS (LNAI), vol. 3476, pp. 183–197. Springer, Heidelberg (2005)

45. SENSORIA. Software engineering for service-oriented overlay computers (2010),
http://www.sensoria-ist.eu

46. Smith, T.J., Hillner, B.E.: Ensuring quality cancer care by the use of clinical practice guidelines and critical pathways. Journal of Clinical Oncology 19(11), 2886–2897 (2001)
47. Terenziani, P., Montani, S., Bottrighi, A., Torchio, M., Molino, G., Correndo, G.: The glare approach to clinical guideline: Main features. Symposium on Computerized Guidelines and Protocols 101, 62–66 (2004)
48. van der Aalst, W., Pesic, M., Schonenberg, H., Westergaard, M., Maggi, F.M.: Declare. Webpage (2010), http://www.win.tue.nl/declare/
49. van der AAlst, W.M.P., Jablonski, S., Jablonski, S.: Dealing with workflow change: identification of issues and solutions. International Journal of Computer Systems Science & Engineering 15(5), 267–276 (2000)
50. van der Aalst, W.M.P., Lohmann, N., Massuthe, P., Stahl, C., Wolf, K.: Multiparty Contracts: Agreeing and Implementing Interorganizational Processes. The Computer Journal 53(1), 90–106 (2010)
51. van der Aalst, W.M.P., Pesic, M., Schonenberg, H.: Declarative workflows: Balancing between flexibility and support. Computer Science - R&D 23(2), 99–113 (2009)
52. van der Aalst, W.M.P., Pesic, M.: DecSerFlow: Towards a truly declarative service flow language. In: Bravetti, M., Núñez, M., Zavattaro, G. (eds.) WS-FM 2006. LNCS, vol. 4184, pp. 1–23. Springer, Heidelberg (2006)
53. van der Aalst, W.M.P.: Inheritance of interorganizational workflows: How to agree to disagree without loosing control? Information Technology and Management 4, 345–389 (2003)
54. Vanderaalst, W., Weske, M., Grunbauer, D.: Case handling: a new paradigm for business process support. Data & Knowledge Engineering 53(2), 129–162 (2005)

Approach and Method for Generating Realistic Synthetic Electronic Healthcare Records for Secondary Use

Kudakwashe Dube[1] and Thomas Gallagher[2]

[1] School of Engineering and Advanced Technology, Massey University, New Zealand
[2] Applied Computing and Electronics, University of Montana, Missoula, USA
K.Dube@Massey.ac.nz, Thomas.Gallagher@UMontana.edu
http://www.massey.ac.nz, http://ace.cte.umt.edu

Abstract. This position paper presents research work involving the development of a publicly available *Realistic Synthetic Electronic Healthcare Record* (RS-EHR). The paper presents PADARSER, a novel approach in which the real *Electronic Healthcare Record* (EHR) and neither authorization nor anonymisation are required in generating the synthetic EHR data sets. The *GRiSER method* is presented for use in PADARSER to allow the RS-EHR to be synthesized for statistically significant localised synthetic patients with statistically prevalent *medical conditions* based upon information found from publicly available data sources. In treating the synthetic patient within the GRiSER method, clinical workflow or *careflows* (Cfs) are derived from *Clinical Practice Guidelines* (CPGs) and the standard local practices of clinicians. The Cfs generated are used together with health statistics, CPGs, medical coding and terminology systems to generate coded synthetic RS-EHR entries from statistically significant observations, treatments, tests, and procedures. The RS-EHR is thus populated with a complete medical history describing the resulting events from treating the medical conditions. The strength of the PADARSER approach is its use of publicly available information. The strengths of the GRiSER method are that (1) it does not require the use of the real EHR for generating the coded RS-EHR entries; and (2) the generic components for obtaining careflow from CPGs and for generating coded RS-EHR entries are applicable in other areas such as knowledge transfer and EHR user interfaces respectively.

Keywords: synthetic data, healthcare statistics, clinical guidelines, clinical workflow, electronic health record, knowledge modeling, medical terminology, ICD10, SNOMED-CT.

1 Introduction

As the healthcare industry continues its transition to the *Electronic Health Record (EHR)*, the rigorous process of obtaining patient records remains a deterrent for clinical trainers, researchers, software system developers and testers. The EHR is a cradle-to-grave systematic collection of a patients health information

J. Gibbons and W. MacCaull (Eds.): FHIES 2013, LNCS 8315, pp. 69–86, 2014.
© Springer-Verlag Berlin Heidelberg 2014

that is distributed across locations and computing platforms and includes a wide range of disparate data types including demographics, medical history, medication, allergies, immunisation status, laboratory test results, radiology images, vital signs, personal measurements (height, weight, age) and billing information, all of which are sharable across healthcare settings [9]. A complete EHR paints a holistic picture of a patient's overall medical history and provides a chronological description of an individual's medical conditions, procedures, tests, and medications.

The problem of generating synthetic data has been widely investigated in many domains [23] [16] [11][3]. Despite the chronic limitations on access to the EHR for secondary use due to privacy concerns, there are very few research efforts to-date directed on developing promising and low cost approaches to generating synthetic EHRs for secondary uses. Only about 5 major works have appeared in literature during the past 12 years [5][15][2][14][21] compared to more than 60 works in other domains. This scenario is not expected in a domain that is characterised by the highly sensitive nature of the information. The work of Buczak et al is of particular significance to this paper due to its comprehensiveness and the ingenuity in the method of generating synthetic EHRs. The method uses clinical care patterns to create a care model that guides the generation of synthetic EHR entries that have realistic characteristics [2]. The major weaknesses of Buczak et al's method are: (1) the use of the real EHR, whose access is still subject to limitations; (2) at a very high-level, the method amounts to the anonymisation of the real EHR still raise concerns from advanced data mining techniques; and (3) the possibility of the existence of an inverse method to re-identify the real EHR used in the method, which could lead to potential privacy breaches.

This paper presents an approach and method that has been developed as part of early work in the investigation of the problem of generating a *Realistic Synthetic Electronic Health Record* (RS-EHR). A key aspect of this problem is the emphasis on no access to the real EHR as well as the use of freely and publicly available health statistics, *clinical practice guidelines* (CPGs) and protocols practiced by clinicians, and medical coding and terminology systems and standards. *Clinical workflow,* also known as *Careflow* (Cf) are the *workflows* (Wf) of a health unit. The Cfs involve steps and processes that a patient goes through in either one clinician-patient encounter or a series of these encounters in the process of disease management and patient care [7]. A CPG is a systematically developed set of statements that guides the clinician and his patient in making decisions and performing tasks as part of managing the patient's health problem [19]. Cfs and CPGs are closely related in that clinical workflow, and hence Cfs, can be derived from CPGs [7]. RS-EHR data that is realistic could be generated from clinically realistic Cf. The hypothesis of our approach and method is that codified RS-EHR skeletons can be generated from publicly available health care statistics while the codified and usually non-codified textual content of these EHR can be derived from the Cf that can be extracted from CPG that is used to manage the disease or clinical problem.

The novelty of the PADARSER approach for generating the RS-EHR presented in this paper is based upon the use of publicly available information. The GRiSER method adopted in this approach involves the creation of a synthetic patient of demographic significance to a region. The generated synthetic patient is iteratively injected with a statistically significant medical condition that is associated with a relevant clinical guideline or protocol. The patient RS-EHR is populated with entries based upon the standardized clinician careflow extracted from the relevant guideline or protocol used in treating the injected medical condition. From the careflow based on clinical guideline or protocols, an associated workflow of treatments, procedures, and lab tests will be generated in order to populate the RS-EHR. The anticipated outcome of PADARSER approach and GRiSER method is the coded RS-EHR that any practising clinician from the location of statistical relevance would deem to be realistic as would be confirmed by using our assessment rubric. Following completion of the generation of the RS-EHR, we have defined a rubric for assessing the realistic characteristics of the RS-EHR that includes comparing the characteristics the clinician would find in an actual EHR.

This paper contributes a new approach and method for generating RS-EHR that incorporates novel techniques for ensuring that the RS-EHR generated is realistic and less costly to produce. The novel techniques are: (1) the statistical generation of the patients and the disease they suffer from; and (2) the generation of RS-EHR entries from clinical guideline-based careflow and medical terminology and coding systems and standards. The statistical basis of the approach takes into account the disease prevalences and probabilities from publicly available information. The benefits of our approach are: (1) no real EHR will be used since content is generated from statistics and clinical guidelines; (2) no anonymization techniques are required since no real EHR is involved; (3) no authorization or obligatory consent are required as no personal patient information will be used; and (4) all acquired information will be obtained through freely and publicly available statistical health data and standardized clinician guidelines, medical codes and terminologies.

This paper begins by examining our motivation for generating RS-EHR data sets. Related works are discussed followed by a high-level analysis of the data sets incorporated for the RS-EHR. We describe our approach in generating RS-EHRs in which we have named PADARSER. GRiSER is introduced as our method in populating RS-EHRs and the iterative algorithm used by GRiSER is documented. Derivation of careflow from CPGs are examined to populate the RS-EHR through coding and textual events. Lastly, before concluding the paper we present our evaluation process and detail the evaluation rubric that include four criteria areas each with multiple components for assessing the realistic aspect of the RS-EHR with the help of domain experts.

2 Background, Problem and Motivation

The rapid adoption of the EHR is taking place throughout the world as one component of a healthcare information technology initiative aimed at improving patient care while reducing costs. In the United States, EHR adoption is being driven by the *Health Information Technology for Economic and Clinical Health* (HITECH) Act (2009) with oversight from the *Office of the National Coordinator* (ONC) for Health Information Technology, while in New Zealand implementation is taking place through the National Health IT Plan with oversight from the IT Health Board and the Ministry of Health. Privacy and confidentiality concerns limit access to actual EHRs for secondary use. Legal protection for patient privacy is addressed in the United States through the *Health Insurance Portability and Accountability Act* (HIPPA) (1996), while in New Zealand patient privacy rights are covered by the *Health Information Privacy Code (1995).* Although secondary use of the patient EHR is permitted, obtaining authorization to access actual records is rigorous and the anonymisation of records can be expensive. Our motivation in generating the RS-EHR is based upon the current challenges associated with obtaining EHR for secondary use, especially research work in *Health Informatics.* These challenges have continued unabated even in the presence of *advances in anonymisation techniques.*

Privacy concerns for the individual restrict the availability of EHRs, limiting secondary use. Addressing the problem of creating synthetic EHRs has been recognised to be the best solution to this limitation. Most works in the literature that address the problem of generating synthetic EHRs use approaches and methods that require access to the real EHR during the process of generating the synthetic EHRs and hence cyclically suffer from the same limitation that they seek to address.

For clinician trainers, the secondary use of the EHR serves as an invaluable teaching tool. The EHR describes all the elements of a successful treatment encounter. As patient careflow takes place in the clinic, the EHR documents details of treatment procedures, tests, and medications. The EHR is a patient case study demonstrating the unique careflow provided to the individual. The EHR can also serve as a knowledge transfer tool. In developed regions of the world, the best practices in careflow are regularly demonstrated by expert clinicians. These careflow practices are documented in the EHR. Sharing the EHR as a training tool to developing regions of the world where expertise is limited serves as a knowledge transfer tool. The knowledge of clinical best practices derived from expertise found in developed regions can be shared through the EHR.

Developing a synthetic EHR with the characteristics of the realistic patient careflow will function as a tool to meet the demands of clinician trainers and serve as a knowledge transfer tool to help developing regions of the world. The synthetic characteristic addresses all privacy concerns associated in obtaining confidential patient records without the expense of anonymisation processing.

3   Related Works

The problem of generating synthetic data for various purposes has been widely recognised and investigated in a wide variety of domains [23][16][11][3]. However, there is the glaring lack of the adequate investigation into addressing this problem for EHRs despite the chronic limitations of access to the EHR due to privacy concerns. For example, following a literature search, limited to four main digital libraries, PubMed, ACM, IEEE and ScienceDirect, for works on synthetic data resulted in the review of 62 published articles of interest which were refined to a list of 42 articles specifically mentioning research involving synthetic data generation, yet only five articles published during the period 2000 to 2012 were identified to have completed work in the EHR domain. From the five articles identified in our search of relevance to synthetic EHR generation, Esteller mentions the use of synthetic and real data in comparing electro-encephalograms (EEG) waveform [5]. Macjewski et al describe a data set developed from emergency room patient data where temporal disease outbreaks can be injected based upon seasonal trends [15]. Lee et al describe exploratory work using synthetic data and real EHRs for use in analytic systems [14]. Raza and Clyde describe synthetic data from work done in developing a test-data creation tool for health data [21]. Buczak et al, in their work on modelling a flu-like epidemic, present two comprehensive methods: one for generating their synthetic background EHR; and another for generating their synthetic epidemic EHR based on the synthetic background EHR [2].

Among the five works that present methods of synthetic EHRs, Buczak et al's work provide the most comprehensive method [2]. By using the real EHR, Buczak et al propose an algorithm for generating EHRs that include a strategy to inject a disease into a synthetic patient who already has an existing background EHR. Buczak et al later realised that the background EHRs also need to be synthetic due to further privacy limitations. Instead of avoiding privacy limitation problem, Buczak et al made their method to require access to the real EHR for deriving the clinical care patterns. A key aspect of Buczak et al's method is the strategy that involves the injection of a disease into the synthetic patient after which care patterns are used to generate the synthetic EHR entries. The care patterns that are associated with the synthetic patient are derived from the real EHR belonging to the patient that has the least similarity or distance measure from the synthetic patient. At a more abstract level, what Buczak et al present for generating their background and epidemic synthetic EHR is another method for the anonymisation of the real EHR, which has not led to the abatement of privacy concerns and resulting limitations to accessing EHRs. The weaknesses of the work of Buczak et al are: (1) the assumption that the real EHR will be accessible for the purpose of generating the synthetic EHR; and (2) the possibility of the existence of an inverse algorithm that uses their similarity or distance measure in reverse to partially or completely re-identify the real EHR and hence the patient using the information in the synthetic EHR. This inverse algorithm could potentially compromise the privacy of the real patient. The ingenuity of the Buczak et al's method is the inherent assurance that the resulting synthetic EHR has realistic characteristics by using clinical care patterns to generate the synthetic entries for the synthetic EHR. This ingenuity in Buczak et al's method inspired the GRiSER method's use of clinical workflow or careflow. The major difference being that the GRiSER method derives the careflow from CPGs from which the RS-EHR entries are generated instead of from the *real EHR*. The PADARSER approach and GRiSER method presented in this paper differ from the work of Buczak et al in that (1) they do not make use of any actual patient data, rather they derive clinical workflow from CPGs; (2) they do not focus on a single disease injection but use health statistics to create a synthetic EHR that has statistically prevalent set of diseases or medical conditions, which could be more than one for each synthetic patient, for instance, diabetes patients may also statistically suffer from renal complications; and (3) as no actual patient data is ever used, the approach used in the GRiSER method is uniquely distinct.

Research works that examine CPGs and clinical workflow have focused mainly on expressing or specifying and executing the process logic in CPGs by using workflow and process languages and technologies [20][8]. Other works have recognised the common process-oriented characteristics and conceptualisations of CPGs with a view towards developing some form of unification of concepts and computational models and formalisms [7]. There is the wide recognition that CPGs can be expressed, at least partially, as clinical workflow [12][17] and that care pathways are goal- and process-oriented and so define the workflow of activities as well as roles and sequencing of activities while also providing a framework for generating data for the EHR [7]. The work presented in this paper seeks to exploit the process nature of CPGs to create the necessary context for the realistic nature of the generated RS-EHR entries.

Healthcare statistics are drawn for the coded aspects of the real EHR [18]. The health statistics contain information on diseases, medical procedures performed, medications and laboratory tests performed. The statistics also usually include the relevant medical codes and terminologies for systems and standards especially the *International classification of Diseases* (ICD) [25] and *Systematized Nomenclature Of Medicine Clinical Terms* (SNOMED-CT) [10]. Therefore, it is possible to extract coded diseases, laboratory tests, observations and medications from statistical information. While CPGs may make use of medical or clinical terms, they are not systematically coded using using medical coding systems such as the ICD-10 [25]. Furthermore, CPGs may also not systematically make use the appropriate terminologies from SMOMED-CT. One of the objectives of this work is to generate coded RS-EHR entries that also systematically make use of terminology systems.

4   Generating Realistic Synthetic E-Healthcare Records

Secondary uses of the EHR such as training clinicians and testing of software under development do not require access to the real EHR. For such forms of secondary use of the EHR, a realistic synthetic EHR would be enough. *Synthetic data is data that is created to simulate real data in the application domain of interest. The synthetic EHR is synthetic data that is generated to simulate the real EHR.* The synthetic EHR can be used in place of the real EHR in scenarios that involve the appropriate forms of the secondary use of the EHR. To be usable, the synthetic EHR must be realistic, which is the single most important characteristic of it whose test would be that a clinician examining the record would not be able to tell that the EHR is synthetic. This work investigates the problem of creating the realistic synthetic EHR (RS-EHR) and this paper presents the approach and method developed in this work for generating the realistic synthetic EHRs (RS-EHRs).The novelty of the approach and method is in (1) the use of publicly available data such as public health statistics, clinical guidelines and protocols, and medical coding and terminology standards and systems, and (2) their assumption that there is no real EHR that would be available for access during the generation of entries that would make up the resulting RS-EHR. Figure 1 presents the relevant aspects that are important in the problem of generating realistic synthetic EHRs.

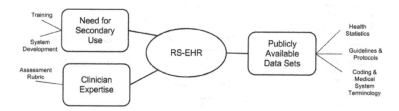

Fig. 1. Relevance diagram presenting the relevant aspects for the creation of the realistics synthetic EHR as investigated in this paper

Publicly available health information and knowledge are important sources that could contribute towards extrapolations that would be used in the generation of data for synthesising the realistic synthetic EHR. For example, health statistics would contribute information for generating patient demographics and disease prevalences as well as medical procedures, medications and laboratory tests. Clinical guidelines and protocols (CPGs) would assist by suggesting the careflow involved in the management of patient problems. Furthermore, the CPGs, when used in an appropriate method to be developed in this work combined with medical coding and terminology systems, would provide the material basis for generating coded textual narrative aspects of the synthetic EHR. Medical experts or clinicians are of significance to this work at the step for the evaluation of the resulting RS-EHR. As pointed out earlier in this section, the resulting RS-EHR must pass the test that establishes the fact that when a practising clinician from the region of statistical significance examines the RS-EHR, its should be that the RS-EHR is indistinguishable from, and have the typical characteristics of, a real EHR that the practising clinician would normally encounter in his or her daily work routine. It would appear from this discussion that the RS-EHR for some secondary use purposes could be generated from publicly available information such that practising clinician could deem the resulting RS-EHR to be realistic.

5   The PADARSER Aproach: *Generating Realistic Synthetic E-Healthcare Records*

The *Publicly Available Data Approach to the Realistic Synthetic EHR* (PADARSER), is the approach presented in this section, whose goal is to exploit publicly available data and information, without access to real EHRs, in generating the RS-EHRs. In particular, the three main types of publicly available data and information that have been selected in the approach for such exploitation are illustrated in Figure 2.

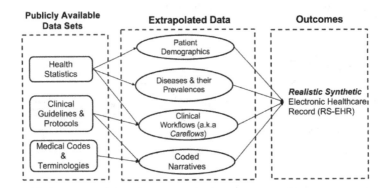

Fig. 2. The PADARSER approach to generating the realistic synthetic EHR from publicly available data and information

As can be seen in Figure 2, the three types of publicly available information that has been selected in this work for use in creating the RS-EHR are: (1) health statistics; (2) clinical guidelines and protocols (CPGs); and (3) medical coding and terminology systems and standards. Figure 2 also illustrates the sub-types of information that can be extrapolated from each of these three main types of information. Figure 2 further elaborates and presents the conceptual approach, from an data and information derivation and extrapolation perspective, for building the RS-EHR. In other words, Figure 2 illustrates the synthetic data for the RS-EHR that would be derived or extrapolated from the publicly available information sources in the approach presented in this paper.

Health statistics for a country or a region within a country provide detailed statistical health information that covers the following aspects of the synthetic EHR: patient demographics, encountered diseases occurring in the population in focus and their prevalences, medications administered to patients, laboratory tests and medical procedures that were performed on patients during the timeframe in focus. Clinical practice guidelines (CPGs) and protocols for specific disease and health problems are useful in the process of generating actual RS-EHR data entries because clinical workflow (Wf) or careflow (Cf) can be derived from these CPGs [7]. The generated Cf contains the appropriate clinical and healthcare events, tasks and procedures that then become the basis for generating the realistic data that goes into the RS-EHR. Synthetic textual narratives to describe the patients clinical conditions, observations and procedures can also be extracted from CPGs for entry into the RS-EHR. Medical codes are important in that most health statistics are based on coded aspects of real EHRs and in that the ideal EHR is one that has extensively coded data [1]. Furthermore, medical coding systems are closely related to, or make use of medical terminologies, which are also implicitly or explicitly used in CPGs. Of particular interest to this paper is the generation of (1) coded synthetic EHR entries and (2) coded synthetic textual narratives in these entries, both of which will make use of medical coding standards, medical terminology systems and CPGs as key data sources in the PADARSER approach.

6   The GRiSER Method for Generating the RS-EHR

This section presents, at a conceptual level, the method for generating the RS-EHR from public available data and information sources. As already pointed out earlier in this paper, all the data that would be required to synthesise the RS-EHR are derived or extrapolated from public health statistics (PHS), clinical guidelines and protocols (CPGs) and medical coding and terminology systems and standards (MCTSS).

6.1   Generating the RS-EHR

The GRiSER Method presented in this section is the method adopted for the PADARSER Approach to generating the RS-EHR. GRiSER stands for Generating the *Realistic Synthetic EHR* (RS-EHR). The GRiSER Method aims at using data from the publicly available data that has been presented in the previous sections to synthesise the RS-EHR. The resulting RS-EHR should be typical of the region from which the publicly available information in obtained. The GRiSER Method seeks to attain this aim without using any information or knowledge from examining the real EHR, which is assumed to be unavailable. The expected outcome of the GRiSER Method is a RS-EHR that would be deemed to be realistic by a practising clinician. Figure 4 presents the conceptual illustration of the method for generating the RS-EHR from publicly available information. In the GRiSER Method, synthetic patients are generated from statistical information. Patient demographics are generated from the statistics and added to the RS-EHR. Each synthetic patient is iteratively injected with a disease extrapolated from publicly available data sources including disease prevalences in the population of interest. Each disease is associated with a specific guideline or protocol from which the clinical workflow for managing the disease is derived. Careflow based on CPGs provide a realistic context for clinical events, which, in turn provide a realistic context for generating synthetic entries for the RS-EHR. Therefore, in the GRiSER Method, CPGs and the careflow that is generated from them are critical in rendering the generated realistics. For each RS-EHR entry synthesised, appropriate codes from the standardised medical coding system are

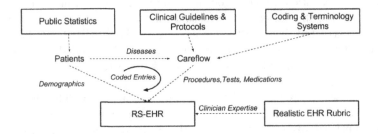

Fig. 3. Conceptual architecture of the GRiSER Method for generating the RS-EHR from publicly available information

attached. The synthetic entrys textual narratives are generated from appropriate textual narratives in the CPG. These narratives are improved by using the appropriate medical terminologies from medical terminology systems and are also coded appropriately. The various types of entries that would be synthesised from careflow events include clinical observations, procedures performed, laboratory test results and medications prescribed. Once the whole RS-EHR for the synthetic patient is fully generated, a RS-EHR rubric for assessing its validity could be applied by a practised clinician to establish that the RS-EHR is indeed realistic.

6.2   Description of the GRiSER Method

Figure 4 presents the activity diagram that illustrates the GRiSER method. The Activity Diagram of Figure 4 illustrates that the GRiSER Method starts with the preparation of the publicly available local health statistics before using the statistics to create synthetic patient demographics, which is then used to create the patient's synthetic EHR. The patient's synthetic EHR holds only the patient demographics at this stage. The demographics are then used to generate a set of health problems that will be reflected in the synthetic EHR for the patient. Figure 4 illustrates a loop to iterate over this set of complaints in order to generate coded synthetic EHR entries for each complaint with the entries covering the same period as that covered by the health statistics. This time period may cover from one year to ten years. The number of complaints to be considered could be limited subject to computation challenges. A model, as illustrated in Figure 4, is generated to guide the temporal aspects of the generated synthetic EHR entries. A part of the Activity Diagram illustrated the selection of a CPG for each health complaint and the generation of the careflow based on the CPG. The careflow then determines the set of events for whose synthetic entries need to be added to the RS-EHR. The activity of generating coded synthetic entries is iterative over all events and makes use of medical terminology and coding systems. Listing 1 presents a high-level algorithm to illustrate the method described here.

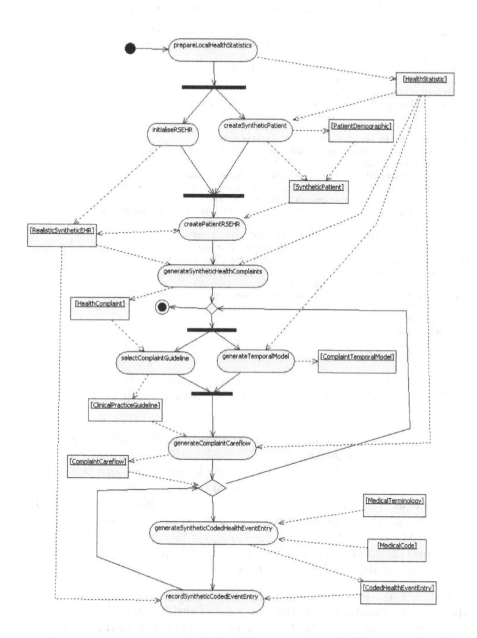

Fig. 4. The UML Activity Diagram illustrating the main activities in the GRiSER method for generating the realistic synthetic EHR from publicly available information.

Listing 1. The GRiSER Algorithm - the high-level algorithm for generating the RS-EHR from publicly available information in the GRiSER Method

```
*0  GRiSER(healthStats, cpgLibrary, medCodes, medTerms, complaintsLimit)
1  // GRiSER - Generating the Realistic Synthetic E-healthcare Record
1  // output: patientRSEHR
2  // input parameters: healthStats, cpgLibrary, medCodes, medTerms, complaintsLimit
3  patientRSEHR  ⟵  initRSEHR();
4  patient  ⟵  initPatient();
*6  patient.demographics  ⟵  genDemographics(healthStats);
7  patientRSEHR.patient  ⟵  patient;
8  complaintsCount  ⟵  0
+9  A: repeat until (complaintCount ≤ complaintsLimit)
10  // iteratively inject patient with statistically significant clinical
11  // complaint or disease
*12    clinicalComplaint  ⟵  genComplaint(healthStats,patient);
*13    cpg  ⟵  selectComplaintCPG(clinicalComplaint, patient, cpgLibrary);
*14    temporalModel  ⟵  initTemporalModel(healthStats);
*15    careflow  ⟵  genClinicalWorkflow(healthStats, cpg, patient, temporalModel);
16    cfEvents  ⟵  careflow.getEvents();
+17    B: repeat until (cfEvents.iter.hasMore()  ==  false)
18  // iteratively generate coded RS-EHR entries from careflow events:
19  // coded textual narratives are generated from CPGs, medical codes and
20  // terminologies
21    cfEvent  ⟵  cfEvents.iter.next();
*22    codedEntries  ⟵  genCodedEventEntries(cfEvent, cpg, medCodes, medTerms);
23    patientRSEHR.entries.add(codedEntries);
+24    B: end
25    complaintsCount  ⟵  complaintsCount + 1;
+26  A: end
27  return patientRSEHR;
```

The GRiSER algorithm presented in Listing 1 creates the RS-EHR for a single synthetic patient. The algorithms returns a RS-EHR accepting the following parameters:

- `healthStats` - the complete set of publicly available health statistics that are relevant for generating RS-EHR;
- `cpgLibrary` - the library of clinical practice guidelines and protocols for diseases that are statistically prevalent in the population;
- `medCodes` - the codes from a standardised medical coding system, e.g., ICD10;
- `medTerms` - the terminology from a standardised medical terminology system, e.g. SNOMED; and
- `complaintsLimit` - ensures that the synthetic patient is injected with a realistic number of clinical complaints.

In Listing 1, the lines marked with the asterisk (*) are the important steps in the GRiSER algorithm while the lines marked with the plus (+) indicate the main iterations. In Line 6, the function, `genDemographics(healthStats)`, generates synthetic patient demographics. Line 9 presents the starting point for the iteration over the patients clinical complaints. In Line 9, the synthetic clinical complaint is generated for the synthetic patient based on statistical information. In Line 13, the clinical practice guideline, cpg, is selected for managing the patients clinical complaint. The GRiSER algorithm, as presented here, assumes that there exists a CPG for every clinical complaint that could arise statistically. This assumption is presented here as a simplification that may not appear in the implementation. In Line 14, a temporal model for each clinical complaint is initialised based on the temporal issues, such as seasonal considerations, that could be deduced from health statistical data. A temporal model that is derived initially from statistical data and enhanced with CPG information for each clinical complaint is important to enhance the realistic characteristics of the generated careflow. In Line 15, the clinical workflow or careflow is generated from the CPG form the synthetic patient taking into account statistical information as well as temporal issues. The careflow will provide the clinical events that would guide the generation of RS-EHR entries. In Line 17 an inner loop is initiated to iterate over the clinical events from the careflow to create all the RS-EHR entries that arise from the event. In Line 22, coded entries for the RS-EHR are synthesised by using CPG narratives, medical codes and terminologies.

There are two major challenges within the GRiSER algorithm that are very significant from the modelling and computational hardness point of view, and of wider applications. The complete and detailed analysis of modelling and computational analysis of these challenges are subjects of currently on-going work and will not be presented in this paper. These challenges are: (1) the derivation of clinical workflow or careflow from clinical practice guidelines and protocols handled by the function, `genClinicalWorkflow(healthStats, cpg, patient, temporalModel)` in the GRiSER algorithm; and (2) the generation of coded synthetic RS-EHR entries from events, CPGs and medical coding and terminology system, handled by the function, `genCodedEventEntries(cfEvent, cpg, medCodes, medTerms)`. The next two subsections, Section 6.2 and 6.3, present and elaborate further on these two challenges without going into the the analysis of the modelling and computational complexity, which will not be presented in this paper as pointed out earlier.

6.3   Deriving Clinical Workflow or Careflow from Clinical Guidelines

Relationship between clinical practice guidelines (CPG) and clinical workflow, also known as careflow, has been identified in the area of CPG computerisation. CPGs structure best practice and clinical workflow while also assisting clinicians in diagnosis and treatment [4]. Laleci and Dogac [13] claims that computerised CPGs could be used to drive computer-based clinical workflow because they communicate with external applications to retrieve patient data and then initiates medical actions in the clinical workflows. Workflow technologies have also been used to computerise CPGs [24][20][8]. It has also been recognised that clinical workflows have demonstrated to be an effective approach to partially model CPGs [12]. As a result of the need to customise CPGs to suite a patient at a specific location,CPGs are known not to completely define clinical workflow. Hence, Juarez et al [12] proposed a workflow fulfilment function to determine the degree of completeness of careflow derived fromm CPGs. More recently, Gonzalez-ferrer et al [6] demonstrated the translation of CPGs into Temporal Hierarchical Task Networks (THTN), which facilitates the automatic generation of time-annotated and resource-based clinical workflow. Thus, it has been shown from the literature that it is feasible to obtain clinical workflow or careflow from CPGs.

Generating clinical workflow or careflow from CPGs is a key feature of the PADARSER approach and the GRiSER method. The derivation of careflow from clinical guidelines is an important part of the GRiSER method that distinguishes it from other methods of generating RS-EHRs found in the literature. For example, in the work of Buczak et al [2], care patterns for generating synthetic is derived from inferences that result from examining entries recorded in the real EHR, which does not apply where there is absolutely no access to the real EHR.

Besides exploiting the process nature of CPGs in generating synthetic entries for the RS-EHR, the GRiSER method for creating careflow from CPGs also has wider applications. For example, Figure 5 details the proposed process of using CPGs to generate careflow and it's proposed application as a knowledge transfer tool.

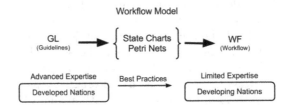

Fig. 5. Careflow knowledge transfer from clinical guidelines

The top part of Figure 5 presents a conceptualisation of the knowledge and technological transfer that is often a key goal for international bodies such as The United Nations and their constituent agencies. Methods, approaches and techniques are being sought by such bodies to facilitate the transfer of advanced expertise from developed regions of the world in forms that encapsulate best practices to developed region of the world where limited expertise is in acute shortage. This conceptualisation of knowledge and technology transfer could be exemplified or instantiated by the computer-assisted extraction of clinical workflow from the text of best practice guidelines as illustrated in the bottom part of Figure 6. Thus, best healthcare practice in the form of CPGs could be captured by using formal models that underlie workflow technology to create clinical workflow that could be customised to suit the conditions of the target developing world.

6.4   Generating Coded Textual Narrative from CPGs and Medical Coding and Terminology Systems and Standard

GRiSER method aims at incorporating a special strategy to extract relevant textual narratives from CPGs and then code them appropriately as well as apply terms from SNOMED-CT. Generating coded entries for the RS-EHR including coded textual narrative is an important component of the GRiSER method that has other applications especially within the area of EHR user interfaces (UIs). Figure 6 illustrates the concept of using codes and coded textual narrative suggestions in EHR user interfaces.

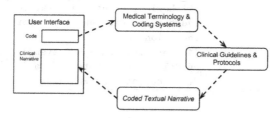

Fig. 6. Coded Textual Narrative for UI

The coded textual narratives are generated from CPGs using medical codes and terminology systems and presented as suggestions to the user, who could be allowed to accept or reject the suggested entries. The suggested coded entries would help the user to enter more accurate information as well as increase the use of medical codes within the EHR entries.

7 Evaluation, Outcomes and Applications

A rubric assessing the realistic aspects of the synthetic EHR has been developed. a high-level summary of this rubric is presented as the table in Table 1. Criteria elements include: (1) patient representation; (2) disease representation; (3) careflow; and (4) clinician acceptance. The record of the synthetic patient will be assessed to match the statistical accuracy of the demographic characteristic found in the regional area of interest. As an example, the synthetic patient in Africa would, in most cases, be of African ethnicity rather than European descent. A limitation on the number of disease injections will be restricted to a maximum value for any given patient. Injecting a patient with an unreasonable number of consecutive diseases will distort the natural prevalence normally found in real patients. Diseases will be limited to those which are reasonably prevalent to a particular region. For instance, the prevalence of malaria would not be considered common to patients in Canada thus unusual to include in the synthetic EHR from this region. The seasonal changes in weather can lead to variation in the prevalence of diseases and will be included in the assessment.

Careflow will be measured for both logical and temporal organization of clinical encounters. The overall completeness of the expected events following diagnosis of a particular disease will be included in the assessment. Lastly the expertise of a clinician reviewer will be used in our assessment. Examination by the expert will be used to determine whether the expected clinical encounters

Table 1. RS-EHR Assessment Rubric

No.	CRITERIA AREA	ASSESSMENT COMPONENT
1	*Patient Representation*	(1) Regional demographic; and (2) Limit maximum injections
2	*Disease Representation*	(1) Regional disease; and (2) Consistent with seasonal changes
3	*Careflow*	(1) Logical event organization; (2) Temporal event placement; and (3) Comprehensive event inclusion
4	*Clinician Acceptance*	(1) Verification – EHR events follow guidelines and protocols; and (2) Verification – RS-EHR as a whole is realistic

found in the RS-EHR match those experienced in an actual patient EHR. Upon reviewing the RS-EHR, the clinician should be able to state that the events and encounters found in the record mimic those expected to be experienced by a real patient. The components of the assessment rubric are presented in Table 1.

An alternative approach in providing assessment for the realistic aspect of the synthetic EHR involves the use of automata learned from the real EHR. Models from automata processes constructed learned or mined from either clinical guidelines [22] or the real EHR provide novelty to assessing the realism characteristic of the RS-EHR. Computer Interpretable Guidelines (CIG) created through machine learning systems are capable of developing patterns of careflow [22]. Using CIG patterns crafted from the actual EHR, a further innovation for assessing the realistic aspect of the synthetic EHR will be worthy of consideration in this on-going work.

8   Summary, Future Work and Conclusion

This paper has presented the results of our early efforts in developing a framework in creating a realistic synthetic EHR for secondary usage. By incorporating publicly available data sets and clinical careflows, this paper has presented a novel strategy in generating EHRs. The RS-EHR alleviates confidentiality concerns and eliminates the use of anonymisation techniques. Proposed application for RS-EHRs include system developers and clinician trainers. The comprehensive medical history found in the patient EHR serves as a new format of teaching tool. It contains the clinical details for delivering rich case studies of patient treatment for training future clinicians.

Adoption of the EHR will continue to drive the desire for secondary use of patient information. Although the associated benefits from secondary use are well documented, the implementation will be slow due to patient privacy concerns, expensive anonymisation techniques, and limited data sets. Our work in developing the RS-EHR can provide highly available data sets of realistic patient information. In addition to standard methodologies employed in education, a new digital medium for case studies will be available in the form of a publicly available EHR. The publicly available EHR data set provides a new medium for training the next generation of clinicians.

This paper provides a general blueprint of our investigative work in developing the RS-EHR. We envision several sub-projects to evolve in our future work. Some examples of future projects include: (1) data extrapolation from public data sources for supporting the PADARSER approach; (2) temporal data population of EHR encounters derived from careflow events; (3) implementation and further refinement of the GRiSER algorithm for RS-EHR; (4) further conceptualisation and implementation of the method for generating careflow from published clinical practice guidelines; and (5) generating coded textual narratives from CPGs and medical coding and terminology systems.

References

1. American Medical Association (AMA). CPT coding, medical billing and insurance (2013), http://www.ama-assn.org/ama/pub/physician-resources/solutions-managing-your-practice/coding-billing-insurance.page?
2. Buczak, A., Babin, S., Moniz, L.: Data-driven approach for creating synthetic electronic medical records. BMC Medical Informatics and Decision Making 10(1), 59 (2010)
3. Daud, H., Razali, R., Asirvadam, V.: Sea Bed Logging Aapplications: ANOVA analysis 2 for Synthetic Data From Electromagnetic (EM) Simulator. In: 2012 IEEE Asia-Pacific Conference on Applied Electromagnetics (APACE), pp. 110–115 (2012)
4. De Backere, F., Moens, H., Steurbaut, K., De Turck, F., Colpaert, K., Danneels, C., Decruyenaere, J.: Automated generation and deployment of clinical guidelines in the ICU. In: 2010 IEEE 23rd International Symposium on Computer-Based Medical Systems (CBMS), pp. 197–202 (2010)
5. Esteller, R., Vachtsevanos, G., Echauz, J., Lilt, B.: A comparison of fractal dimension algorithms using synthetic and experimental data. In: Proceedings of the 1999 IEEE International Symposium on Circuits and Systems, ISCAS 1999, vol. 3, pp. 199–202 (1999)
6. GonzáLez-Ferrer, A., Teije, A.T., Fdez-Olivares, J., Milian, K.: Automated generation of patient-tailored electronic care pathways by translating computer-interpretable guidelines into hierarchical task networks. Artif. Intell. Med. 57(2), 91–109 (2013)
7. Gooch, P., Roudsari, A.: Computerization of workflows, guidelines, and care pathways: a review of implementation challenges for process-oriented health information systems. J. Am. Med. Inform. Assoc. 18, 738–748 (2011)
8. Grando, M.A., Glasspool, D., Boxwala, A.: Argumentation logic for the flexible enactment of goal-based medical guidelines. J. of Biomedical Informatics 45(5), 938–949 (2012)
9. Grimson, J.: Delivering the electronic healthcare record for the 21st century. International Journal of Medical Informatics 64(2-3), 111–127 (2001)
10. International Health Standards Development Organization (IHSDO). Systematized nomenclature of medicine clinical terms, SNOMed-CT (2013), http://www.ihtsdo.org/snomed-ct/

11. Jeske, D.R., Lin, P.J., Rendon, C.: Rui Xiao, and B. Samadi. Synthetic data generation capabilities for testing data mining tools. In: IEEE Military Communications Conference, MILCOM 2006, pp. 1–6 (2006)

12. Juarez, J.M., Martinez, P., Campos, M., Palma, J.: Step-Guided Clinical Workflow Fulfilment Measure for Clinical Guidelines. In: Moreno-Díaz, R., Pichler, F., Quesada-Arencibia, A. (eds.) EUROCAST 2009. LNCS, vol. 5717, pp. 255–262. Springer, Heidelberg (2009)

13. Laleci, G.B., Dogac, A.: A semantically enriched clinical guideline model enabling deployment in heterogeneous healthcare environments. IEEE Transactions on Information Technology in Biomedicine 13(2), 263–273 (2009)

14. Lee, N., Laine, A.F.: Mining electronic medical records to explore the linkage between healthcare resource utilization and disease severity in diabetic patients. In: 2011 First IEEE International Conference on Healthcare Informatics, Imaging and Systems Biology (HISB), pp. 250–257 (2011)

15. Maciejewski, R., Hafen, R., Rudolph, S., Tebbetts, G., Cleveland, W.S., Grannis, S.J., Ebert, D.S.: Generating synthetic syndromic-surveillance data for evaluating visual-analytics techniques. IEEE Computer Graphics and Applications 29(3), 18–28 (2008)

16. Margner, V., Pechwitz, M.: Synthetic Data for Arabic OCR System Development. In: Proceedings of the Sixth International Conference on Document Analysis and Recognition, pp. 1159–1163 (2001)

17. Milla-Millán, G., Fdez-Olivares, J., Sánchez-Garzón, I., Prior, D., Castillo, L.: Knowledge-driven adaptive execution of care pathways based on continuous planning techniques. In: Lenz, R., Miksch, S., Peleg, M., Reichert, M., Riaño, D., ten Teije, A. (eds.) ProHealth 2012 and KR4HC 2012. LNCS, vol. 7738, pp. 42–55. Springer, Heidelberg (2013)

18. New Zealand Ministry of Health (NZ-MoH). New Zealand Health Statistics: Classificiation and Terminology (2011),
http://www.health.govt.nz/nz-health-statistics/
classification-and-terminology (accessed: May 21, 2013)

19. Institute of Medicine (IOM). Guidelines for Clinical Practice: From Development to Use. National Academy Press, Washington DC (1992)

20. Peleg, M., Tu, S.W.: Design patterns for clinical guidelines. Artif. Intell. Med. 47(1), 1–24 (2009)

21. Raza, A., Clyde, S.: Testing health-care integrated systems with anonymized test-data extracted from production systems. In: 2012 International Conference on Cyber-Enabled Distributed Computing and Knowledge Discovery (CyberC), pp. 457–464 (2012)

22. Riaño, D.: Ordered Time-Independent CIG Learning. In: Barreiro, J.M., Martín-Sánchez, F., Maojo, V., Sanz, F. (eds.) ISBMDA 2004. LNCS, vol. 3337, pp. 117–128. Springer, Heidelberg (2004)

23. Stark, E., Eltoft, T., Braathen, B.: Performance of Vegetation Classification Methods Using Synthetic Multi-Sspectral Satellite Data. In: International Geoscience and Remote Sensing Symposium (IGARSS 1995). Quantitative Remote Sensing for Science and Applications, vol. 2, pp. 1276–1278 (1995)

24. Tsai, A., Kuo, P.-H., Lee, G., Lin, M.-S.: Electronic clinical guidelines for intensive care unit. In: 2007 9th International Conference on e-Health Networking, Application and Services, pp. 117–124 (2007)

25. World Health Organisation (WHO). International Classificiation of Diseases (ICD), Web, http://www.who.int/classifications/icd/en/ (accessed: May 21, 2013)

Insulin Pump Software Certification

Yihai Chen[1,*], Mark Lawford[2,**], Hao Wang[2,***], and Alan Wassyng[2,**]

[1] School of Computer Engineering and Science, Shanghai University, Shanghai, China
[2] McMaster Centre for Software Certification
McMaster University, Hamilton, Ontario, Canada

Abstract. The insulin pump is a safety-critical embedded medical device used for treatment of type 1 and insulin treated type 2 diabetes. Malfunction of the insulin pump will endanger the user's life. All countries impose some regulation on the sale and use of medical devices. The purpose of such regulation is to protect the public by imposing standards of *safety* for medical devices, including insulin pumps. The regulator in the USA, the USA Food and Drug Administration (FDA), actually goes further, and includes *efficacy* in the regulatory requirement. Until recently, regulatory approval was dependent on *process based* guidance. However, this has proven to be inadequate in some (most) cases where the device depends on software for its safe and effective operation, and the FDA recently changed its approval process for infusion pumps (including insulin pumps), so that the production of an assurance case that demonstrates that the device is safe and effective is now a strongly suggested regulatory requirement. However the current regulatory guidance does not recommend any particular software development methodology, and does not include definitive guidance on the evaluation component of the certification process. In this paper, we briefly review the related USA regulatory standards for insulin pumps, highlight development and certification challenges, briefly discuss attributes of a safe, secure and dependable insulin pump, and propose an effective certification process for insulin pumps.

Keywords: insulin pump, safety critical system, software certification, standards compliance.

1   Introduction

Diabetes mellitus is one of the major noncommunicable diseases (NCDs) facing modern society today. Type 1 diabetes results from the inability of the pancreas to create the insulin required to constrain the blood glucose levels in the body. Type 1 diabetes is fatal unless insulin can be introduced into the bloodstream. Type 2 diabetes is also characterized by high blood glucose levels, but in this case the lack of insulin in the body is not absolute. Type 2 diabetes can be treated through other means, but sometimes

* Supported by National Natural Science Foundation of China (NSFC) under grant No. 61170044 and China Scholarship Council.
** Partially supported by IBM SOSCIP Project, and Ontario Research Fund - Research Excellence.
*** Supported by IBM Canada R&D Centre and Southern Ontario Smart Computing Innovation Platform (SOSCIP) project.

J. Gibbons and W. MacCaull (Eds.): FHIES 2013, LNCS 8315, pp. 87–106, 2014.
© Springer-Verlag Berlin Heidelberg 2014

the use of insulin is necessary. Diabetes is directly responsible for 3.5% of NCD deaths. Type 1 and insulin treated type 2 diabetes patients must inject insulin daily for their survival. Historically, this has been achieved by the patient injecting insulin at particular times in the day, typically at meal time.

For some years now, an alternative has been available. Continuous subcutaneous insulin infusion (CSII) has been successfully used to treat type 1 and insulin treated type 2 diabetes patients. This subcutaneous infusion of insulin is achieved through the use of an *insulin pump*.

An insulin pump is a pager sized electronic device that continuously delivers insulin using a catheter. The first reported insulin pump system was developed by Dr. Arnold Kadish in the early 1960s. Since then people have explored using CSII therapy to treat diabetes. The Diabetes Control and Complication Trial [28] in 1993, showed that sustained lowering of blood glucose slows diabetes complications. The insulin pump can imitate physiological insulin secretion, and a recent study showed that it results in significant improvement in glycated hemoglobin levels as compared with injection therapy [4]. These research findings and improvements in the design and function of insulin pumps motivated their increased usage in recent years. More than 300,000 patients around the world use insulin pumps today [26].

An insulin infusion pump is a safety-critical software-intensive medical device (SMD). Flaws in the pump software can cause serious injury or even loss of life. Until recently, regulatory approval of SMDs was dependent on *process based* guidance, e.g., in Europe, IEC 62304 regulates the development processes of medical device software. Process based guidance has proven to be inadequate: The USA Food and Drug Administration (FDA)[1] received nearly 17,000 insulin pump-related adverse-event reports from Oct. 1, 2006 to Sept. 30, 2009 [8] and 41 of the 310 death reports were associated with blood-sugar levels being too high or too low, suggesting the device may not have been working properly.

The FDA recently changed its approval process for infusion pumps, so that the production of an *assurance case* that demonstrates that the device is safe and effective is now a *recommended* regulatory requirement in the USA. However the current regulatory guidance does not recommend any particular software development methodology, and does not include definitive guidance on the evaluation component of the certification process. In this paper, we briefly review the related USA regulatory standards for insulin pumps, discuss development and certification challenges for such medical devices, and propose an effective certification process for insulin pumps.

The remainder of this paper is organized as follows: section 2 introduces the domain knowledge of an insulin pump system and the challenges for development and certification. Section 3 gives an overview of related regulatory requirements and standards for insulin pumps. Section 4 discusses required quality attributes, and Section 5 presents a suggested certification process based on our understanding of those software attributes and assurance cases. The final section provides conclusions.

---

[1] In this paper, we use the FDA as representative of a government regulatory agency for medical devices because we are more familiar with their regulatory standards and guidelines and their certifying practices, and, more importantly, FDA approval is an important benchmark for marketing medical devices globally.

2   The Insulin Pump System

2.1   A Generic Insulin Pump

Typically, in modelling such devices, and in discussion related to their development and certification, we need to be specific regarding the features and components of the devices. This paper discusses a *generic* insulin pump, which is a pump that is not marketed and not manufactured. The reason we have done this is so that we are able to describe a pump that is typical of pumps on the market, and exhibits behaviour representative of most pumps that we know about. The idea is to remove this from the baggage that is often associated with analysis of an existing, physical pump, manufactured by a specific company. The paper is concerned with principles, rather than with the certification of a specific pump.

Throughout the remainder of this paper, when we talk about the insulin pump, we are talking about the *generic insulin pump*. The structure of such a pump is presented in the following section.

2.2   Insulin Pump Structure

The basic components of an insulin pump include (see Figure 1):

- a user interface;
- the controller;
- the pumping mechanism;
- the insulin reservoir; and
- wireless input/output.

Note that the infusion set, the complete tubing system to connect an insulin pump to the pump user, is assumed to be outside of the system boundary for the purpose of this paper. This affects any modelling of physical links and the hazards analysis, but has no other effect. We have excluded discussion related to it simply to reduce the complexity of the system dealt with in the paper. Similarly, although the battery is shown in Figure 1, we are not going to include battery behaviour in our analysis other than to recognize that power may be on or off. The last item missing from Figure 1, is the environment. For the sake of simplicity in the presentation of this paper, we assume that the environment, which is everything outside of the system, relates almost entirely to the user – whether it be infusion of insulin into the user's body, or data focused interaction with the pump. In actual practice, of course, we would include the hardware, all relevant aspects of the environment, and their interaction with the software, in the development of convincing proof that the insulin pump is safe and secure.

The remainder of this section will provide a brief description of the components of the insulin pump system.

The *user interface* includes the capability to input data, and also to choose actions. In addition, the pump is able to display information to the user. In our case, the input and output are kept very simple and not specific as to whether they are textual or audible.

The *controller* is the digital control unit that we are able to program. Again, this is assumed to be as general as feasible. We are not interested (in this paper) in the different faults that are introduced by digital computers compared with field programmable gate arrays, e.g., The (pump) controller can be programmed to administer basal (periodic) or bolus (extra) insulin according to a patient's request.

The *pumping mechanism* is the hardware pump that moves the insulin from the reservoir into the user's body (through the infusion set). It is also generic in that we do not distinguish between the different types of pumps.

The *insulin reservoir* holds the insulin cartridges. The reservoir needs to have the capability of signalling when the remaining amount of insulin is low (below a threshold), or empty.

Some of the latest insulin pumps can communicate *wirelessly* with a remote computer, a continuous glucose monitor (CSM), or even the cloud [17].

The pump that we are considering is referred to as an *"open loop" system* in that it does not use any form of automated feedback to determine the amount of insulin to administer. Compared with open loop insulin pumps, a *closed-loop system* or "artificial pancreas" can monitor glucose levels 24/7, and automatically delivers an appropriate dose of insulin without a patient's intervention. These pumps are just appearing, or are about to appear, on the market. They are much more complex than the open loop pumps, and since this complexity does not contribute to the principles and approaches we want to present, and because we have not yet managed to develop even the simpler open loop pumps to the appropriate level of dependability, we have excluded them from further discussion in this paper.

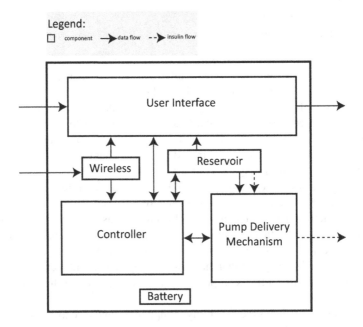

Fig. 1. Structure of a Generic Insulin Pump

2.3   Challenges for Development

Developers of medical devices face many challenges, and software intensive systems certainly add to these. The following challenges have to be dealt with if we are to be able to produce dependably safe and secure, software dependent insulin pumps.

- *Medical software is subject to government laws and regulations*
  In the USA, the FDA requires the manufacturers to submit a premarket notification[2] [510(k)] [14]. The submission process requires the insulin pump to be in compliance with guidelines including *General Principles of Software Validation* [12] and *Guidance for the Content of Premarket Submissions for Software Contained in Medical Devices* [13], etc. More discussion on regulatory requirements can be found in Section 3.
- *Process based regulation – yet there is no recommended software development life cycle*
  In spite of the perceived burdensome regulation imposed on medical device manufacturers, in terms of the software embedded in the device, the regulation and referenced international standards do not mandate the usage of a specific software development life cycle.
- *Safety*
  This is a safety critical device and there are a large number of safety requirements. Below are examples of some safety concerns related directly to the components of the insulin pump.
    - The user interface is critical in that the user cannot be assumed to be as skilled as a nurse would be in interfacing with other types of infusion pumps
    - The pump delivery mechanism must not allow free-flow, and must not allow air bubbles to form in the liquid insulin
    - The controller must deliver 24/7 service outside of routine maintenance, and so must be proven to be deadlock free, and robust in the event of hardware failures
- *Security*
  Modern insulin pumps have wireless capabilities (see Figure 1) that bring additional security challenges for insulin pump software development. It has been reported that insulin pumps are vulnerable to hackers [2,7]. This security problem leads directly to a safety concern. Some research work has been done to address the problem, but it is far from being solved [19,27].

2.4   Challenges for Certification

The goal of certification is to systematically determine, based on the principles of science, engineering and measurement theory, whether an artifact satisfies accepted, well defined and measurable criteria [15]. Maibaum and Wassyng pointed out that process oriented software process quality does not necessarily translate into good software product quality [21]. The certification of insulin pump software poses some additional challenges:

---

[2] A stricter premarket approval (PMA) process is required for closed-loop insulin pumps.

- *Lack of clear definition of evidence and how to evaluate it [15]*
  What evidence would convince the FDA that the insulin pump is safe, secure and dependable? In general, the FDA provides very little definitive guidance on what evidence to provide. This results in huge unpredictability for the manufacturers, because they are not sure how to document or structure the evidence they have produced. Of course, in many cases they have not even developed the evidence that the FDA may be expecting. In addition to this, different staff at the FDA may have different lists of 'essentials'. In the case of the insulin pump, in particular, what will convince the regulator? Do they want/need to see that the manufacturer has defined the smallest air bubble that can be detected in the pump, and that bubbles over a threshold size can be prevented from being injected into the user?

- *Do not provide any guidance on how to evaluate assurance cases and hazard analysis results*
  Currently relevant standards and guidance recommend assurance cases and talk about mitigating hazards, but do not necessarily provide guidance on how to demonstrate that all hazards have been mitigated. So, the FDA recommends that assurance cases should be submitted – but it does not explicitly require that assurance cases should have a structure that argues over all identified hazards [14].

- *What do the FDA need to know about the battery?*
  The battery must be safe, i.e., it must not spontaneously combust. It needs to provide sufficient power and must provide n hours of continuous use. There should be accurate warnings to the user when battery life is low. What evidence should be presented to the FDA to support all of these 'claims'?

- *Integrating with third-party components*
  Insulin pump software usually integrates with third-party software components, called *Software Of Unknown Provenance* (SOUP) components in IEC 62304. For example, the insulin pump software may interface to WiFi radio software developed by another company. SOUP components impede certification efforts.

- *Insulin pump systems are becoming part of Medical Cyber-Physical Systems*
  A modern insulin pump system is not a stand-alone device anymore. It is connected with a continuous glucose management system, blood glucose monitor, and other associated devices and health information systems. These interconnections make the certification more difficult and more challenging.

- *Minimizing certification time and effort*
  Under the Medical Device User Fee Act (MDUFA), the FDA is under pressure to finish 510(k) reviews quicker than they do now. Failure to follow guidance document(s) or recognized standards, inadequate software documentation will delay the review process [10].

3   Overview of Regulatory Requirements for Insulin Pumps (Software Focus)

Many years ago, the FDA included a way of grandfathering devices onto the market with the so-called "510(k) Guideline". Its introduction was supposed to have been temporary, and was made at the time the U.S. started to regulate medical devices. It has never been removed. Infusion pumps in general have been remarkably prone to error, and so the FDA has published new guidance on the 510(k) process, the *infusion pump premarket notification 510(k) guidance* (FDA 510K Guideline) [14]. The guideline requires that the manufacturer show *substantial equivalence* with an existing device on the market, and show that no new hazards are introduced in the device submitted for approval. The guideline also encourages the manufacturers to take advantage of any recognized software standards and provide statements or declarations of conformity as described in the FDA guidance *Use of Standards in Substantial Equivalence Determinations* [11]. In addition, in reaction to the poor dependability and safety record of infusion pumps, the new guideline recommends that manufacturers demonstrate substantial equivalence by using an *assurance case* to structure the claim [14]. In Section 5.2, we discuss assurance cases in detail and present a partial assurance case template as part of our proposed certification process.

Figure 2 shows international standards relevant to the development of medical device software. The IEC 62304 standard provides a framework of life cycle processes and requirements for each life cycle process. The standard requires that the manufacturer use a *quality management system*, for which ISO 13485 is recommended, and a *risk management process* complying with ISO 14971. In particular, IEC 62304 addresses the usage of SOUP.

Risk management is undoubtedly vital to the development and certification of insulin pumps, but the hazard analysis methods recommended by ISO 14971 do not reflect more recent established methods for software-intensive systems like the STAMP-based Analysis[3] (STPA) [20]. More importantly, the European Committee for Standardization (CEN) identified[4] all content deviations of ISO 14971 compared with the requirements of EU Directives 93/42/EEC. One deviation is that:

> ISO 14971 ... contains the concept of reducing risks "as low as reasonably practicable"...(while) Directive 93/42/EEC and various particular Essential Requirements require risks to be reduced "as far as possible" without there being room for *economic considerations*.

We can see that the majority of related standards are concerned with the development process of medical device software, with the exception of IEC 60601-1[5]. However, IEC 60601-1 is for general medical devices, so it does not cover all aspects of medical device software. The FDA 510K Guideline recommends the insulin pump meet IEC 60601-1 as to the alarms/warnings and environmental safety requirements

4   The Quality Attributes of Insulin Pump Software

This section discusses some of the quality attributes important to insulin pump software. It is not a comprehensive list, but covers several key elements that can be used as

---

[3] STAMP stands for *Systems-Theoretic Accident Model and Processes*, an accident model by the same MIT group

[4] when the ISO 14971:2007, Corrected version 2007-10-01 was taken over as a European Standard EN ISO 14971:2012

[5] The other product standard – IEC 61010-1 – is for electrical equipment for measurement, control and laboratory use, which is not relevant to insulin pumps.

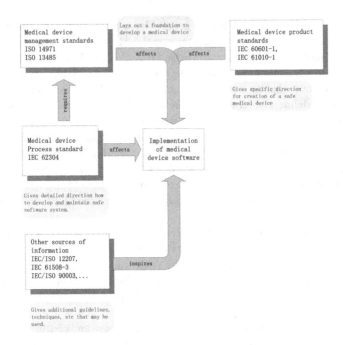

Fig. 2. Relationship of key MEDICAL DEVICE standards to IEC 62304 [18]

acceptance criteria to evaluate insulin pump software. We divide the quality attributes of the insulin pump into three sets: functional attributes, 'design' attributes ('design' in the conceptual sense, which includes requirements specifications as well), and software development process attributes. We have listed functional and design attributes in the remainder of this section. We have not included process attributes in order to save space, and also because process attributes form the mainstay of current certification processes and we do not have anything significantly new to say on the subject.

4.1 Functional Quality Attributes

Safety. The safety challenge was described briefly in Section 2.3. What evidence do we look for in this regard, and use in the certification? Brief list: global safety and liveness properties satisfied; hazards mitigated (includes fail-safe behaviour); completeness checks satisfied; Human machine interface (HMI) testing report. Figure 3 provides an excerpt from a table detailing the system hazards and proposed mitigations.

Security. The security challenge was also described briefly in Section 2.3. Brief list of evidence: hazards mitigated; completeness checks satisfied; freedom from coding defects.

Availability. This was also discussed in Section 2.3, and straddles the safety attribute. Evidence to consider includes: global safety and liveness properties satisfied; fail-safe hazards mitigated; completeness checks satisfied; freedom from coding defects.

Hazard	Contributing Factor	Mitigation
Failure in the pump causes the flow rate to be incorrect	Backflow through the pump	Use a pump which prevents flow when not being powered by the system
	Free flow through the pump	
	Efficiency fatigue over time	Require user to replace or perform maintenance after given period of time
	Cracking/damage to the pump	Use a pump that is composed of resilient materials
	Blockage	Pressure sensing included in the pump
	Not enough power provided	Regulate the power source and ensure the correct voltage outputs from system to pump
	Too much power provided	
Failure in reservoir provides incorrect volume of insulin	Cracking/damage	Use a reservoir that is composed of resilient materials
	Empty reservoir	Include volume sensing in the reservoir to alert when low
	Blockage	Pressure sensing included to ensure insulin is exiting the reservoir
Failure in the delivery line provides incorrect flow rate	Cracking/damage	Use a delivery line that is composed of resilient materials
	Line not attached to the user	Medical professional provides training on how to set up the infusion set
	Blockage	Pressure sensing included to ensure insulin flowing
	Air in line	Force user to prime the line before use and include sensing capabilities for air gaps

Fig. 3. Hazards and mitigations corresponding to infusion rate not matching requested value [29]

Usability. ([34]) Straddles safety and availability and is also discussed in Section 2.3. Evidence is primarily HMI related validation test reports.

Maintainability. The lifespan of insulin pumps may be years, requiring updates and safety/security enhancements as more usage data becomes available, and the science of insulin pumps further develops. Evidence to consider includes: requirements-traceability forward and backward; *information hiding* modularization (see 4.2); a documented uses hierarchy.

4.2 Design Attributes

Requirements Consistent, Complete and Unambiguous. If this is not true, then the software design loses its context. Evidence includes: completeness checks satisfied; verification reports that include consistency, completeness, etc.

No Dead Code. 'Dead code' affects both safety and security, and many regulatory domains have statements to the effect that it must be avoided. The question is what evidence do we need to show that it has been avoided? The most effective evidence in our opinion is a code (formal) verification report that demonstrates that the code faithfully implements the software design.

Code Free from Common Defects. Reports from two or more static code analysis tools are excellent evidence in this regard. We suggest two or more since different tools tend to find different errors [5].

Information Hiding. The objective of information hiding is to identify requirements or design decisions that are likely to change and to encapsulate the essence of what would change in a single module/class. This results in excellent modularity and clearly facilitates maintainability [23,24]. Evidence of effective information hiding includes lists of requirements and design decisions that are likely to change in the future, and traceability of those 'secrets' down into the software design level.

Design Facilitates Verification. Verification means confirmation through provision of objective evidence that specified requirements have been fulfilled [18]. The IEC 62304 [18] guided process requires planning for software verification. Borrowing from the nuclear domain, the design output "should facilitate the establishment of verification criteria and the performance of analyses, reviews, or tests to determine whether those criteria have been met"[22]. Evidence of this should be visible in project planning procedures, and in the design itself.

One task the certifier must then perform is to understand what quality attributes are used in claims in the assurance case, and evaluate the evidence associated with them. In the following section we describe the certification process.

5   A Suggested Certification Process

We have briefly described the current regulatory (certification) process for medical devices in the USA (Section 3). It is not remarkably different, we believe, in most countries that have equivalent oversight of medical devices. We also briefly described the major challenges faced by manufacturers of medical devices (Section 2.3), as well as certifiers of medical devices (Section 2.4). In this section we present an overview of a certification process for medical devices, focused on the evaluation of the software attributes in those devices.

It is important to note that we are considering the certification of a medical device that is safety critical – the insulin pump saves lives, but can also take them.

There is an old maxim that the certification of software intensive systems should depend on a tripod – *people, process and product*. Currently, the regulatory regime in most domains that deal with software intensive safety critical systems is predominantly process based. As we have seen, the certification of medical devices is no different. Our contention is that people (the developers and certifiers) and process are undoubtedly important, but the certification process should be as *product-focused* as possible. This section presents ways in which we think we can achieve this.

5.1   People and Process

Before we describe the product-focused aspects of the certification process, we deal with the essentials that relate to people and process.

People. The developers of the insulin pump must be competent in a variety of domains in order to develop a safe, secure, effective and dependable pump. In terms of software expertise, the developers need to be able to document knowledge and experience in the crucial aspects of safety critical software development. If the company/division is too small to be able to perform some of the activities, they will need to contract others to help them. Their expertise will also need to be documented. We are not certain that the FDA or other medical device regulators currently conduct checks of this nature – but they should. In particular, development teams must be able to document relevant expertise in: hazard analysis; software requirements elicitation and specification; software design; coding; hardware interfacing; security; testing; configuration management; and assurance cases. The acceptance criteria by which the regulator can evaluate this knowledge and expertise is currently problematic. The body of knowledge in these areas is not universally accepted. However, accreditation by various professional bodies, degrees in relevant disciplines, and so on, are all useful in this regard.

Development Process and Tools. Safe, secure and dependable software needs to be developed using a development process approved by the regulator. This is often achieved by showing compliance with a process standard, such as IEC 62304. Alternative standards usually exist within the relevant regulatory framework. The FDA, for example, has process guidance in their set of regulatory guidelines [11]. Any tool support for the process should not represent a potential "single point of failure" that either introduces an error or result in an error going undetected. In many standards such reliance upon a tool requires that the tool itself be developed to the same level of rigour as the system under development. Thus the process and supporting tools must support each other to eliminate any potential "single point failures".

5.2   Product

As indicated in Sections 1 and 3, the FDA now recommends the submission of an assurance case for insulin pumps. An assurance case should have substantial product evidence to support the claims and arguments included in the case, and so is one way in which we can focus our certification regime more on the product under scrutiny, rather than on the process used to build it.

A Brief Introduction to Assurance Cases. An assurance case (originally developed as safety cases) is a structured document that presents a claim about the product and also demonstrates the validity of the claim through a series of connected arguments, sub-claims and evidence [6].

Hawkins et al. [16] recently compared the two approaches to certification of software safety: *prescriptive certification*[6] and assurance cases. They argue that the two approaches are complementary and could lead to "a better solution than either approach on its own".

---

[6] Some standards prescribe specific processes and techniques that must be followed.

Assurance Case Template. We believe that the quality of the evaluation of the assurance case by a regulator (or certification authority) is just as important as the quality of the development of the assurance case by the manufacturer. This would seem to contradict our belief (shared by most proponents of assurance cases) that the act of developing the assurance case is more beneficial than the resulting assurance case, but it does not. For the manufacturer, the act of developing the assurance case forces the development team to consider gaps and the validity of their claims, continually. This assumes, of course, that the assurance case is developed with honest intent, and that it drives development, rather than serve as documentation after the fact. Sincerity and skilled work are not sufficient though. We are probably all familiar with the effect of reading and critiquing our own work ("own work" here includes other members of the team or members of another team within the same company). We need an objective check on this, and it makes sense that the relevant regulators (or certifying authority) are the ones to do it. Not only is it within their mandate, but they are (almost always) aware of issues that have plagued other manufacturers in the same domain. Thus, their evaluation of the assurance case is also vital.

Now that we have established the importance of the regulatory evaluation of the assurance case, we need to examine aspects of the development and evaluation of the assurance case that are likely to affect the quality of the evaluation. This has only recently generated interest. One of our concerns for some time now [32], has been that if each assurance case submitted to the FDA is a *one-off* example, then the FDA is not likely to build sufficient expertise in evaluating these assurance cases, and they are likely to struggle to find subtle flaws in these cases in the time that they have available for the evaluation. It is mainly for this reason, that we think that frameworks/patterns/templates for assurance cases within an application domain, make excellent sense. *Sufficiency* of the safety argument is also of interest, and there have been a few different approaches in this regard. One recent approach is described in [3]. There are a number of assurance case frameworks that have been suggested for medical device certification [1,30,33]. We would go a little further, and suggest that a reasonably prescriptive template be provided to insulin pump manufacturers, and that the manufacturers be given guidelines on how (and why) to use the template. This introduces some problems – political and technical. The political problems all stem from the fact that *prescription* seems to be a dirty word in software. However, we need to come to terms with the fact that most branches of engineering are quite prescriptive and conservative in their approved approaches to the development of safety critical systems, that they do this for good reasons, and that they often do manage to keep just behind the curve of innovation, so that there is progress as new methods pass the stage from *radical* to *normal* design. We should also realize that there are good ways and bad ways of mandating prescriptive approaches. The technical problems relate to having to know more about our domain than we think we do. Our belief is that we do know enough to get started. This paper presents one approach to getting started on more prescriptive approaches to assurance cases for insulin pumps.

Most assurance cases that we have seen have used a hazards analysis to drive and structure the assurance case. We do not believe that this is the best way to structure the case. It is difficult to determine and show that any hazard analysis is complete, in the sense that all relevant hazards have been identified. If we use the structure of the hazard analysis to structure the assurance case, we are then going to find it very difficult to argue that the assurance case is sound. We could, of course, add a claim that deals with the case that not all hazards were identified, but that seems to lead into having to then show the argument we could have used if the hazard analysis was not the driver of the structure. It seems clear to us then, that hazard analyses should be included at lower levels of the arguments. Our suggested template has three claims at the top level:

- The requirements accurately and consistently specify the behaviour of the insulin pump, such that the pump, if built in compliance with these requirements, will maintain the user's insulin levels so that they are within a safe range for the user
- The pump is built so that its behaviour is compliant with the behaviour specified in the requirements, within specified tolerances
- It will be possible to maintain and operate the pump over its projected lifetime without adversely affecting the safety, security and effectiveness of the pump

A fourth top level claim, *fail-safe*, is a possibility. If fail-safe behaviour is included explicitly in the requirements specification, then we have an option to deal with evidence related to fail-safe behaviour in the verification claim regarding compliance with requirements. We could also separate it out as a separate claim. If details of the fail-safe behaviour are not explicitly included in the requirements, then we definitely need a fourth top level claim regarding fail-safe behaviour.

The real idea behind an assurance case template is to provide guidance to both manufacturers and regulators of the assurance case in a way that directs the manufacturers to develop arguments that are important in that domain, but are not so detailed as to make it a mindless exercise performed solely to convince the regulators.

An idea of what this may look like is presented in Figure 4, in which we have shown the claims and sub-claims for just one of the three top claims, since it is not possible to show the other two claims in the space available. The claims are shown but the strategies, context, and other types of possible nodes are not shown, again because of space limitations. Also, because they are not really relevant to the point we are making. The evidence at the end of the argument chain is blank here, but in an actual template we would include a description of acceptable evidence for each of these paths. We would also use context nodes to describe the rationale for the choice of claims, sub-claims, strategies, etc.

So, how does this help us? It actually helps us in a number of ways.

First of all, for the regulator/certification authority:

- It conveys to the manufacturers, in a very explicit way, the type of argument and supporting evidence required in order to obtain approval for marketing an insulin pump;
- The main structure of the assurance case is pre-determined (not the specific content of a node in many cases), and the regulator should have (must have) done sufficient analysis to determine that arguments based on this structure, with relevant content in the nodes, should produce adequate arguments;
- The consistency of the structure will allow the regulator to develop expertise in what content leads to adequate assurance cases, and will be able to audit submissions to determine if there is something important lacking, whether the specific evidence presented does not adequately support a specific argument, etc.

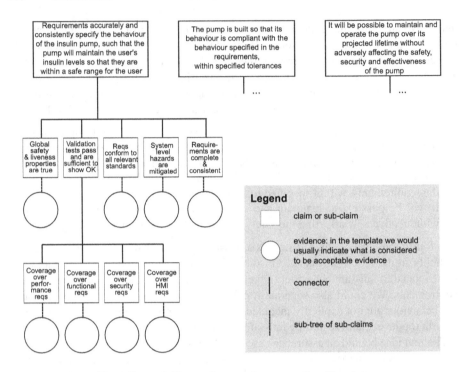

Fig. 4. Example Extract from an Assurance Case Template

Secondly, for the manufacturer:

- There should be much better predictability of the regulatory evaluation process, and this is one of the major concerns of manufacturers;
- It provides guidance based on the regulator's experience and knowledge of problems that are common in a specific domain;
- Manufacturers need to develop products knowing that they will be safe, not prove that they are safe after development. Templates like this can help direct development so that the product will be safe, secure and dependable.

We already presented an overview in graphical form of the top level claim *"The requirements accurately and consistently specify the behaviour of the insulin pump, such that the pump, if built in compliance with these requirements, will maintain the user's insulin levels so that they are within a safe range for the user"* in Figure 4. Now, as another example, we show a template in text form[7] that supports the claim that *"The pump is built so that its behaviour is compliant with the behaviour specified in the requirements, within specified tolerances"*. Possible sub-claims are as follows:

---

[7] Although most assurance case research uses graphical representations of the case, we are not yet convinced that this is effective for large, practical assurance cases. Tabular text form for cases may be more appropriate in that we may be able to design the layout so that it facilitates views of the 'big picture' more effectively than graphical layouts can.

- The pump's behaviour is compliant with the behaviour specified in the requirements, within specified tolerances
  - All requirements in the system requirements spec (REQ) are present and equivalent in the system level design (DGN)
    * *Evidence:* DGN review report that shows all requirements from REQ are present in DGN
    * *Evidence:* DGN verification report shows equivalence of requirements in REQ with their representation in DGN [may be omitted if model and notation in REQ and DGN are the same]
  - All behaviour specified in DGN that is not in REQ has been justified, and DGN is correct, complete, unambiguous and consistent
    * *Evidence:* DGN review report documents this justification
  - All software related behaviour in DGN is represented equivalently in the software requirements (SRS), and
  - All hardware related behaviour in DGN is described in M-I or O-C mappings (as in the 4 variable model [25], and transfer events [31])
    * The software design (SDD) correctly includes all behaviour in the SRS
      · *Evidence:* SDD verification report shows equivalence of requirements in SRS with their representation in the SDD, within tolerance
    * All behaviour specified in the SDD that is not in the SRS has been justified, and the SDD is correct, complete, unambiguous and consistent
      · *Evidence:* SDD review report shows justification
      · *Evidence:* SDD verification reports demonstrates SDD is complete, unambiguous and consistent
  - All behaviour in the SDD is equivalently implemented in code
    * *Evidence:* Code verification report shows equivalence of behaviour in code with its representation in the SDD
    * *Evidence:* Test reports demonstrate that no tests fail
  - All behaviour implemented in code and not in the SDD has been justified
    * *Evidence:* Code review report shows justification
  - Code is complete, unambiguous and *"free from coding defects"*
    * *Evidence:* Code verification report shows complete and unambiguous
    * *Evidence:* Reports from two independent static code analysis tools show code is *"free from coding defects"*

There are clearly some claims missing from this template – they are missing simply because we do not want to complicate the claim/argument structure for the purpose of this illustration. In particular, all the claims related to hazard analysis are missing. Similarly, fail-safe items are also ignored. However, there is enough detail here to see that there is some obvious prescription implicit in this template.

1. Required documents tell us something about the process – system level requirements, system level design, software requirements, software design, system level design review report, software requirements review report, software design review report, software design (mathematical) verification, code verification, testing (lots of it), static analysis;
2. Mathematical verification is required;

3. The above point implies that the software requirements and software design must be mathematically specified;
4. More subtly, it gives the manufacturer the option to form the SRS directly from the DGN without rewriting the behaviour in any way.

c_InfuFlRt

Inputs:

Name	Description	Initial Value	Reference
M_BolAmt	A request for an amount of bolus	N/A	–
f_BasProf	The current basal profile in the system	N/A	–
c_SysOp$_{-1}$	The previous value of the system operation indicator	NoOp	4.3
c_BolInProg$_{-1}$	The previous value of the bolus administration notification	NoBolInProg	4.4
c_BadDelivNotif$_{-1}$	The previous value of the bad delivery notification	NoBadDelivNotif	4.7

Output:

Name	Description
c_InfuFlRt	The flow rate of the insulin to be delivered

Function Table:

				Result
		Condition		c_InfuFlRt
c_SysOp$_{-1}$ = Op	c_BadDelivNotif$_{-1}$ $\neq$ MaxDose	c_BolInProg$_{-1}$ = BolInProg	f_BasProf + M_BolAmt $* \Delta t \leq$ k_MaxTotFlRt	f_BasProf(t_{now}) + M_BolAmt $* \Delta t$
			f_BasProf + M_BolAmt $* \Delta t >$ k_MaxTotFlRt	k_MaxTotFlRt
		c_BolInProg$_{-1}$ = NoBolInProg		f_BasProf(t_{now})
	c_BadDelivNotif$_{-1}$ = MaxDose			0
c_SysOp$_{-1}$ = NoOp				0

Fig. 5. Example tabular requirements specification from [29]

This paper is about insulin pumps, yet if we examine the suggested items in the template that we have presented, other than some very high-level claims we cannot actually see anything specific to insulin pumps – it is reasonably general. This is an excellent demonstration of why such a template is useful. It is possible to structure the assurance case in a way that reviewers/certifiers build expertise in what should be presented in particular sections, and it will still **not** be a mindless *fill-in the blanks* exercise. The reason we can *claim* this, is that the domain and problem specific claims, arguments and evidence will be necessary and visible at lower levels. They are essential to the overall argument. The fact that a template is used to say what should be proved, in no way diminishes the intellectual burden on the developers to provide the appropriate, problem specific sub-claims, arguments and evidence.

For example, in order to support the sub-claim "Requirements are complete & consistent" from the template in Figure 4, once the system's monitored and controlled variables have been identified, the developers may choose to use tabular specifications for the SRS such as the one in Figure 5. Part of the evidence to support the claim that the requirements are complete and consistent would be that that the value of every controlled variable is determined by a single table (or composition of tables) and each table is complete (no missing input cases) and disjoint (no ambiguities). Figure 5 defines the behaviour of the infusion flow rate which is given by the flow rate output to the pump based on the current basal profile and any requested bolus. Due to space limitation we refer the reader to [29] for a more detailed description of the requirement. The important thing to note from the example is that it is easy to inspect that the table is complete and disjoint. Further, these properties of the table can be easily formally verified by using a tool such as [9].

Another low level sub-claim in the assurance case may be that no insulin will be delivered when the maximum dosage has already been reached. The evidence to support this could be a reference to appropriate test cases, as well as a reference to the tabular expression in Figure 5, in which we see that when $c\_BadDelivNotif_{-1} = MaxDose$, the value of $c\_InfuFlRt$ is 0.

Evaluation of the Assurance Case. Although the assurance case template is used by the manufacturer, it is presented in this section since it is developed by the regulator. The regulator's task is not finished though - the regulator has to evaluate the submitted assurance case.

There are a number of ways to achieve this, and some of these have been presented in the literature already [3,33]:

- The regulator audits one or more *slices* of the assurance case. A 'slice' may be defined by following a path of claim, sub-claim, evidence. It is likely that the regulator will know that specific claims are problematic for the insulin pump (or whatever other device is being evaluated), and will want to audit those claim-slices. If the audit is close to perfect, it is likely that the regulator will simply then go through a check-list of items, such as the safety requirements documented by the manufacturer. If the audit uncovers problems, the regulator may immediately halt the evaluation and inform the manufacturer, or they may start looking for more detailed evidence that the submission is poor so as to have an overwhelming case for denial.
- Another way of evaluating the assurance case would be to go through the entire assurance case, comparing the submission with the regulator's model case (documented or un-documented).
- Yet another process that could be followed is for the regulator to make an *approval assurance case* (or a *denial assurance case*). This would document the claims for approval (or denial) in a claim, sub-claim, evidence structure. Regulators do this now, but it is implicit. Many people believe that assurance cases are effective simply

because they force us to make our arguments explicit, and this should work equally well for evaluation as it does for development.

All of these involve *confidence* as a major component of the decision process. Some of the literature already cited deals with this, and it is a growing research topic in assurance cases. However, we (personally) do not have enough evidence yet to draw conclusions about how confidence should be presented (as a separate case, for example), or how it should be evaluated.

Our current preference for an assurance case evaluation process would be the audit or the approval (denial) case – or a combination of the two.

6   Conclusion

In this paper we described some of the challenges in developing and certifying a generic insulin infusion pump. We then outlined ways in which to address these challenges, including a partial assurance case template, justifying a product focused approach to the certification evidence and evaluation, and taking into account one of the main certification challenges – reducing the variation in submitted assurance case structure. An important point is that a prescriptive template provides structure that is useful and appropriate in multiple domains and for multiple specific applications, and that, if carefully constructed, it should not lead to mindless completion of the template, since the lower levels of the template require specific claims and evidence that depend on the specific application. There is still important work to be done in identifying the form of evidence required, how to evaluate the evidence (how to 'measure' the degree to which specific attributes have been achieved), and how to evaluate the assurance case itself. The important aspect of *confidence* in assurance cases will be central to some of this research.

References

1. Ankrum, T.S., Kromholz, A.H.: Structured Assurance Cases: Three Common Standards. In: HASE 2005: 9th IEEE International Symposium on High-Assurance Systems Engineering, pp. 99–108 (2005)
2. Associated Press: Insulin Pumps Vulnerable to Hacking, http://www.foxnews.com/tech/2011/08/04/insulin-pumps-vulnerable-to-hacking/
3. Ayoub, A., Chang, J., Sokolsky, O., Lee, I.: Assessing the Overall Sufficiency of Safety Arguments. In: SSS 2013: 21st Safety-critical Systems Symposium. LNCS. Springer (2013)
4. Bergenstal, R.M., Tamborlane, W.V., Ahmann, A., Buse, J.B., Dailey, G., Davis, S.N., Joyce, C., Peoples, T., Perkins, B.A., Welsh, J.B., et al.: Effectiveness of Sensor-augmented Insulin-pump Therapy in Type 1 Diabetes. New England Journal of Medicine 363(4), 311–320 (2010)
5. Black, P.E.: Samate and Evaluating Static Analysis Tools. Ada User Journal 28(3), 184–188 (2007)
6. Bloomfield, R., Bishop, P.: Safety and Assurance Cases: Past, Present and Possible Future–an Adelard Perspective. In: Making Systems Safer, pp. 51–67. Springer (2010)
7. Carollo, K.: Can Your Insulin Pump Be Hacked?, http://abcnews.go.com/blogs/health/2012/newline04/10/can-your-insulin-pump-be-hacked/

8. Dooren, J.C.: FDA Sees Increasing Number Of Insulin Pump Problems, http://online.wsj.com/article/SB10001424052748703862704575099961829258070.html

9. Eles, C., Lawford, M.: A Tabular Expression Toolbox for Matlab/Simulink. In: Bobaru, M., Havelund, K., Holzmann, G.J., Joshi, R. (eds.) NFM 2011. LNCS, vol. 6617, pp. 494–499. Springer, Heidelberg (2011)

10. FDA: Analysis of Premarket Review Times Under the 510(k) Program, http://www.fda.gov/AboutFDA/CentersOffices/OfficeofMedicalProductsandTobacco/CDRH/CDRHReports/ucm263385.htm

11. FDA: Use of Standards in Substantial Equivalence Determinations, http://www.fda.gov/MedicalDevices/DeviceRegulationandGuidance/GuidanceDocuments/ucm073752.htm

12. FDA: Guidance – General Principles of Software Validation (2002)

13. FDA: Guidance for the Content of Premarket Submissions for Software Contained in Medical Devices (2005)

14. FDA: Guidance – Total Product Life Cycle: Infusion Pump-Premarket Notification Submissions [510(k)] Submissions (2010)

15. Hatcliff, J., Heimdahl, M., Lawford, M., Maibaum, T., Wassyng, A., Wurden, F.: A software certification consortium and its top 9 hurdles. Electronic Notes in Theoretical Computer Science 238(4), 11–17 (2009)

16. Hawkins, R., Habli, I., Kelly, T., McDermid, J.: Assurance Cases and Prescriptive Software Safety Certification: A Comparative Study. Safety Science 59, 55–71 (2013)

17. Horowitz, B.T.: Cellnovo's Cloud System Monitors Diabetes in Real Time, http://www.eweek.com/c/a/Health-Care-IT/Cellnovos-Cloud-System-Monitors-Diabetes-in-Real-Time-520914/

18. International Electrotechnical Commission: IEC 62304: 2006 Medical Device Software–Software Life Cycle Processes (2006)

19. Klonoff, D.C., Paul, N.R., Kohno, T.: A Review of the Security of Insulin Pump Infusion Systems. Journal of Diabetes Science and Technology 5(6) (2011)

20. Leveson, N.: Engineering a Safer World: Applying Systems Thinking to Safety. MIT press (2012)

21. Maibaum, T., Wassyng, A.: A Product-Focused Approach to Software Certification. Computer 41(2), 91–93 (2008)

22. NRC: Guidance on Software Reviews for Digital Computer-Based Instrumentation and Control Systems, http://pbadupws.nrc.gov/docs/ML0525/ML052500547.pdf

23. Parnas, D.L.: On the Criteria to be Used in Decomposing Systems into Modules. Communications of the ACM 15(12), 1053–1058 (1972)

24. Parnas, D.L., Clements, P.C., Weiss, D.M.: The Modular Structure of Complex Systems. In: 7th International Conference on Software Engineering, pp. 408–417. IEEE (1984)

25. Parnas, D.L., Madey, J.: Functional documents for computer systems. Science of Computer programming 25(1), 41–61 (1995)

26. Potti, L.G., Haines, S.T.: Continuous subcutaneous insulin infusion therapy: a primer on insulin pumps. Journal of the American Pharmacists Association 49(1), e1–e17 (2009)

27. Raghunathan, A., Jha, N.K.: Hijacking an Insulin Pump: Security Attacks and Defenses for a Diabetes Therapy System. In: IEEE 13th International Conference on e-Health Networking, Applications and Services, pp. 150–156. IEEE (2011)

28. Siebert, C.: Diabetes control and complications trial (DCCT): Results of the feasibility study and design of the full-scale clinical trial. Controlled Clinical Trials 7 (1986)

29. Stribbell, J.: Model Based Design of a Generic Insulin Infusion Pump. M.Eng. Report, McMaster University (2013)

30. Sujan, M.-A., Koornneef, F., Voges, U.: Goal-Based Safety Cases for Medical Devices: Opportunities and Challenges. In: Saglietti, F., Oster, N. (eds.) SAFECOMP 2007. LNCS, vol. 4680, pp. 14–27. Springer, Heidelberg (2007)

31. Wassyng, A., Lawford, M.: Lessons Learned from a Successful Implementation of Formal Methods in an Industrial Project. In: Araki, K., Gnesi, S., Mandrioli, D. (eds.) FME 2003. LNCS, vol. 2805, pp. 133–153. Springer, Heidelberg (2003)

32. Wassyng, A., Maibaum, T., Lawford, M., Bherer, H.: Software Certification: Is There a Case against Safety Cases? In: Calinescu, R., Jackson, E. (eds.) Monterey Workshop 2010. LNCS, vol. 6662, pp. 206–227. Springer, Heidelberg (2011)

33. Weinstock, C.B., Goodenough, J.B.: Towards an Assurance Case Practice for Medical Devices. Tech. rep., DTIC Document (2009)

34. Zhang, Y., Jones, P.L., Klonoff, D.C.: Second insulin pump safety meeting: summary report. Journal of Diabetes Science and Technology 4(2), 488 (2010)

An Ontology for Regulating eHealth Interoperability in Developing African Countries

Deshendran Moodley[1], Christopher J. Seebregts[1,2],
Anban W. Pillay[1], and Thomas Meyer[1]

[1] UKZN/CSIR Meraka Centre for Artificial Intelligence Research and
Health Architecture Laboratory, School of Mathematics, Statistics and Computer Science,
University of KwaZulu-Natal, Durban, South Africa
[2] Jembi Health Systems NPC,
Cape Town and Durban, South Africa

Abstract. eHealth governance and regulation are necessary in low resource African countries to ensure effective and equitable use of health information technology and to realize national eHealth goals such as interoperability, adoption of standards and data integration. eHealth regulatory frameworks are under-developed in low resource settings, which hampers the progression towards coherent and effective national health information systems. Ontologies have the potential to clarify issues around interoperability and the effectiveness of different standards to deal with different aspects of interoperability. Ontologies can facilitate drafting, reusing, implementing and compliance testing of eHealth regulations. In this regard, we have developed an OWL ontology to capture key concepts and relations concerning interoperability and standards. The ontology includes an operational definition for interoperability and is an initial step towards the development of a knowledge representation modeling platform for eHealth regulation and governance.

Keywords: eHealth regulation, Interoperability, Standards.

1   Introduction

Health information technology and eHealth are increasingly being used in an effort to improve health service delivery in low and middle-income countries (LMICs) despite significant challenges, risk and limited proven benefits [3,6,24,25]. The need to improve interoperability [19] and the adoption of eHealth and interoperability standards in low resource settings have been identified as fundamental challenges to build coherent and sustainable national health information systems [13,9,33,1]. In these settings national health information systems are expected to evolve incrementally with systems maturing in line with available funding and regional priorities. The middle-out architecture approach proposed by Coeira [5] for developed countries also appears to be the most appropriate approach for developing countries [20]. The approach entails providing leadership, policies and regulations at the

J. Gibbons and W. MacCaull (Eds.): FHIES 2013, LNCS 8315, pp. 107–124, 2014.

national level, but delegating autonomy to provincial or regional levels for system selection, procurement, deployment and maintenance [20]. Health information exchanges, similar to the recent deployment in Rwanda [7,2], are essential to bridge the gap between disparate regional systems. For countries adopting a middle-out architecture approach, an effective governance framework and regulatory environment, including appropriate strategies, policies, guidelines and legal structures are central to the effective and equitable implementation and integration of health information systems within the country [16,27,32].

An effective regulatory environment and governance framework is also crucial to manage the complex relationships and dependencies between national government and the different stakeholders, including international donors, private sector, commercial software development organizations and non-governmental organisations. Such a framework must protect the rights, privacy and safety of patients and allow the national government to maintain control but must simultaneously promote innovation, open architectures and systems while discouraging closed technologies that result in vendor lock-in, whether proprietary or open source. eHealth regulations can provide a powerful legal mechanism to help developing countries encourage interoperability and harmonization of health information systems with a national computing platform that support common standards and data interchange formats.

The need for an overarching legal and regulatory framework for eHealth has recently been articulated by, among others, the Agenda for Action on Global E-Health [9,18], the World Health Assembly [33], the International Telecommunications Union [15], and the World Health Organization (WHO) together with the International Telecommunications Union (ITU) in their eHealth Strategy Toolkit [34]. Governments in developing countries such as South Africa, Ghana, Kenya, Uganda and Rwanda have responded to these calls and many now have eHealth strategies in place[1]. Most of these eHealth strategies identify the need for appropriate legal structures and an eHealth regulatory framework. However, the development of appropriate eHealth guidelines and regulations is still under-developed in sub-saharan Africa [12] and often limited to general provisions in the national health act supplemented with a few telecommunications regulations. Usually, there is little or no legal or regulatory framework specifically targeting eHealth or health information and HIS. Few other examples of eHealth regulations exist and examples from developed countries are not necessarily appropriate in low resource settings where the healthcare priorities, resourcing and capacity to adopt technology are often different [30].

The lack of appropriate governance has contributed to the uncoordinated implementation of electronic medical record systems and mobile phone pilot applications outside of the national HIS in several developing countries. To alleviate concerns regarding interoperability with existing public health systems and wastage of scarce government and donor resources some national governments have

---

[1] http://www.HingX.org/eHealthStrategy

established moratoria to curtail new implementations and/or have implemented eHealth-specific regulations to try and curtail this practice. Several developing countries in Africa have embarked on intiatives to develop national enterprise architectures, interoperability frameworks and related technologies [8,11,29,21,7] with several examples of interoperability guidelines and policy documents being developed at national level[2].

In recognition of this need, the WHO convened an international working group to develop guidelines aimed at improving data standardization and interoperability [35] and international standards organizations, e.g. HL7 and the International Standards Organization (ISO) have begun to consider ways to make standards more accessible in low resource countries. More recently, the WHO [33] and others, e.g. [1] have begun to research and develop guidelines for the selection of relevant standards that are appropriate in LMICs from among the plethora of overlapping standards that are available from a number of international standards development organizations. Regulations will play an important role in entrenching an agreed set of standards within a particular legislative domain.

In this paper, we present our initial eHealth governance ontology that focuses on interoperability and standards. The ontology aims to clarify core concepts in this domain and is part of a broader project to develop a knowledge representation and modeling platform for eHealth governance and regulation. The platform aims to facilitate greater coordination between government needs and eHealth implementations and to assist with drafting, refining, reusing, implementing and compliance testing of eHealth regulations and other instruments of eHealth governance.

2   Developing an Ontology for Regulating eHealth Interoperability

The ontology for regulating eHealth interoperability is envisaged as a core component of a modelling platform for facilitating the drafting of policies for the regulation of standards, assessing their impact on interoperability and allow for a better understanding of the choices of standards available. We have approached the development of the ontology from three usage viewpoints.

(i) Policy and Legal

Policies and legal instruments must be consistent with existing policies and laws as well as international best practice. Language needs to be harmonized and, in the case of technical regulations, such as those for interoperability and standards, sufficient technical detail is required to ensure that the provisions can be effectively implemented and enforced. The ontology should provide legislators with a clear understanding of the core technical issues and approaches around interoperability and the impact of regulations on the design and implementation of software systems.

---

[2] http://www.HingX.org/interoperability

(ii) *Regulation and Compliance*

The ontology should provide support for evaluating different vendor proposals during the software procurement process and determining compliance of final implementations. It should also support the evaluation of existing systems for compliance to standards and provide a clear upgrade path to mature systems to advanced levels of compliance.

(iii) *System and Software Development*

The ontology should allow for the translation of regulations into concrete technical software requirements that can feed into software design, development and deployment.

2.1 Ontology Design Approach

In order to clarify the issue of interoperability in the eHealth domain, we developed an OWL ontology of the key concepts and the relationships between them. Our focus was on eHealth regulations, systems and standards. Ontology development followed a middle out design [31], i.e. a combination of a bottom up and top down approach.

In developing the interoperability regulation ontology, we analysed a real world regulation from Brazil, viz. *Ordinance # 2.073/11 - GM: standards and interoperability* [4], as a case study to ground our ontology. This ordinance is one of five regulations pertaining to eHealth in Brazil. Other ministerial acts regulate the national health card system, the use of the national health number and funding for the development of interoperability solutions.

The ordinance deals specifically with interoperability and standards. In this work, we only considered the standards part of the ordinance. Table 1 shows English language extracts (direct translations from the Portuguese) from the ordinance as well as the concepts that refer to standards, to be modelled in the ontology. Even though it is clear that the intent is towards adopting specific standards to deal with certain aspects of interoperability, these aspects are not explicitly stated. In general interoperability is loosely used and not qualified. One exception is Section 4.3 where "semantic interoperability" is associated with the use of SNOMED-CT. It is not clear what types or levels of interoperability exist. Even though systems can be evaluated in terms of the standards which they implement, one cannot infer from this what level of interoperability they will support.

Higher level abstract concepts (top down) was informed by our previous work in designing interoperability solutions in developing African countries [7,19], the Interoperability Framework developed by the Australian National eHealth Transition Authority (NEHTA) [22], the European Commission report on ICT standards for health [17] and a recent survey on standards and interoperability of African health information systems [1].

Table 1. Example extracts dealing with eHealth Standards in the Brazilian eHealth Ordinance (translated from the Portuguese)

Ordinance # 2,073 of 31 August 2011 - TRANSLATED		
ANNEX		
Chapter I	Standard	Translated extract from CATALOG SERVICES
Article 1	SOAP	For **interoperability between systems** will be used the SUS Web Service technology, the standard SOAP 1.1 (Simple Object Access Protocol) or higher
CHAPTER II		
Section 4.1	OpenEHR	For the definition of the Electronic Health Record (EHR) will use the openEHR reference model
Section 4.2	HL7	To establish **interoperability between systems**, aiming at integrating the results of examinations and inquiries, we will use the standard HL7 - Health Level 7
Section 4.3	SNOMED-CT	In terms of clinical coding and mapping of national and international terminologies in use in the country, aiming **support semantic interoperability** between systems, will be used terminology SNOMED CT, available at http://www.ihtsdo. org / SNOMED-CT
Section 4.5	CDA	To define the clinical document architecture is used standard HL7 CDA
Section 4.6	DICOM	For information relating to representation of imaging will be used DICOM standard
Section 4.7	LOINC	For coding of laboratory tests will use the standard LOINC (Logical Observation Identifiers Names and Codes).
Section 4.9	ISO 13606-2	Towards **interoperability of knowledge models**, including archetypes, templates and management methodology, we will use the standard ISO 13606-2.
Section 4.10	IHE-PIX	To the intersection of identifiers of patients of different information systems, will be used to specify integration IHE-PIX (Patient Identifier Cross-Referencing).

3   An Ontology for eHealth Interoperability: Regulations, Systems and Standards

This section describes the key concepts, relations and modeling decisions taken when developing the ontology. The ontology is represented in OWL and was developed using the Protégé software tool.

3.1   Overview of the Ontology

Figure 1 shows the high level concepts and relations between regulations, the health system and software. Each country has a health system, e.g. the Brazilian Health System, which provides health services and which, in turn, are supported by one or more health software system services. This distinction between health service and software service is important in the health domain as there is often confusion between the service from the health perspective and the service from the computer system (IT) perspective. Furthermore, different health services may deal with different data elements, which use different data standards, e.g. a lab service may use LOINC, while a radiology service may use DICOM (see Sections 4.6 and 4.7 in Table 1).

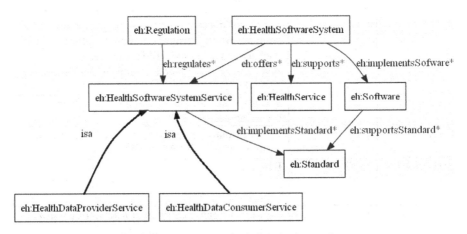

Fig. 1. Key concepts and relations in the ontology

A health software system supports one or more software system services, regulated by one or more regulations. Since the current focus is on interoperability and health data exchange, we broadly categorize services as being either data provisioning or data consuming. Other types of services may be added to the ontology in future. A health software system service implements one or more eHealth standards. We are more concerned with the interaction between services rather than the internal data model of the software system. This allows for wrapping legacy systems with a standards compliant service interface, without having to completely re-engineer the legacy system.

3.2   Interoperability

In broad terms, we define interoperability as the ability of a sub-system to effectively interact with other sub-systems. Classification or levels of interoperability are usually linked to the types of heterogeneity that exists between systems. From a Computer Science perspective, early classifications differentiated between system, syntactic, structural and semantic interoperability [28]. As systems evolved toward open systems, and technologies that adequately deal with lower levels, e.g. XML and web-services, mature and are more pervasive, new levels of interoperability are being identified and older levels no longer prove challenging. A more recent classification suggests differentiating between syntactic, semantic, pragmatic and social world interoperability [26]. An investigation into interoperability issues specific to health information systems [10] identified three levels of interoperability, i.e. technical, semantic and process. A recent survey on interoperability and standards in African HIS can be found in [1]. What is clear is that multiple types of interoperability exist and even though specific types of heterogeneity have been emphasized in the health domain, there is still no consensus on the types of interoperability.

Drawing from our experience in developing architectures to facilitate interoperability in low resource settings [7,19] and the pragmatic approach taken in Australia's NEHTA Interoperability Framework [22] we note three pragmatic characteristics concerning interoperability:

- *Allow for different perspectives for different systems and settings*: Depending on the nature and maturity of the eHealth system, different countries will have different requirements and types of interactions between health software services. As such, countries will have their own interpretation of interoperability, which may differ.
- *Dynamic*: A country's health information system continuously evolves to increasing levels of maturity. New subsystems will appear, functionality will change and increase and new versions of data exchange and standards will be adopted to support improved interactions. Different subsystems will be at different levels of maturity and it is naive to assume that the system will ever reach a complete level of stasis. The degree of interoperability of a sub-system, in terms of its interaction with other sub-systems, is fundamentally affected by this dynamism.
- *Measurable along a continuum*: interoperability should be considered as a measure along a continuum, i.e. different sub systems could have different degrees of interoperability. Each country will define its own measures and levels and allow

for evolution of these as their health information system evolves and matures. This is similar to the five interoperability maturity levels identified in the Australian NEHTA Interoperability Framework [22, 23].

We use the concept "CompliantHSS" to allow for custom definitions of compliance for software services. The current compliancy types represent different levels of interoperability. For illustration, we define five interoperability levels in the ontology, i.e. technical, syntactic, partially semantic, semantic and organization (adapted from the 4 levels in [1]). We split semantic into partially semantic, i.e. the service has some support to enable semantic interoperability, but cannot be said to be fully semantically interoperable. The levels are incremental, e.g. any service that is semantically interoperable is also syntactically and technically interoperable. As such technical interoperability is modeled as the superclass of syntactic interoperability, which is a superclass of semantic interoperability, which in turn is a superclass of organization interoperability (Figure 2). Our approach measures the level of interoperability of a service based on which data exchange standards are implemented by a software service.

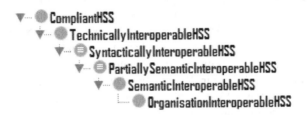

Fig. 2. Interoperability levels of software services

The five levels of interoperability defined above are used to illustrate compliance, but a country may define their own levels and these can differ between countries.

3.3   Standards

The level of interoperability of a software system is determined by the standards implemented by the service interfaces that it exposes. A standard is managed by a standards organization and follows different processes for its development. The definition is shown in figure 3.

Different categories of eHealth standards have been modeled. Categories have been adapted from a European Commission report on ICT standards in the health sector [17, page 15, exhibit 2-1]. The report identifies seven categories of eHealth standards. Table 2 shows these categories and their mappings to concepts in the ontology, and the class hierarchy and sample instances are shown in figure 4.

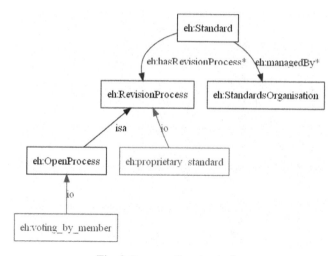

Fig. 3. Representing standards

Table 2. Categories of standards and equivalent concepts in the ontology (instances in bold are examples from the Brazilian Ordinance)

Standard category [17]	Equivalent concept in ontology	Example instances
Architecture	eHealthArchitectureStandards (expanded)	***OpenEHR, DICOM, ISO13606-2, IHE-PIX*** HL7
Modeling	ModelingStandard	CEN TR 15300 Framework for Formal Modelling of Healthcare policies ISO 10746 ODP
Communication	CommunicationStandard (expanded)	SOAP1.1, XML
Infrastructure	InfrastructureStandard	***GeneralSOA*** CanadaHealthInfoWay ESB, OpenHIM
Data security	DataSecurityStandard	WSSecurity
Safety	SafetyStandard	CEN TR 13694 Safety and Security Related Software Quality Standards for Healthcare
Terminology and ontology	TerminologyAndOntologyStandard	***CID, LOINC, SNOMED-CT***

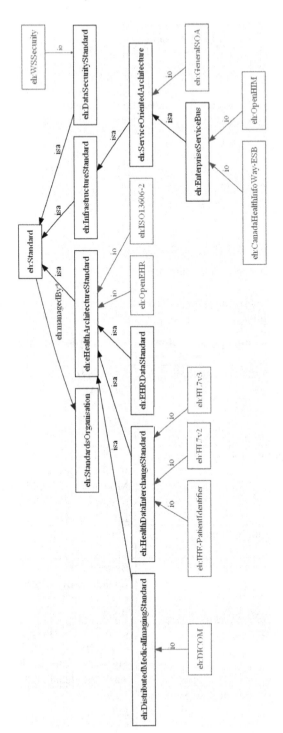

Fig. 4. Categories (types) and instances of standards

Table 3. Categorization of standards and mappings to levels of interoperability [1]

Standard	Interoperability level			
	technical	syntactic	semantic	organizational
Identifiers				
ISO/TS 22220:2011		X	X	
ISO/TS 27527:2010		X	X	X
Messaging / information exchange				
HL7 V2.X		X	X	
HL7 V3		X	X	
DICOM		X	X	
SDMX-HD		X		
Structure and content				
ASTM E2369-12		X	X	
HL7 CDA		X	X	
HL7/ASTM CCD		X	X	
HL7 CRS		X	X	
ISO 21090		X	X	
Clinical terminology and coding				
SNOMED		X	X	
LOINC		X	X	
ICD		X	X	
ICPC-2		X	X	
CPT		X	X	
Electronic health record				
ISO 18308:2011		X	X	X
System functional models				
HL7 EHR-System Functional Model, Release 1.1	X	X	X	X
Security and access control				
ISO/TS 22600				X

The ontology can support alternate and even multiple categorizations of standards and interoperability. For example a recent mapping between eHealth standards and levels of interoperability [1] (see Table 3) can be easily modelled in the ontology.

3.4   Knowledge Representation, Reasoning and Compliance Checking

A further benefit of the ontology, in addition to the consistent and explicit definition of concepts such as interoperability, is the ability to use algorithms for reasoning over ontologies to assist in matters such as compliance testing. More precisely, given an ontology that specifies different levels of compliance in a particular country, such algorithms (amongst other functions) can be used to:

- check whether a given health service meets a specific level of compliance;
- explain why a given health service does or does not meet that level of compliance;
- suggest measures for meeting that level of compliance, if it does not.

As an example, suppose that we have three levels of compliance for health software system services (HSS):

1. We define a service that is *syntactically interoperable* to be associated with the implementation of at least one syntactic interoperability standards, e.g. HL7v2 or HL7v3
2. We define a service that is *partially semantic interoperable* to be associated with the implementation of at least one semantic interoperability standard e.g. HL7v3 which supports the use of clinical terminologies and coding systems.
3. We define a service that is *semantically interoperable* to be associated with the implementation of the HL7v3 standard, as well as the medical ontology standard SNOMED CT.

The following statements, represented in the Manchester OWL Syntax for the Web Ontology Language OWL 2 (http://www.w3.org/TR/owl2-manchester-syntax/), represent a syntactically interoperable HSS (1), by defining the class `SyntacticInteroperableHSS` as:

```
Class: SyntacticInteroperableHSS
    EquivalentTo:
            HealthSoftwareSystemService and
            implementsStandard some
            SyntacticInteroperabilityStandard
```

Now, suppose we are told that X and Y are health software system services, and that X implements HL7v2 (we are not told whether or not Y implements some standard)

```
Individual: HL7v2
    Types: SyntacticInteroperabilityStandard

Individual: HL7v3
    Types: SyntacticInteroperabilityStandard

Individual: X
    Types: HealthSoftwareSystemService
    Facts: implementStandard HL7v2

Individual: Y
    Types: HealthSoftwareSystemService
```

A reasoning algorithm would then be able to give us the following information:

- X complies with a syntactic compliance level and since it is a health software systems service, it is therefore also a syntactic health software system service.
- We don't know if Y complies with a syntactic compliance level. But we know that if Y is made to implement either HL7v2 or HL7v3, it would become a syntactic health software system service.

The notions of partial semantic interoperability can similarly be represented in OWL 2. However, semantic interoperability is a little more complex as it can be achieved by implementing two standards and is defined as:

```
Class: SemanticallyInteroperableHSS
EquivalentTo:
    HealthSoftwareSystemService  and  (implementsStandard
    some  SemanticInteroperabilityStandard  or  (imple-
    mentsStandard  value  HL7v3  and  implementsStandard
    value SNOMEDCT))
```

Another example is to query for syntactically interoperable standards that are open:

```
SyntacticInteroperabilityStandard  and  hasRevisionProcess
some OpenProcess
```

Consider the ontology fragment in figure 5 below that represents software platforms. Two widely used software platforms OpenMRS and DHIS are shown as instances of EMR and health management information system software respectively. OpenMRS supports both the HL7 version 2 and version 3 standards.

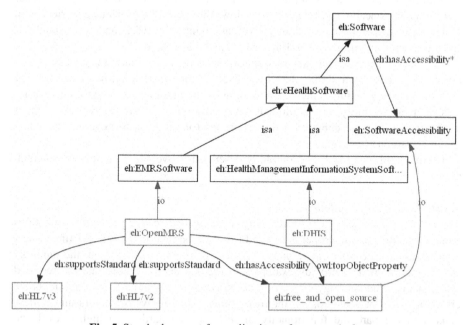

Fig. 5. Standard support for application software or platforms

Now suppose that we wanted to find all EMR software platforms that provides supports for partial or full semantic interoperability then:

EMRSoftware and supportsStandard some (PartialSemanticIn-
teroperabilityStandard   or   SemanticInteroperabilityStan-
dard)

will return OpenMRS since it supports HL7v3 which is an instance of PartialSe-
manticInteroperabilityStandard.

Similarly a query to find only those platforms that are free and open source:

EMRSoftware and supportsStandard some (PartialSemanticIn-
teroperabilityStandard   or   SemanticInteroperabilityStan-
dard) and (hasAccessibility value free_and_open_source)

will also return OpenMRS.

4   Discussion

We developed an initial ontology to regulate eHealth interoperability and standards.
The design was informed by both a bottom up approach, by analyzing real world
eHealth regulations in a developing country, in this case Brazil and modeling higher
level abstract concepts and relations (top down) informed by previous experiences in
designing interoperability solutions in African countries [7,19,1] and other standards
and interoperability initiatives in Europe [17] and Australia [22].

The ontology provides an abstract conceptual model containing the necessary pri-
mitives for a country to define their own levels of interoperability. It is expected that
each country will maintain their own version of the ontology, defining their own levels of interoperability, and additional categorization of standards. However, upper
level concepts will be common across countries (ontologies), to facilitate reuse and
sharing between countries.

The modeling approach and ontology described above has a number of potential
uses.

Assist with drafting regulations
The ontology can assist with developing, refining and re-using eHealth regulations
around standards and interoperability and may also be used to analyze existing or new
regulations in order to identify gaps and areas of overlap. In addition, the ontology
can be interrogated to provide examples of regulations to demonstrate the required
functionality. The ontology provides a categorisation of standards and highlights the
effect of different standards on interoperability. This allows regulators and policymakers to compare the functionality of different standards at a higher level and
evaluate the level of functionality and compliance required.

Bridge the gap between regulators and policy makers and software developers.
The ontology provides a more rigorous specification of regulated functionality which
can potentially be converted directly into system specifications. Regulators and

software developers can agree on a common interpretation of interoperability and compliance to standards, resulting in more pragmatic regulations which balance patient and national health interests with pragmatic software design, development and deployment concerns.

Compliance and evaluation of software
The ontology will be useful for testing compliancy to eHealth interoperability regulations and for developing specifications for compliance testing. Existing systems and new software products can be objectively evaluated and developed to fulfill interoperability requirements. As described in section 3.4 the model can be used to automatically measure the interoperability of software systems and to identify paths for improving the interoperability of sub-systems

Contribute to the evolution of standards
The usage of standards can be evaluated in terms of its tangible benefit in enabling aspects of interoperability, identification of gaps to develop new standards or to enhance existing ones for specific settings and provides a more meaningful discussion on adoption and promotion of standards

Measuring Interoperability
The ontology and future models will assist national governments and regulators in low resource settings to control and strengthen their national Health Information Technology infrastructure in a more positive way. Although moratoria are effective at limiting the explosion of eHealth application variability, the ideal situation would likely be to regulate the industry at the level of the standards and functionality (eg interoperability) that systems are expected to achieve in order to be considered part of the national system and then leave it up to market forces to determine which applications are deployed in-country. This will potentially allow poor facilities to make use of low-cost systems and more top-end facilities to support applications with richer functionality to support their needs.

5   Conclusion and Future work

The ontology and conceptual model presented in this paper aim to provide a common interpretation and to bring clarity to the issue of interoperability in national health information systems. The ontology is a first step towards a broader knowledge representation and modeling platform for eHealth governance and regulation. Such a platform can facilitate greater coordination between government needs and eHealth implementations and to assist with drafting, refining, reusing, implementing and compliance testing of eHealth regulations and other instruments of eHealth governance.

We plan to test the ontology in the field by making it available for use in other African countries that are currently in the process of developing and applying eHealth regulations and, e.g. in Rwanda where an initial version of an health information exchange [7] has been deployed to facilitate interoperability between individual HIS and applications. Feedback from these processes will allow us to refine the current model.

There are many possible directions for further extension of the ontology. The ontology can be extended by incorporating existing legal ontologies such as LKIF [14] to capture other richer aspects of regulations, e.g. their intent and consequences.

The current ontology and case study deals specifically with interoperability as an example of a software system concern and its relationship to governance and regulations. The ontology can be expanded to incorporate regulations that deal with other eHealth system concerns such as information security, data access, patient identifiers, patient confidentiality and privacy.

Acknowledgements. This work originates from a study on regulatory aspects commissioned by the European Space Agency (ESA) and its Telemedicine Task Force (TTF) with sponsorship from Luxembourg Development (LuxDev) and the Government of Luxembourg (http://iap.esa.int/projects/health/ehsa). The authors acknowledge productive discussions with Mr Gonzalo Martín-de-Mercado and Prof Alexander Horsch (ESA), Sean Broomhead and Tom Jones (Greenfield Management Solutions), Carl Fourie and Daniel Futerman (Jembi Health Systems).

The Health Architecture Laboratory (HeAL) at the University of KwaZulu-Natal is funded by grants from the Rockefeller Foundation (Establishing a Health Enterprise Architecture Lab, a research laboratory focused on the application of enterprise architecture and health informatics to resource-limited settings, Grant Number: 2010 THS 347) and the International Development Research Centre (IDRC) (Health Enterprise Architecture Laboratory (HeAL), Grant Number: 106452-001).

References

1. Adebesin, F., Foster, R., Kotzé, P., Van Greunen, D.: A review of interoperability standards in e-Health and imperatives for their adoption in Africa. South African Computer Journal 50, 55–72 (2013)
2. Biondich, P., Grannis, S., Seebregts, C.J.: Open Health Information Ex-change (OpenHIE): An International Open-Source Initiative in Support of Large Scale Data Interoperability for the Underserved. In: American Medical Informatics Association Annual Symposium (accepted 2013)
3. Black, D., et al.: The Impact of eHealth on the Quality and Safety of Health Care: A Systematic Overview. PLoS Med. 8(1), e1000387 (2011)
4. Brazil Ministry of Health. ORDINANCE No 2073 of August 31, 2011. Brazil Ministry of Health (2011),
   http://www.brasilsus.com.br/legislacoes/gm/109456-2073.html
5. Coiera, E.: Building a National Health IT System from the Middle Out. Journal of the American Medical Informatics Association 16(3), 271–273 (2009)
6. Coiera, E., Aarts, J., Kulikowski, C.: The dangerous decade. Journal of the American Medical Informatics Association 19(1), 2–5 (2012)

7. Crichton, R., Moodley, D., Pillay, A., Gakuba, R., Seebregts, C.J.: An Architecture and Reference Implementation of an Open Health Information Mediator: Enabling Interoperability in the Rwandan Health Information Exchange. In: Weber, J., Perseil, I. (eds.) FHIES 2012. LNCS, vol. 7789, pp. 87–104. Springer, Heidelberg (2013)
8. eGhana Enterprise Architecture Project, Ghana Health Service Enterprise Architecture (The eHealth Architecture). Deliverable of the eGhana Enterprise Architecture Project (2009),http://wiki.healthmetricsnetwork.info/wiki-kigali/lib/exe/fetch.php?media=ghs_enterprise_architecture_final_vs.2.pdf
9. Gerber, T., Olazabal, V., Brown, K., Pablos-Mendez, A.: An Agenda for Action on Global E-Health. Health Affairs 29(2), 233–236 (2010)
10. Gibbons, P., Arzt, N., Burke-Beebe, S., Chute, C., Dickinson, G., Flewelling, T., Stanford, J.: Coming to terms: Scoping interoperability for health care. HL7 HER Interoperability Working Group White Paper (2007), http://www.hln.com/assets/pdf/Coming-to-Terms-February-2007.pdf
11. Government Information Technology Officer's Council (GITOC) of South Africa, 'Government-Wide Enterprise Architecture (GWEA) Framework: Implementation Guide.Rev 1.2'. eGWEA-00002. GITOC Standing Committee on Architecture. (2010), http://www.gissa.org.za
12. Greenfield Management Solutions, Satellite-Enhanced Telemedicine and eHealth for Sub-Saharan Africa (eHSA) Programme Study on Regulatory Aspects: Summary Report (2013), http://www.greenfield.org.za/downloads/eHSA%20Reg%20Study%20Summary%20Report.pdf
13. Hammond, W.E.: The role of standards in creating a health information infrastructure. International Journal of Bio-Medical Computing 34(1-4), 29–44 (1994)
14. Hoekstra, R., Breuker, J., Di Bello, M., Boer, E.: The LKIF Core Ontology of Basic Legal Concepts. In: Casanovas, et al. (eds.) Proceedings of the Workshop on Legal Ontologies and Artificial Intelligence Techniques (2007)
15. International Telecommunication Union, 'Implementing e-Health in De-veloping Countries: Guidance and Principles.' ITU (2008), http://www.itu.int/ITU-D/cyb/app/docs/e-Health_prefinal_15092008.PDF
16. Khoja, S., Durrani, H., Nayani, P., Fahim, A.: Scope of Policy Issues in eHealth: Results From a Structured Literature Review. Journal of Medical Internet Research 14(1), e34 (2012)
17. Lilischkis, S., Austen, T., Jung, B., Stroetmann, V.: ICT standards in the health sector: current situation and prospects. A Sectoral e-Business Watch Study. European Commission, DG Enterprise & Industry. Special Study 1:2008 (2008), http://www.empirica.com/themen/ebusiness/documents/Special-study_01-2008_ICT_health_standards.pdf
18. Mars, M., Scott, R.E.: Global E-Health Policy: A Work In Progress. Health Affairs 29(2), 237–243 (2010)
19. Moodley, D., Pillay, A.W., Seebregts, C.J.: Position Paper: Researching and Developing Open Architectures for National Health Information Systems in Developing African Countries. In: Liu, Z., Wassyng, A. (eds.) FHIES 2011. LNCS, vol. 7151, pp. 129–139. Springer, Heidelberg (2012)
20. Mudaly, T., Moodley, D., Seebregts, C.J., Pillay, A.: Architectural Frameworks for Developing National Health Information Systems in Low and Middle Income Countries. In: The First International Conference on Enterprise Systems (ES 2013), Cape Town, South Africa, November 7-8 (to appear in 2013)

21. Mwanyika, H., et al.: Rational Systems Design for Health information Systems in Low-Income Countries: An Enterprise Architecture Approach. Journal of Enterprise Architecture 7(4), 60–69 (2011)
22. National E-Health Transition Authority, NEHTA Interoperability Framework, version 2.0. National E-Health Transition Authority Ltd. NEHTA-1146:2007 (2007), http://www.nehta.gov.au/implementation-resources/ehealth-foundations/EP-1144-2007
23. National E-Health Transition Authority, 'NEHTA Maturity Model version 1.0'. National E-Health Transition Authority Ltd. NEHTA-0062:2007 (2007b), http://www.nehta.gov.au/implementation-resources/ehealth-foundations/EP-1143-2006/NEHTA-0062-2007
24. Noormohammad, S.F., et al.: Changing course to make clinical decision support work in an HIV clinic in Kenya. International Journal of Medical Informatics 79(3), 204–210 (2010)
25. Oluoch, T., et al.: The effect of electronic medical record-based clinical decision support on HIV care in resource-constrained settings: A systematic review. International Journal of Medical Informatics 81(10), e83–e92 (2012)
26. Ouksel, A.M., Sheth, A.: Semantic interoperability in global information systems. ACM Sigmod Record 28(1), 5–12 (1999)
27. Scott, R.E., Jennet, P.: Access and authorization in a Global e-Health Policy context. International Journal of Medical Informatics 73(3), 259–266 (2004)
28. Sheth, A.P.: Changing focus on interoperability in information systems: from system, syntax, structure to semantics. In: Interoperating Geographic Information Systems, pp. 5–29. Springer US (1999)
29. Shvaiko, P., Villafiorita, A., Zorer, A., Chemane, L., Fumo, T., Hinkkanen, J.: eGIF4M: eGovernment Interoperability Framework for Mozambique. In: Wimmer, M.A., Scholl, H.J., Janssen, M., Traunmüller, R. (eds.) EGOV 2009. LNCS, vol. 5693, pp. 328–340. Springer, Heidelberg (2009)
30. Stroetmann, K.A., Artmann, J., Dumortier, J., Verhenneman, G.: United in Diversity: Legal Challenges on the Road Towards Interoperable eHealth Solutions in Europe. European Journal for Biomedical Informatics 8(2), 3–10 (2012)
31. Uschold, M., Gruninger, M.: Ontologies: Principles, Methods and Applications. Knowledge Engineering Review 11(2) (1996)
32. World Health Organization. International Health Regulations. 2nd edn. WHO (2005), http://www.who.int/ihr/9789241596664/en/index.html
33. World Health Organisation, Resolution of the World Health Assembly WHA58.28 eHealth. WHO (2005), http://www.who.int/healthacademy/media/WHA58-28-en.pdf
34. World Health Organization and International Telecommunication Union, 'National eHealth Strategy Toolkit'. WHO & ITU (2012), http://www.itu.int/dms_pub/itu-d/opb/str/D-STR-E_HEALTH.05-2012-PDF-E.pdf
35. World Health Organization, eHealth standardization and interoperability: Agenda item 10.5, WHO 132nd session: EB132.R8. WHO (2013), http://apps.who.int/gb/ebwha/pdf_files/EB132/B132_R8-en.pdf

Use of XML Schema Definition for the Development of Semantically Interoperable Healthcare Applications

Luciana Tricai Cavalini[1] and Timothy Wayne Cook[2]

[1] Department of Health Information Technology, Medical Sciences College,
Rio de Janeiro State University, Brazil
[2] National Institute of Science and Technology –
Medicine Assisted by Scientific Computing, Brazil
`lutricav@lampada.uerj.br, tim@mlhim.org`

Abstract. Multilevel modeling has been proven in software as a viable solution for semantic interoperability, without imposing any specific programming languages or persistence models. The Multilevel Healthcare Information Modeling (MLHIM) specifications have adopted the XML Schema Definition 1.1 as the basis for its reference implementation, since XML technologies are consistent across all platforms and operating systems, with tools available for all mainstream programming languages. In MLHIM, the healthcare knowledge representation is defined by the Domain Model, expressed as Concept Constraint Definitions (CCDs), which provide the semantic interpretation of the objects persisted according to the generic Reference Model classes. This paper reports the implementation of the MLHIM Reference Model in XML Schema Definition language version 1.1 as well as a set of examples of CCDs generated from the National Cancer Institute – Common Data Elements (NCI CDE) repository. The set of CCDs was the base for the simulation of semantically coherent data instances, according to independent XML validators, persisted on an eXistDB database. This paper shows the feasibility of adopting XML technologies for the achievement of semantic interoperability in real healthcare scenarios, by providing application developers with a significant amount of industry experience and a wide array of tools through XML technologies.

Keywords: semantic interoperability, electronic health records, multilevel modeling.

1 Introduction

The implementation of electronic health records has been proposed to increase the effectiveness of healthcare, but the expectations in this field are yet to be met. Since 1961, when the first computerized health record system was installed at the Akron General Hospital [1], and over the more than 50 years since that time, software companies of all types have sought the ability to integrate various systems in order to provide a coherent healthcare information platform [2] [3].

J. Gibbons and W. MacCaull (Eds.): FHIES 2013, LNCS 8315, pp. 125–145, 2014.
© Springer-Verlag Berlin Heidelberg 2014

The challenges related to recording clinical information in computer applications are primarily associated to the fact that healthcare is a complex and dynamic environment. Regarding complexity, it is known, for instance, that the Systematized Nomenclature of Medicine – Clinical Terms (SNOMED-CT), the most comprehensive terminology for healthcare, has more than 311,000 terms, connected by more than 1,360,000 links [4]. The dynamism observed in healthcare information is essentially related to the speed of scientific evolution and technology incorporation, which is a main feature of the field [5] [6].

Furthermore, the healthcare system is by definition hierarchical and decentralized; thus, it is expected that the patients will access the system through primary care settings and then ascend to higher complexity levels of care [7]. For historical and economic reasons, primary care settings are located closer to the user's household, while more complex healthcare institutions (such as hospitals) are usually built in central areas [8]. The functions of primary care and hospitals are clearly different, which determines a high level of variability regarding their architectural format and structure and, in consequence, each healthcare institution will adopt specific workflows that are adapted to its form and function [9]. This process will reflect on the specificity of information collected, stored and processed inside a given facility [10].

However, no healthcare institution is isolated from the others. Because of the configuration of the healthcare system, patients circulate across more than one setting [11]. This is particularly true of patients with chronic conditions that see more than 80 different physicians in the course of their disease [12]. Thus, ideally, every patient's record should be kept longitudinal, since any piece of information might be important at any moment of the patient's life [13].

The achievement of such levels of interoperability between electronic health records still remains as a challenge [14] [15]. Currently, there is a multiplicity of companies and governmental institutions whose mission is to develop healthcare applications, each one of them implementing its own data model, which is specific for that application [16] [17]. Such data models are not only different from system to system, but they are also ever changing as the scope of the applications change, which includes the continuous changes in medical science, insurance company regulations and government policies [18] [19].

This constant change is a costly component of managing healthcare information [20] and creates a situation in which much of the semantic context of the healthcare data is embedded into the structure of the database, as well as in the programming language source code. Thus, when sharing data between healthcare applications is attempted, even in the simplest situation (when the data types are the same), the complete context in which the data was recorded remains unknown to the receiving system. This happens due to the fact that the semantics are locked up in the database structure and the source code of the application [21].

Many solutions have been proposed to the problem of interoperability in healthcare information systems, which include a vast and variable set of knowledge representation models, especially terminologies and ontologies [22] [23]. Nevertheless, the high implementation and maintenance costs of the available electronic health records have slowed down their widespread implementation; even some throwbacks have been observed over the last years [24] [25]. Until this date, the only development method that has achieved semantic interoperability is the multi (or dual)-level modeling approach originally proposed by the *open*EHR Foundation [26] and evolved by two projects based on the same principles: the ISO 13606 family of standards [27] and the Multilevel Healthcare Information Modeling (MLHIM) specifications [28].

Although the ability to achieve semantic interoperability between electronic health records has been already proven in multilevel modeling-based software [29], there are relatively few known implementations of the *open*EHR specifications or the ISO 13606 standards. This can be attributed to the complexity of the *open*EHR specifications [30] or to the fact that the ISO 13606 standard does not provide for data persistence, but only message exchange between systems [31].

Another significant barrier to the wider adoption of the multilevel modeling principles, as implemented in *open*EHR and ISO 13606, is the use of a domain-specific language, the Archetype Definition Language (ADL), for defining the data models. In both approaches, ADL was adopted for the definition of constraints to the information model (known as Reference Model) classes, for each healthcare concept [27]. Some authors have expressed their concerns about the technical barriers of using ADL for the widespread development of applications to run on real healthcare settings, when concepts will have a high level of complexity [32] [33].

Given the fact that semantic interoperability is such a key issue for the successful adoption of information technologies in healthcare, and multilevel modeling is a solution for it, there is a need for making such principles implementable in real life applications. This was achieved in the MLHIM specification by adopting XML technologies for its implementation, which are an industry standard for software development [34] and information exchange. This paper presents the development of a demo application based on version 2.4.2 of the MLHIM specifications.

2   Method

The methodological approach adopted in this study included: (a) the implementation of the basic components of the MLHIM specifications (the Reference Model and the Domain Models) in XML Schema 1.1; (b) the generation of simulated data based on a set of selected Domain Models for demographic and clinical concepts and (c) the demonstration of persistence and querying procedures implemented in two demo applications, using the simulated data produced.

2.1   Overview of the MLHIM Specifications

The MLHIM specifications are published (https://github.com/mlhim) as a suite of open source tools for the development of electronic health records and other types of healthcare applications, according to the principles of multilevel modeling. The specifications are structured in two Models: the Reference Model and the Domain Model.

The conceptual MLHIM Reference Model is composed of a set of classes (and their respective attributes) that allow the development of any type of healthcare application, from hospital-based electronic medical records to small purpose-specific applications that collect data on mobile devices. This was achieved by minimizing the number and the residual semantics of the Reference Model classes, when compared to the original *open*EHR specifications. The remaining classes and semantics were regarded as *necessary and sufficient* to allow any modality of structured data persistence. Therefore, the MLHIM Reference Model approach is minimalistic [34], but not as abstract as a programming language.

The reference implementation of the MLHIM Reference Model is expressed in a XML Schema 1.1 document. Each of the classes from the Reference Model are expressed as a complexType definition, arranged as 'xs:extension' [34]. For each complexType there is also an 'element' definition. These elements are arranged into Substitution Groups in order to assist with the concept of class inheritance defined in the conceptual Reference Model.

The MLHIM Domain Model is defined by the Concept Constraint Definitions (CCDs), expressed in XML Schema 1.1, being conceptually equivalent to the *open*EHR and ISO 13606 archetypes. Each CCD defines the combination and restriction of classes and class attributes of the (generic and stable) MLHIM Reference Model that are *necessary and sufficient* to properly represent a given healthcare concept. In general, CCDs are set to allow wide reuse, but there is no limitation for the number of CCDs allowed for a single concept in the MLHIM ecosystem. Each CCD is identified by a Type 4 Universal Unique Identifier (UUID) [28]. This provides permanence to the concept definition for all time, thus creating a stable foundation for instance data established in the temporal, spatial and ontological contexts of the point of recording. This is a very important concept, in order to preserve the original semantics at the time of data capture so that any future analytics will not be skewed into unknown directions. This is a common problem when data is migrated from one database format to another and source code in the application is modified [35]. Since this is where the semantics exist in typical applications, the data no longer represents those semantics after such a migration.

The key innovation in the MLHIM specifications is the use of complexType definitions in the CCD based on restrictions of the Reference Model types. Giving the fact that the majority of medical concepts are multivariate, for the majority of CCDs, a n ($n > 0$) number of complexTypes will be included. For instance, since it is likely to have a CCD with more than one complexType, each one of them will be also associated to a Type 4 UUID, which is similar to the complete CCD identification process described above [28]. This allows the existence of multiple complexTypes of the same nature (for instance, a CCD may have more than one ClusterType or more than one DvStringType) in the same CCD without a conflict of the restrictions. This approach also enables data query, since it creates a universally unique path statement to any specific MLHIM based data.

CCDs have the capability to accommodate any number of medical ontologies and terminologies [27]. All complexTypes may include links as computable application information ('xs:appinfo'), which can be used to include any amount of specific semantics by linking into any ontology or terminology. These are created as part of the CCD in an 'annotation' element and allow the inclusion of Resource Description Framework (RDF) content for further improvement of the concept's semantics, based on any relevant ontology.

The second key innovation is in the approach in handling missing data or data that is outside the expected range or type. This is not an uncommon occurrence in health-care applications. All data types in MLHIM (descendants of DvAny) carry an 'ev' element for exceptional value semantics [36]. This approach is similar to what ISO 21090 calls Null Flavours. However, the approach in ISO 21090 is brittle and does not allow for expansion, creating the probability for missing, incomplete or incorrect missing data semantics. MLHIM solves this issue by providing a tree based on the 'ev-meaning' and 'ev-name' elements of the ExceptionalValue complexType, being the values for these elements fixed for each complexType.

For example, with the INVType; 'ev-name' is "Invalid" and 'ev-meaning' is "The value as represented in the instance is not a member of the set of permitted data values in the constrained value domain of a variable"; which are taken from ISO 21090. An example of an extension to ISO 21090 is the ASKRType, representing the prevalent (yet underreported) "Asked But Refused" value. Thus, in addition to the extensions for exceptional values in the Reference Model, any CCD can extend the ExceptionalValue complexType to create context specific missing or exceptional value data semantics with no loss of interoperability.

It is important to note that the MLHIM specifications are concerned with semantic interoperability of all biomedical applications. This means that many application development requirements that are specific to any particular type of application are not included. This includes very important concepts such as; how to persist CCDs in meaningful and useful ways, authentication and authorization, Application Programming Interfaces (APIs) and query processing. These are all outside the scope of the MLHIM specifications. These other requirements are well defined in other industry specifications and standards, and attempts to include them inside MLHIM would only serve to confuse the core issue of semantic interoperability.

2.2   Description of the MLHIM Reference Model

The implementation of the MLHIM Reference Model version 2.4.2 was produced as a single XML Schema Definition (XSD) file according to the XML W3C standards version 1.1 (source code available at https://github.com/mlhim/specs). The implementation approach in XML was based on extensions and substitutions, in order to maintain the hierarchical structure of the conceptual model.

The MLHIM Reference Model data types are defined as the Datatypes package and are originally based on ISO 21090 with modifications to reduce unnecessary complexity and semantic dependency. For any Element of a CCD, the 'Element-dv' attribute must be constrained to one of the concrete complexTypes of this package.

The ordered data types from the MLHIM specifications comprise any type of data whose instances can be ordered; such are all complexTypes under the abstract DvOrdered complexType. The DvOrdered children complexType allow the persistence of ordinal values such as ranks and scores (DvOrdinal), dates and times (DvTemporal) and true numbers (all complexTypes under DvQuantified) (Table 1).

Table 1. MLHIM Reference Model: Ordered complexTypes

Parent complexType	complexType	Usage
DvAny	DvInterval ReferenceRange	Intervals of DvQuantitifed data types Normal or abnormal intervals
DvOrdered[a]	DvOrdinal	Ranks or scores
DvQuantified[b]	DvQuantity DvCount DvRatio	Quantities in units Count data Ratios, rates and proportions
DvAny	DvTemporal	Complete or incomplete dates or times Durations

[a] DvAny child complexType. [b] DvOrdered child complexType.

The unordered data types from the MLHIM specifications comprise any type of string, Boolean or parsable data. Some of those complexTypes inherit directly from the abstract DvAny complexType and do not have any other inheritance relationship (DvBoolean and DvURI). On the other hand, the DvString and DvCodedString complexTypes defines a data type set that might contain characters (as well as DvIdentifier), line feeds, carriage returns, and tab characters, and the DvEncapsulated children complexTypes define the common metadata and allow persistence of all types of parsable or multimedia data (Table 2). A UML diagram of the Datatypes package is shown in Figure 1. For improved usability, a ZIP compressed package of all UML diagrams of the MLHIM Reference Model, in SVG format, is available at https://docs.google.com/file/d/0B9KiX8eH4fiKQVpHbmNmQ1pZS1U/edit?usp=sharing.

Table 2. MLHIM Reference Model: Unordered complexTypes

Parent complexType	complexType	Usage
DvAny	DvBoolean DvURI DvString	Truly boolean data (e.g. true/false) Uniform Resource Identifiers (URIs) Alphanumeric characters
DvString	DvCodedString DvIdentifier	Controlled vocabulary terms Identities of DemographicEntry
Dv Encapsulated[a]	DvMedia DvParsable	Multimedia types and their metadata Encapsulated parsable strings

[a] DvAny child complexType. [b] DvOrdered child complexType.

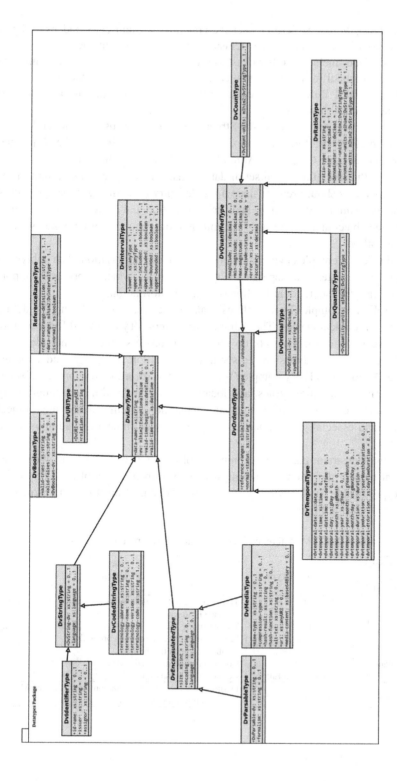

Fig. 1. UML diagram of the MLHIM Reference Model – Datatypes package

The Reference Model Structures package contains the Item class and its children complexTypes; Element and Cluster. Clusters are structural containers of any Item child complexType (including other Clusters), which allows the definition of any size or shape of data model for a given healthcare concept. Elements are the finest granularity of the MLHIM Reference Model structure, where data types are assigned for each variable of a healthcare concept.

The complexTypes that compose the Structures package are used to model the data structure of the Entry children complexTypes, which are defined in the Reference Model Content package: CareEntry, AdminEntry and DemographicEntry.

An Entry is the root of a logical set of data items. It is also the minimal unit of information any query should return, since a whole Entry (including sub-parts) records spatial structure, timing information, audit trail definition and contextual information, as well as the subject and generator of the information, required for complete semantic interoperability.

Each Entry child complexType has identical attribute information. The subtyping is used to allow persistence to separate the types of Entries, which is primarily important in healthcare for the de-identification of clinical information.

The CareEntry complexType defines data structure, protocol and guideline attributes for all clinical entries. The AdminEntry complexType is used for recording administrative information that sets up the clinical process, but it is not clinically relevant itself, such as admission, episode, ward location, discharge and appointments. The DemographicEntry complexType is used to record demographic information, such as name structures, roles, and locations. It is modeled as a separate Entry child complexType in order to facilitate the separation of clinical and non-clinical information, and especially to support de-identification of clinical and administrative data.

Finally, the Constraint package is composed of the CCD complexType, which has one element named 'defintion', which must be constrained to any of the Entry child complexTypes (Table 3). A UML Diagram of the Content, Constraint and Structures packages are shown in Figure 2.

Table 3. MLHIM Reference Model: Content and Structures packages

Parent complex-Type (Package)	complexType	Function
Item (Structures)	Element	The leaf variant of Item class, to which a data type instance is attached
	Cluster	The grouping variant of Item class, which may contain further instances of Item in an ordered list
Entry (Content)	CareEntry	Container of healthcare data
	AdminEntry	Container of administrative data
	DemographicEntry	Container of demographic data
CCD (Constraint)	CCD	Defining the further constraints on the Reference Model for a given healthcare concept

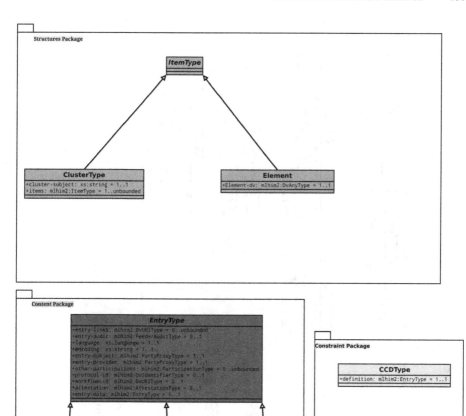

Fig. 2. UML diagram of the MLHIM Reference Model – Structures, Content and Constraint packages

Table 4. MLHIM Reference Model: Common package

Parent Type	complexType	Usage
PartyProxyType	PartySelfType	Representing the subject of the record
	PartyIdentifiedType	Proxy data for an identified party other than the subject of the record
xs:anyType	ParticipationType	Modeling participation of a Party in an activity
	AttestationType	Recording an attestation of item(s) of record content by a Party
	FeederAuditType	Audit and other meta-data for software applications and systems in the feeder chain
	FeederAuditDetailsType	Audit details for any system in a feeder system chain
ExceptionalValueType	Please refer to [36]	Please refer to [36]

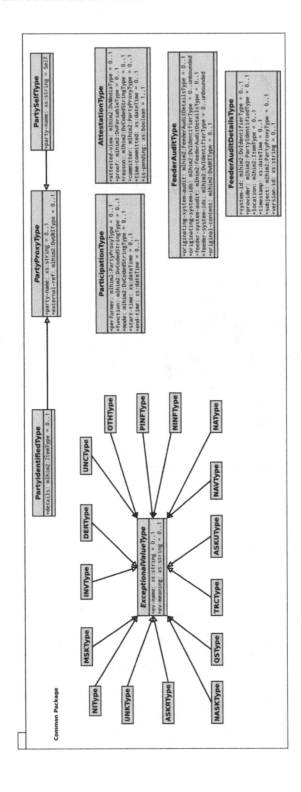

Fig. 3. UML diagram of the MLHIM Reference Model – Common package

The Common package is composed by complexTypes that inherit directly from the 'xs:anyType' from the XML Schema 1.1 specifications, containing all of the components required for all CCDs such as subject of care, provider and other participants as well as audit trail and exceptional value information (Table 4). A UML diagram of the Common package is shown in Figure 3.

2.3   Demo Application Development

Two demo applications were developed using the MLHIM Demo EMR, an eXist-db based application development framework of the MLHIM specifications (code available at https://github.com/mlhim/mlhim-emr). The demo application data models were based on a set of selected Common Data Elements (CDE) developed by the National   Cancer   Institute,   available   at   the   NCI   CDE   Browser (https://cdebrowser.nci.nih.gov/CDEBrowser/), related to Demographic and Vital Signs (Demo 1) and Demographic and Basic Metabolic Panel (BMP) (Demo 2) data. The CDEs were mapped to the admin interface of the Concept Constraint Definition Generator   (CCD-Gen),   a   web-based   MLHIM   CCD   editor (https://github.com/twcook/ccdgen-public), which generated the code for the Pluggable ComplexTypes (PCT) for each CDE. Some CCDs pre-dated the CCD-Gen and were hand developed using an XML Schema editor. A mixture of MLHIM 2.4.1 and 2.4.2 CCDs were used to demonstrate the continued validity of MLHIM based instance over time, even as the Reference Model may be modified for future versions. The CCDs were validated and simulated XML data instances were generated for each CCD by the use of the XML editor oXygen version 14.2 and persisted in the eXist-db database.

A minimalist application design was used on the demo applications in order to demonstrate the interoperability provided by MLHIM and does not represent the industrial implementation of a fully functional, robust Electronic Medical Record (EMR) or other healthcare application. Two instances of both applications were installed with some instance data from different CCDs in each. The patient record identifiers and demographics were identical, since it was not the purpose of this paper to address the issue of patient record linking. Again, that is outside the scope of semantic interoperability. The CCDs used are available from the Healthcare Knowledge Component Repository at: http://hkcr.net/ccd_sets/mlhim_emr_demo.

3   Results

The achievement of semantic interoperability between the two demo applications was based on two core elements: the data model definitions as CCDs, and the backwards validation chain, from the data instance to the CCD schema, the MLHIM Reference Model Schema and finally to the W3C XML specifications.

3.1   Data Modeling

The 'Demographics' CCDType was constrained to DemographicEntry complexType, which contained a ClusterType including ElementTypes for person details and address data. The 'Vital Signs' and 'BMP' CCDTypes were constrained to CareEntry complexTypes. The 'Vital Signs' CCD included blood pressure, heart and respiratory rate and temperature measurements; the 'BMP' CCD defined the data model for the recording of sodium, potassium, glucose, urea and creatinine measurements.

The data modeling process defined the type of each data element, according to the MLHIM Datatypes package, as defined in Tables 1 and 2 and Figure 1. For instance, for the definition of the data element 'Gender', DvStringType was chosen, and restrictions were made to its correspondent 'enumeration' facet, to constrain the permissible values to 'Male', 'Female', 'Unknown' and 'Unspecified'. The same process was repeated to each one of the data elements included in the CCDs by following the specific requirements of each data type defined on the MLHIM specifications.

After the definition of the data types for all ElementTypes, they were combined into a ClusterType (see Table 3). In the CCD-Gen, the procedure requires the selection of the ElementTypes that will compose a given ClusterType. For this demo application, one ClusterType was defined for each one of the CCDs, which included all correspondent ElementTypes as seen on Table 5.

The ClusterType that contains all the ItemTypes is associated to an EntryType that corresponds to demographic (DemographicEntry), administrative (AdminEntry) or clinical (CareEntry) data (Table 3).   In the CCD-Gen, this association is made by the selection of the containing Cluster that will be included in the chosen Entry child type as the value for the 'entry-data' element. In this example, the Demographic CCD was modeled as a DemographicEntry, and Vital Signs and BMP were modeled as CareEntry types. To complete the generation of the CCD, Dublin Core Metadata Initiative (DCMI) information was included in the correspondent section of the CCDs.

The Demographic, Vital Signs and BMP CCDs defined the simulated XML data instances for 130 fictitious patients, each of them with one Demographic data instance and n (n = 1, 2, 3...) Vital Signs and BMP data instances, resulting, as an example, in 1,531 data instances of Diastolic Blood Pressure from the Vital Signs CCD. All data instances were valid according to the correspondent CCDs, and those were valid according to the MLHIM Reference Model Schema (either 2.4.1 or 2.4.2), which is valid according to the W3C XML Schema Definition 1.1 and to the W3C XML Language specification; thus, the MLHIM specifications achieved a complete backwards validation chain, from the data instance to the W3C XML specifications. That was repeated for all data instances, with a success rate of 100%. Figure 4 shows an XQuery performed on the database using the web-based XQuery IDE eXide.

Table 5. Results of the data modeling for the concepts of Demograhics, Vital Signs and Basic Metabolic Panel (BMP) as MLHIM CCDs

CCD	Data Element	Data Type
Demograhic	Gender	DvString with enumeration
	Zip Code	DvIdentifier
	State	DvCodedString
	City	DvCodedString
	Driver License no.	DvIdentifier
	Social Security no.	DvIdentifier
	Phone no.	DvString
	Email address	DvURI
	First Name	DvString
	Last Name	DvString
Vital Signs	Systolic Pressure	DvQuantity
	Diastolic Pressure	DvQuantity
	BP Device Type	DvString with enumeration
	Cuff Location	DvString with enumeration
	Patient Position	DvString with enumeration
	Heart Rate	DvCount
	Respiration	DvCount
	Body Temperature	DvQuantity
	Temperature Location	DvString with enumeration
	Temperature Device	DvString with enumeration
BMP	Sodium	DvQuantity
	Potassium	DvQuantity
	Glucose	DvQuantity
	Urea	DvQuantity
	Creatinine	DvQuantity

The Basic Metabolic Panel CCD based on RM 2.4.2 (id=ccd-f8dada44-e1e9-4ea9-8e7e-46af767ccc66) also demonstrates the use of 'xs:assert' elements. These assertions are XPath statements that are added to complexTypes to provide more fine grained control or permissible data such as the requirements for a valid geographical latitude;

```
<xs:asserttest="matches(mlhim2:DvString-dv,'^-?([1-
8]?[0- 9]\.{1}\d{1,6}$|90\.{1}0{1,6}$)')"/>
```

as well as to provide a level of built-in decision support. The assertions can function as business rules on one complexType, or across multiple complexTypes in a CCD, to insure that if a certain type of data is chosen for one entry then it may restrict the available entries for another choice. For example, if the Gender was chosen as Male, then it might restrict a selection of test options from including Pap Smear. This is a key benefit of the internal semantics of a CCD. In current application design approaches there is no way to share this concept with other applications. In MLHIM, it is shared by default.

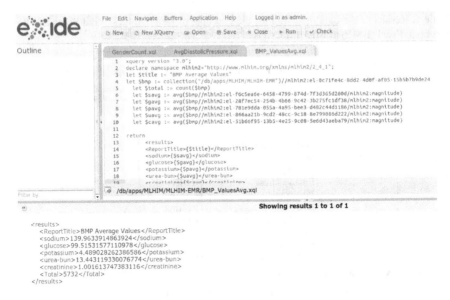

Fig. 4. eXide XQuery for BMP average (detail)

3.2   The Proof of Concept

The proof of concept of the achievement of semantic interoperability across the MLHIM-based demo applications developed for this study is shown in the ability to exchange instance data between applications and those instance data components having the ability to point to the specific semantics for the concept, as well as adhere to the exact syntactic constraints that were designed for those semantics at CCD modeling time. The demos are quite small, but this proof of concept was kept small so that the entire system can be seen at one time without the analysis being too arduous.

Since the unit of exchange is the concept as defined by a CCD and the representation in XML is available across all platforms, it is therefore proven that any type of healthcare information application can be accommodated in the MLHIM ecosystem.

4   Discussion

This study presented the process of development of an open source, industry-standard based multilevel modeling specification. The results have shown that the adoption of XML technologies implemented in a multi-level approach, allowed the establishment of a backward validation chain from the data instance to the original W3C XML specifications.

The real advantage of adopting XML technologies for the development of the MLHIM specifications is the potential of having semantically interoperable applications being developed for real healthcare settings completely independent of the application size or use. Since XML is a universal industry standard and every major programming language has binding tools for XML Schema, this allows developers to work in their preferred language, using their preferred persistence models and yet not build data silos [37]. MLHIM-based applications can persist data on native XML and other types of NoSQL databases as well as SQL databases. It is also common to generate GUIs through XForms tools and other language specific frameworks as required for each application.

Using XML technologies also allows use of emerging semantic web tools and technologies by allowing CCDs to be marked up with common use RDF and other tags for semantic reasoning across conforming instance data [38]. The uniqueness in the MLHIM approach is to *not markup the instance data*, but the CCDs that the instance data refers to for its syntactic and semantic constraints. This approach reduces the size and overall overhead of data querying and exchange processes.

The knowledge modeling process adopted in this study was based on the MLHIM specifications. The process of modeling CCDs was a simple task for the domain expert, only responsible for selecting the NCI CDE concepts and defining their data types according to the MLHIM Datatypes package, and then defined the constraint for each variable on the CCD-Gen. It is important to notice that there have been reports in literature that found the elaboration of openEHR archetypes quite complex [30], but that has not being the case for MLHIM CCDs.

It is important to note that systems that use MLHIM concepts do not have to have the Reference Model in source code or even the CCD for that matter. That is why the validity chain is important. It is considered best practice for new applications to be written based on the MLHIM Reference Model; however, this is not required for effective semantic interoperability, which is ensured by the exchange of documents containing valid instance data and their correspondent CCDs. Since MLHIM is based on a widely adopted and well supported industry standard, the XML Schema representation can be used with virtually any application in any programming language. The only requirement will be that the application can import and export valid instance data when compared with the CCD. This provides a complete validation chain that no other approach can provide; from the data instance to the CCD, to the MLHIM RM Schema, to the W3C XML Schema and finally to the W3C XML specification.

4.1   Relationship to Model-Driven Architecture

There are some conceptual similarities between multi-level modeling in MLHIM and Model Driven Architecture, also known as model-driven engineering or meta-modeling; however, there are distinct differences. The MDA approach is concerned with the overall architecture and development of a specific software application or specific system of applications developed around a set of requirements. This approach improves software quality and ease of maintenance. These are generally implemented using a domain specific language (DSL) and a specific technology platform [39].

While MLHIM incorporates those same advantages, it extends the MDA approach to achieve syntactic and semantic interoperability at the concept level, across every development platform. This is accomplished by using XML technologies, because of the ubiquity of XML [40]. While DSLs provide a significant level of power and control when used in a closed environment, this is not the case in healthcare, where a multitude of software and hardware platforms must be accommodated. This has been proven by the *open*EHR Foundation specifications where they initiated the multi-level interoperability concepts but used ADL, a DSL that lacks broad uptake and reusable tooling. After more than 15 years it has achieved very little penetration across the global healthcare community, in spite of also being part of the ISO 13606 standard.

During the development of MLHIM the MDA approach, using the Eclipse Modeling Framework (EMF), was investigated, which showed that the EMF locks the developer into that technology; even the XML Schema export process includes EMF dependencies. In addition to this the Eclipse system did not fully support XML Schema 1.1. This lack of support for multiple substitution groups and assertions negated the ability to export the models into a format that was usable outside of the EMF.

4.2   Relationship to OWL and RDF

As there is often confusion in the purposes of the Web Ontology Language (OWL) and the Resource Description Framework (RDF) in building semantic web applications [41], it is important to address them. Our investigation of those technologies has shown that both OWL and RDF have been extensively used to markup or define a structure for metadata (in the case of OWL) [42] and instance data (in the case of RDF) [43]. However, we did not find implementations where syntactic data model structures were marked up with either to create concept models for interoperability.

OWL is intended as an ontology language for the Semantic Web with formally defined meaning. OWL ontologies provide classes, properties, individuals, and data values and are stored as Semantic Web documents. OWL ontologies can be used along with information written in RDF, and OWL ontologies themselves are primarily exchanged as RDF documents using one of several syntaxes.

Since RDF is an implementation for graph networks of information and can also represent OWL constructs it is useful for MLHIM in having one representation syntax for all MLHIM metadata. A major representation for RDF is XML and therefore can exploit the plethora of XML tools for processing. We decided that it is a natural fit for MLHIM to use RDF/XML to represent CCD metadata and provide the semantic links for that metadata. However, RDF lacks the expressiveness, syntactic structure and completeness as well as the relationship to XPath and XQuery that XML Schema provides. Because of these and other missing features of these two concepts as well as the complexity in expressing relationships in them, a number of syntaxes have evolved for each. This leads to wide open challenge to interoperability.

Therefore, the MLHIM specifications use RDF as it was intended, as a link to expanded semantics, by including the ability to add these links into the CCD so that it represents the semantics of all data instances generated against it, without the requirement to include that code and data overhead in every instance. However, it is important to keep studying those technologies; there is a possibility that, with maturity in the specifications and the tooling, MLHIM 3.x may be developed using OWL semantics, using the RDF/XML representation. At that time there will be tooling that can translate MLHIM 2.x instances (that will remain valid) to MLHIM 3.x instances without loss of semantic integrity.

4.3   Relationship to other Standards

MLHIM can be seen, in a general way, as the harmonization of the Health Level Seven version 3 (HL7v3) standard and the *open*EHR specifications, without the limitations they each introduce. For instance, in *open*EHR, there is a requirement that the entire Reference Model be included in each application, since there is no independent validity chain for *open*EHR; all validation is based on the human eye or internal *open*EHR Reference Model parser or validator. This is not the case with MLHIM because it uses standard XML technologies that are available on all platforms in both open source and proprietary packages.

A similar comparison can be made with the Health Level Seven version 3 (HL7v3) standard. Although HL7v3 is not a restriction-based multi-level model standard, it is also XML-based. The challenge for the achievement of semantic interoperability with HL7v3 is that, since it is not fully restriction-based, there is no validity chain to insure conformance back to a known valid model. The HL7v3 Reference Information Model-based data models are all independently designed as can be seen by the update, simplify and re-expand process that has gone on through its history, which poses maintenance issues for HL7v3-based applications. Although the HL7v3 Common Definition Architecture (CDA) has been partially adopted as a reference document and there is now a tendency to use it as a base reference model, it is too large and has unnecessary requirements for many applications, such as mobile applications or devices using only a push data approach.

MLHIM 1.x began as an XML Schema implementation of the *open*EHR model, to which additional HL7v3 benefits were added, such as closer alignment with ISO 21090, finally having all of the semantics that directly relate to specific applications (such as EMRs) extracted. Also, there is the semantic integrity issue developed in the *open*EHR eco-system by non-reviewed archetypes being created, outside of the centralized control required by the *open*EHR specifications; that creates the risk that multiple archetypes with the same archetype ID (that may actually define different syntactic and semantic structures) to appear in that eco-system. This issue causes instance data to, in the best case, be invalid and, in the worst case, create unknown and undetectable errors. This issue was solved in MLHIM with the CCD identification by Type 4 UUID and by making CCDs non editable. This also resulted in a much simpler eco-system since there is no need to track CCD modifications and versioning.

The Integrating the Healthcare Enterprise (IHE) profiles that actually define data structures are implementable in MLHIM. However, the majority of IHE work is based around standardized work-flow, which is not a semantic interoperability issue, being solved at the application implementation level.

The Standards and Interoperability (S&I) Framework is analogous to the HL7v3 CDA and the NCI CDE initiatives. It can be defined as a top-down, document-centric approach attempting to gain consensus on modeling concepts. The documents available from the S&I Content Browser can be modeled as MLHIM CCDs or collections of CCDs without requiring global consensus, still keeping semantic interoperability among distributed, independently developed applications.

4.4   Disadvantages of the MLHIM Approach

The adoption of any technological solution to a social problem requires trade-offs and the healthcare domain is not different. The first major hurdle for the adoption of a technology such as MLHIM is a shift in the thinking from one level to multi-level modeling. There are anecdotal comments that (within the healthcare informatics domain) this shift is similar to that required from geo-centric to helio-centric awareness in the study of cosmology. This is a challenge for many software developers that have been taught how to develop one-level modeled systems.

Another challenge is the complexity of the XML Schema reference model implementation and the rules around CCD development. Many of the one-level model XML experts are not familiar with this innovative use of the XML Schema specifications, which is similar to the geo-centric versus helio-centric debate described above.

The last and likely the most difficult issue is the need for domain experts to participate in the development process. Though there is enough evidence showing healthcare providers should be included in the design process, this is not yet regarded as a formal part of the work for most of the healthcare professionals. In order to overcome this obstacle, there is a need for the emergence of a new area of expertise in biomedical sciences: knowledge modeling. A healthcare knowledge modeling expert should be specifically trained to take the domain knowledge from healthcare providers and turn it into computer-readable concept models such as MLHIM CCDs.

5   Conclusion

The results of this study showed that semantic interoperability in healthcare information systems is achievable by the adoption of the multilevel modeling approach, which is implementable by the XML technology-based MLHIM specifications. While the broad goal of the MLHIM specifications is to foster long-term, semantic and syntactic interoperability across all healthcare related applications on a global scale, even self-contained applications can benefit from MLHIM technologies (e.g., a software company, a locality, a state). Even in such cases, it is possible to build applications that are already interoperable and require less maintenance overhead as the science of healthcare changes, in the temporal, spatial and ontological dimensions.

A key concept in any interoperability solution is that there is an eco-system that must grow and permeate the industry. As long as the information technology businesses benefit from the lack of interoperability, government policies and user requirements must demand it, since the technological solution exists. The MLHIM eco-system model approach has learned from decades of research on a global basis. The MLHIM approach allows developing application requirements capability, at any level, to suit the local needs, across all time; along with maintaining interoperability and freedom for developers' choices.

Ongoing and future work requires improved tools to engage domain experts. As the functionality of the Eclipse Modeling Framework matures it may be suitable to use for a more solid model-driven engineering approach.

References

1. ACMI, electronic medical records, `http://www.youtube.com/watch?v=t-aiKlIc6uk` (last accessed: April 1, 2013)
2. De Leon, S., Connelly-Flores, A., Mostashari, F., Shih, S.C.: The business end of health information technology. Can a fully integrated electronic health record increase provider productivity in a large community practice? J. Med. Pract. Manage 25, 342–349 (2010)
3. Javitt, J.C.: How to succeed in health information technology. Health Aff. (Millwood) (2004); Suppl. Web Exclusives:W4-321-4
4. U.S. National Library of Medicine. 2011AA SNOMED CT Source Information, `http://www.nlm.nih.gov/research/umls/sourcereleasedocs/current/SNOMEDCT` (last accessed: April 28, 2013)
5. Maojo, V., Kulikowski, C.: Medical informatics and bioinformatics: integration or evolution through scientific crises? Methods Inf. Med. 45, 474–482 (2006)
6. Fitzmaurice, J.M., Adams, K., Eisenberg, J.: Three decades of research on computer applications in health care: medical informatics support at the Agency for Healthcare Research and Quality. J. Am. Med. Inform. Assoc. 9, 144–160 (2002)
7. Preker, A., Harding, A.: The economics of hospital reform from hierarchical to market-based incentives. World Hosp. Health Serv. 39, 3–10 (2003)
8. Harris, N.M., Thorpe, R., Dickinson, H., Rorison, F., Barrett, C., Williams, C.: Hospital and after: experience of patients and carers in rural and remote North Queensland, Australia. Rural Remote Health 4, 246 (2004)
9. Zusman, E.: Form facilitates function: innovations in architecture and design drive quality and efficiency in healthcare. Neurosurgery 66, N24 (2010)
10. Ward, M.M., Vartak, S., Schwichtenberg, T., Wakefield, D.: Nurses' perceptions of how clinical information system implementation affects workflow and patient care. Comput. Inform. Nurs. 29, 502–511 (2011)
11. Jung, M., Choi, M.: A mechanism of institutional isomorphism in referral networks among hospitals in Seoul, South Korea. Health Care Manag (Frederick) 29, 133–146 (2010)
12. Hoangmai, H.P., O'Malley, A.S., Bach, P.B., Saiontz-Martinez, C., Schrag, D.: Primary care physicians' links to other physicians through medicare patients: the scope of care coordination. Ann. Intern. Med. 150, 236–242 (2009)
13. Sittig, D.F., Singh, H.: A new sociotechnical model for studying health information technology in complex adaptive healthcare systems. QualSaf Health Care (suppl. 3), i68–i74 (2010)
14. Hyman, W.: When medical devices talk to each other: the promise and challenges of interoperability. Biomed. Instrum. Technol. (suppl.), 28–31 (2010)
15. Charters, K.: Home telehealth electronic health information lessons learned. Stud. Health Technol. Inform. 146, 719 (2009)
16. Raths, D.: Shifting away from silos. The interoperability challenges that hospitals face pale in comparison to the headaches plaguing State Departments. Healthc Inform. 27, 32–33 (2010)

17. Achimugu, P., Soriyan, A., Oluwagbemi, O., Ajayi, A.: Record linkage system in a complex relational database: MINPHIS example. Stud. Health Technol. Inform. 160, 1127–1130 (2010)
18. Metaxiotis, K., Ptochos, D., Psarras, J.: E-health in the new millennium: a research and practice agenda. Int. J. Electron. Healthc 1, 165–175 (2004)
19. Hufnagel, S.P.: Interoperability. Mil. Med. 174, 43–50 (2009)
20. Kadry, B., Sanderson, I.C., Macario, A.: Challenges that limit meaningful use of health information technology. Curr. Opin. Anaesthesiol. 23, 184–192 (2010)
21. Blobel, B., Pharow, P.: Analysis and evaluation of EHR approaches. Stud. Health Technol. Inform. 136, 359–364 (2008)
22. Rodrigues, J.M., Kumar, A., Bousquet, C., Trombert, B.: Using the CEN/ISO standard for categorial structure to harmonise the development of WHO international terminologies. Stud. Health Technol. Inform. 159, 255–259 (2009)
23. Blobel, B.: Ontologies, knowledge representation, artificial intelligence: hype or prerequisites for international pHealth interoperability? Stud. Health Technol. Inform. 165, 11–20 (2011)
24. National Health Service Media Centre. Dismantling the NHS national programme for IT, http://mediacentre.dh.gov.uk/2011/09/22/dismantling-the-nhs-national-programme-for-it (last accessed: May 15, 2013)
25. Lohrs, S.: Google to end health records service after it fails to attract users. The New York Times (June 24, 2011), http://www.nytimes.com/2011/06/25/technology/25health.html?_r=3&. (last accessed: April 28, 2013)
26. Kalra, D., Beale, T., Heard, S.: The open EHR Foundation. Stud. Health Technol. Inform. 115, 153–173 (2005)
27. Martinez-Costa, C., Menarguez-Tortosa, M., Fernandez-Breis, J.T.: Towards ISO 13606 and open EHR archetype-based semantic interoperability. Stud. Health Technol. Inform. 150, 260–264 (2009)
28. Cavalini, L.T., Cook, T.W.: Health informatics: The relevance of open source and multilevel modeling. In: Hissam, S.A., Russo, B., de Mendonça Neto, M.G., Kon, F. (eds.) OSS 2011. IFIP AICT, vol. 365, pp. 338–347. Springer, Heidelberg (2011)
29. Dias, R.D., Cook, T.W., Freire, S.: Modeling healthcare authorization and claim submissions using the openEHR dual-model approach. BMC Med. Inform. Decis. Mak. 11, 60 (2011)
30. Kashfi, H., Torgersson, O.: A migration to an open EHR-based clinical application. Stud. Health Technol. Inform. 150, 152–156 (2009)
31. Eichelberg, M., Aden, T., Riesmeier, J., Dogac, A., Laleci, G.: A survey and analysis of electronic healthcare record standards. ACM Comput. Surv. 37, 277–315 (2005)
32. Yu, S., Berry, D., Bisbal, J.: Clinical coverage of an archetype repository over SNOMED-CT. J. Biomed. Inform. 45, 408–418 (2012)
33. Menezes, A.L., Cirilo, C.E., Moraes, J.L.C., Souza, W.L., Prado, A.: Using archetypes and domain specific languages on development of ubiquitous applications to pervasive healthcare. In: Proc. IEEE 23rd Int. Symp. Comput. Bas. Med. Syst., pp. 395–400 (2010)
34. Cavalini, L.T., Cook, T.: Knowledge engineering of healthcare applications based on minimalist multilevel models. In: IEEE 14th Int. Conf. e-Health Networ. Appl. Serv., pp. 431–434 (2012)
35. Sanderson, D.: Loss of data semantics in syntax directed translation. PhD Thesis in Computer Sciences. Renesselaer Polytechnic Institute, New York (1994)
36. Cook, T.W., Cavalini, L.: Implementing a specification for exceptional data in multilevel modeling of healthcare applications. ACM Sighit Rec. 2, 11 (2012)

37. Lee, T., Hon, C.T., Cheung, D.X.: Schema design and management for e-government data interoperability. Electr. Je.-Gov., 381–391 (2009)
38. Daconta, M.C., Obrst, L.J., Smith, K.T.: The Semantic Web. Wiley, Indianapolis (2003)
39. Rutle, A., MacCaull, W., Wang, H.: A metamodelling approach to behaviouralmodeling. In: Proc. 4th Worksh. Behav. Mod. Foundat. Appl., vol. 5 (2012)
40. Seligman, L., Roenthal, A.: XML's impact on databases and data sharing. Computer, 59–67 (2001)
41. Fenton, S., Giannangelo, K., Kallem, C., Scichilone, R.: Data standards, data quality, and interoperability. J. Ahima (2007); extended online edition
42. Hitzler, P., Krötzsch, M., Parsia, B., Patel-Schneider, P.F., Rudolph, S.: OWL 2 Web Ontology Language Primer, 2 edn., http://www.w3.org/TR/owl2-primer/ #Modeling_Knowledge:_Basic_Notions (last accessed: October 17, 2013)
43. Manola, F., Miller, E.: RDF Primer, http://www.w3.org/TR/ rdf-primer/#dublincore (last accessed: October 17, 2013)

A Bayesian Patient-Based Model for Detecting Deterioration in Vital Signs Using Manual Observations

Sara Khalid, David A. Clifton, and Lionel Tarassenko

Institute of Biomedical Engineering, Old Road Campus, University of Oxford,
Oxford, UK, OX3 7DQ
{Sara.Khalid,David.Clifton,Lionel.Tarassenko}@eng.ox.ac.uk

Abstract. Deterioration in patient condition is often preceded by deterioration in the patient's vital signs. "Track-and-Trigger" systems have been adopted in many hospitals in the UK, where manual observations of the vital signs are scored according to their deviation from "normal" limits. If the score exceeds a threshold, the patient is reviewed. However, such scoring systems are typically heuristic. We propose an automated method for detection of deterioration using manual observations of the vital signs, based om Bayesian model averaging. The proposed method is compared with an existing technique - Parzen windows. The proposed method is shown to generate alerts for 79% of patients who went on to an emergency ICU admission and in 2% of patients who did not have an adverse event, as compared to 86% and 25% by the Parzen windows technique, reflecting that the proposed method has a 23% lower false alert rate than that of the existing technique.

Keywords: Intelligent patient monitoring, Track-and-Trigger, novelty detection, Bayesian inference.

1   Introduction

It has been recognised that deterioration in patient condition is often preceded by physiological deterioration in vital-sign data [1], and that adverse events can be prevented by detecting this deterioration early. However, continuous monitoring of patient vital signs is not always possible; typically a patient's vital signs are monitored by clinical staff every four hours on a general ward [2], with each nurse attending several patients. This often causes physiological deviation in vital signs to go unnoticed [3]. According to the UK National Confidential Enquiry on post-operative care [4], current systems of care fail to detect signs of patient deterioration sufficiently, or to elicit the necessary response from the clinical staff, possibly due to a lack of clearly defined response procedures.

1.1   Track-and-Trigger System

In the UK, the conventional system of assessing patient condition using vital signs is known as the Track-and-Trigger (T&T) system, which follows guidelines issued by

J. Gibbons and W. MacCaull (Eds.): FHIES 2013, LNCS 8315, pp. 146–158, 2014.

the National Institute of Clinical Excellence (NICE) for assessing patient status [5]. Nurses record vital-sign observations at regular intervals (typically on paper charts, or in a Personal Digital Assistant, PDA), enabling a patient's vital signs to be "tracked" through time. An individual score is assigned to each vital sign, and an aggregate is calculated by summing the individual scores. If either the individual scores or the aggregate score exceeds some pre-defined thresholds, an alarm is "triggered" and the patient's condition is reviewed. T&T systems have received mixed reviews in the clinical literature, where some have criticised their effectiveness [6], while others have encouraged use of modified T&T in hospitals after modifications [7]. A common limitation of these systems is that they are based on manual checks performed by clinical staff, and that these observations, and hence escalations, only occur intermittently.

1.2   Automatic Alarm Generation

More recently, the focus has shifted towards developing "intelligent" early warning systems which are aimed at improving the clinical decision-making process by enabling automated and continuous monitoring of patients, and generating an alarm in the event of deterioration.

The problems associated with manual scoring systems are addressed by automated monitoring systems. However most of these automated alarm systems are designed for use in the ICU and cannot be used in wards outside the ICU where continuous monitoring is not carried out, such as the step-down ward or the general ward. Here the level of care is less intensive than in the ICU which means that monitoring is manual and intermittent instead of being continuous. Furthermore, these are wards in which patients are mobile. This further complicates the use of continuous monitoring in these wards because telemetry systems remain unreliable [18]. Continuous data recorded from ambulatory patients is far more susceptible to noise and data dropouts than that recorded for ICU patients. Hence there is a need for automated systems calibrated for intermittently recorded low-frequency T&T data which forms part of standard care in most hospitals.

1.3   Limitations of Existing Methods

Automated systems for patient monitoring are generally designed to perform novelty detection. Novelty detection may be defined as the identification of data that is aberrant with respect to some definition of normality [8]. A typical density-based novelty detection system for patient vital-signs involves the construction of a "model of normality" based on the probability density function (pdf) of samples of vital-sign data considered to be "normal". Any sample whose probability density lies below some threshold is considered to be "abnormal".

There are several examples of the use of novelty detection-based systems for the detection of deterioration using continuously monitored vital-sign data in the current literature [8]. However, designing such a model for a dataset comprising manually-acquired T&T data which does not contain a large number of "normal" samples, such as the dataset considered in this work, poses a challenge. In previous work [9], we have shown that a population-based [1]model of normality can be constructed using the same dataset as we consider in this work. However, the population-based approach, which was non-Bayesian, does not account for any uncertainty in modelling that may occur due to the low sampling rate of T&T data. A population-based approach is suitable for use when a large number of training data are available, which is not the case when data are recorded intermittently. Therefore we propose an alternative model which copes with the limitation of small quantity of "normal" data being available.

In sections 2 and 3, the construction of a patient-based model of normality is discussed. Section 4 describes an existing population-based approach. In Section 5 the dataset acquired from a clinical study is described, and the challenge in performing novelty detection with intermittently-recorded data is discussed. The proposed patient-based method was applied to the dataset with results presented in   Section 6, which are compared with those obtained using an existing population-based method.

2   Uncertainty in Parameter Estimation

Let us assume that the uni-dimensional dataset $X = \{x_1 \ldots x_N\}$ is associated with an underlying Gaussian distribution. A non-Bayesian approach would be to find point-estimates of $\theta = \{\mu, \sigma^2\}$ from the N samples using, for example, the maximum likelihood estimation (MLE) approach, which results in the standard formulae $\mu = \frac{1}{N}\sum_{n=1}^{N} x_n$ and $\sigma^2 = \sum_{n=1}^{N}(x_n - \mu)^2$, where μ is simply the arithmetic mean of the N samples. While the arithmetic mean of a large number of samples may be expected to converge to some expected value, in keeping with the central limit theorem, the same may be not necessarily be true for a small sample size, such as when $N \ll \infty$. In the latter case, the point-estimates of μ and σ^2 may or may not be accurately representative of the underlying distribution to which the samples belong, as shown in [14]. In the Bayesian approach, the "uncertainty" in the estimation of the parameters θ of a distribution is taken into account explicitly. We have a distribution over the parameters $\theta = \{\mu, \sigma^2\}$, which for the case of a uni-dimensional dataset, can be expressed by a Normal-Gamma (NG) distribution

$$(\mu, \lambda) \sim N(\mu | \mu 0, \kappa\lambda - 1)G(\lambda | \alpha, \beta) \tag{1}$$

where μ_0 and $(\kappa\lambda)^{-1}$ are the mean and the variance of the distribution of μ which takes the form of a Gaussian distribution (N), and κ is the hyperparameter which governs the dependence of μ on λ (where $\lambda = \frac{1}{\sigma^2}$, used here instead of σ^2 for ease of computation). Hyper-parameters α and β are the shape and scale, respectively, of the distribution of λ, which takes the form of a Gamma (G) distribution. Figure 1 illustrates how recursive Bayesian inference is used to learn $p = (\mu, \lambda | X)$ for an artificial dataset $x \in X$, which is generated from a Gaussian distribution, with

---

[1]   Here, a population-based model refers to one which is trained using "normal" samples contributed by the entire "normal" population, considering each sample to be independent. To which patient the "normal" samples belong is irrelevant for constructing such a population-based model of normality.

$p(X) \sim N(0,1)$. In the dataset described later in Section 5, there are $N = 5.3$ HR samples per patient. Hence if we assume that the $N = 5.3$ HR samples are associated with a Gaussian distribution, the distribution of θ would resemble that shown in Figure 1 (b).

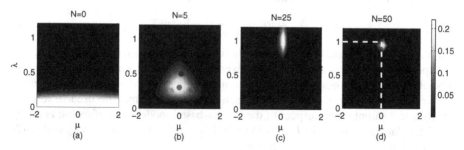

Fig. 1. An example of learning the NG distribution over the parameters $\theta = \{\mu, \lambda\}$ using recursive Bayesian inference. (a) to (d) show the posterior distribution $p = (\mu, \lambda | x_1 \ldots x_N)$ upon the arrival of data, for $N = 0$, $N = 5$, $N = 25$, and $N = 50$, respectively. The artificial dataset $x \in X$, and $p(X) \sim N(0,1)$. In (b), five sample points on $p = (\mu, \lambda | x_1 \ldots x_N)$ are shown by the coloured dots. In (d), MLE point-estimates $\mu_{MLE} = 0$ and $\lambda_{MLE} = 1$ are marked by dashed lines in white.

3   Constructing a Patient-Based Model

We now define a hypothesis H_i and its associated vector of parameters θ_i. According to Bayes' Theorem [12], hypothesis H_i may be described by a prior probability distribution $p(\theta_i | H_i)$, a conditional distribution $p(X | \theta_i, H_i)$, and a posterior probability distribution $p(\theta_i | X, H_i)$, where $X = \{x_1 \ldots x_N\}$. Let X now represent the data from patient i in the training set. We then define a patient-based model such that it contains hypotheses H_i $_{=1 \ldots 154}$ over all 154 patients.

3.1   Evidence for a Hypothesis

The evidence p($X | H_i$) for hypothesis H_i is defined as

$$p(X|H_i) = \int p(X|\theta_i, H_i)p(\theta_i|H_i)d\theta_i \tag{2}$$

and is in effect the likelihood of X considering only hypothesis H_i to be true.

The evidence for all hypotheses in the patient-based model may be combined to generate the posterior predictive distribution [15] of new test data, X_{new}, given previously observed data X, as

$$p(X_{new}|X) = \sum_{i=1}^{I} p(X_{new}|H_i, X)p(H_i|X) \tag{3}$$

where $p(X_{new}|X)$ is an average of the posterior distributions under each of the candidate hypotheses, weighted by their posterior probability (or their evidence). This is based on the notion that a weighted average of candidate models has a better predictive ability than any single model [17]. In the context of our problem, it addresses the limitation posed by having only a small number of training data per patient by taking the associated modelling uncertainty into account.

Considering X_{new} to be a sample from a test patient, and abbreviating $p(X_{new}|X)$ as $p(X_{new})$ for clarity, we may then express a novelty score z as

$$z(X_{new}) = \log \frac{1}{p(X_{new})} = -\log p(X_{new}) \tag{4}$$

If X_{new} is associated with a hypothesis within the patient-based model, the corresponding novelty score $z(X_{new})$ is expected to be low; conversely, if X_{new} is associated with a hypothesis that is not within the patient-based model, then the corresponding novelty score should be high. Hence this method may be used to test the novelty a test sample with respect to the patient-based model. Classification is determined by placing a threshold T on $z(X)$ such that if $z(X_{new}) \geq T$, then X_{new} is considered "abnormal", and "normal" otherwise.

Here it is important to clarify that the proposed method is not an example of model combination. Indeed, in the limit $N \to \infty$, $\theta_i \to \theta_{MLE}$; i.e., the estimate of θ tends to resemble the estimate of θ achieved using the maximum likelihood (MLE) approach. As $N \to \infty$, a single hypothesis H_i in the patient-based model would resemble a single Gaussian kernel H_i in a mixture model, such as in the case of a Parzen windows model (described below in Section 4), but this is not the case in our problem where N is small ($N \approx 5$).

The proposed method is a "first approach" towards Bayesian model averaging (BMA) [16] for novelty detection. We note that BMA assumes that competing hypotheses belong to different parametric forms so that they may have different orders of model complexity [17].

4   Parzen Windows Model

Parzen windows is a popular density-estimator which can be considered as a "equi-weight" mixture model, in that a hyper-spherical kernel is placed on each training sample. It involves forming an estimate of the distribution of vital-sign data $p(x)$, where $X = \{x_1 \dots x_N\} \in \mathbb{R}^d$ are N vectors of vital-sign data in the d-dimensional space defined by the vital signs (e.g., $d = 4$ when considering the heart rate, breathing rate, blood pressure, and oxygen saturation levels), and where σ is the "bandwidth" parameter, defining the probability density function (pdf) $p(x)$ for a model of normality

$$p(x) = \frac{1}{N} \sum_{i=1}^{N} \frac{1}{\sigma^d} \frac{1}{(2\pi)^{d/2}} \exp \left\{ -\frac{|x - \mu_i|^2}{2\sigma^2} \right\} \tag{5}$$

In previous work [19], we have shown that a probability, $\tilde{P}$, may be defined such that $\tilde{P}$ is an estimate of how "normal" x may be considered to be. We also define a probability P to be the probability for novelty or "abnormality" of vector x with respect to the model of normality (or more simply, $P = 1 - \tilde{P}$). From our model of normality, a highly "normal" pattern (i.e., one with a high $p(x)$), would be highly probable and thus have a high probability, $\tilde{P}$ and low P. Conversely, a highly "abnormal" pattern would take a low value of $\tilde{P}$ and a high value of P.

The probability $\tilde{P}$ may then be calculated. For unidimensional x, the probability that x lies within a certain interval $[a,b]$ is given by :

$$\tilde{P}(x \in (a,b)) = \int_a^b p(x)dx \qquad (6)$$

Which is the cumulative distribution (cdf) for pdf $p(x)$. However if the cdf is undefined for multidimensional distributions, such as a 4-D pdf $p(x)$, we use the probability of a vector lying within the region bounded by some threshold T_{pdf} on probability density, given by

$$\tilde{P}(\{p(x) \geq T_{pdf}\}) = \int_\gamma^\tau p(x)dx \qquad (7)$$

where $\gamma = \arg \, {}_x^{max}p(x)$, which is the mode of the pdf, and where $\tau = \{x : p(x) = T_{pdf}\}$, which is the level set on the pdf at T_{pdf}. Thus $\tilde{P}(\{p(x) \geq T_{pdf}\})$ is the probability mass contained by integrating the pdf from its location of highest density γ to the probability density contour T_{pdf} at τ. Finally, we define a threshold T (which is not the same as T_{pdf}) such that, if $P(x) \leq T$, then x is "normal", and if $P(x) > T$, then x is "abnormal" with respect to the model of normality. As $0 \leq P(x) \leq 1$, therefore $0 \leq T \leq 1$. However at $T = 0$, all x would be considered "abnormal", and at $T = 1$, x would be considered "normal", therefore we sue the the range $0.1 \leq T \leq 0.9$. For example, if $T = 0.9$ (as shown in Figure 2), then any sample whose $P(x) > 0.9$ and correspondingly whose $p(x) < 0.026$ is "abnormal".

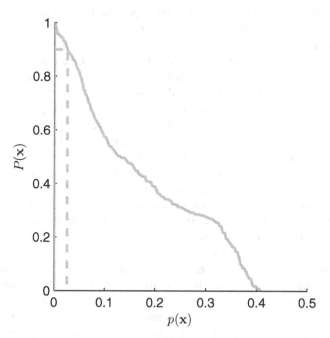

Fig. 2.   P(x) plotted against the $p(x)$ for the Parzen window models of normality. $p(x) = 0.026$ corresponding to $P(x) = 0.9$ is shown by a dashed line.

5   Clinical Study

5.1   Data Collection

The Computer ALerting and Monitoring System-2 (CALMS-2, Oxford, UK) study[2] was conducted in Oxford, UK in 2010-12. Vital-sign data were acquired from 200 patients recovering from upper-gastrointestinal (GI) surgery at the upper-GI ward of the Oxford University Hospitals NHS Trust, Oxford, UK. These patients have a high risk ($\approx$ 20%) of post-operative complications, which often results in an emergency re-admission to the ICU, and a correspondingly high mortality rate.

Out of a total of 233 patients initially consented, 200 remained in the study. The remainder were removed from the study due to revoked consent, transferral to a different ward, early discharge, or due to cancellation of surgery. The median age was 64 years (with an inter-quartile range of 15 years), and the median length-of-stay (LOS) was 10 days (with an inter-quartile range of 7 days). All patients remaining in the study were recovering from upper-gastro intestinal surgery, ranging from whipples (30%), liver resection (10%), hemi-hepatectomy (4%), total gasterectomy (8.5%), and others (28%) including pancreatectomy and splenectomy.

Heart rate (HR), breathing rate (BR), systolic blood pressure (SBP), oxygen saturation (SpO_2), and temperature data were recorded by nurses on the ward, typically every 4 hours using T&T paper charts. A recording was typically made every four hours, and the frequency of recording increased if the patient required greater medical attention. 16,503 T&T observations were recorded on paper charts and were transcribed into two separate electronic databases by two separate research nurses in order to minimise human error during transcription. The first transcription was carried out on a daily basis by a research nurse who would enter data from the previous 24 hours (or 72 hours if following a week-end) into a PDA. The second transcription was carried out when a patient was discharged from the ward. It was performed by a second research nurse who entered the data into a second database without seeing the first PDA database. The two databases were merged by a computer program into a third database, and any transcriptional discrepancies between the two databases were automatically identified. If a discrepancy was too large (i.e., above a certain threshold), a third research nurse corrected the entry by consulting the patient notes. The reconciled database contained the vital-sign values as recorded by the duty nurse, and the individual and aggregate T&T scores as recorded by the duty nurse. It also contained the time of entry to ward and discharge from ward (or time of death for any patient who died on the ward), as well as the times of any pre-scheduled or emergency admissions to ICU, and subsequent return to ward.

176 patients were considered to have had "normal" recovery (with a median LOS in the ward of 8.6 days) and were placed in to a "normal-recovery" group. A normal recovery was deemed to have occured when the patient was discharged from the hospital without any emergency ICU re-admission, and was alive 30 days after discharge. Patients for whom LOS < 4 days or > 30 days were removed from the

---

[2]   Approved by the Oxford Research Ethics Committee, OxREC No. 08/H0607/79.

normal-recovery group. A total of 23 patients had post-surgery emergency ICU admissions or died on the ward, and were placed into an "adverse-event" group.

5.2   Training and Test Sets

We assume that patients in the adverse-event group were most unwell in the hours prior to their adverse event, which may be an emergency ICU admission or death, and that their vital signs at this time were "abnormal". We therefore created a test set containing the last day's vital-sign data from the 23 abnormal patients belonging to the "adverse event" group. Furthermore, we assume that patients in the normal-recovery group were most healthy at the time of discharge from the hospital, and that their vital signs for the 24 hours preceding discharge were "normal". 23 patients from this group were added to the test set. A training set was created which included vital-sign data from the last day in hospital of the remaining 154 patients in the normal-recovery group. We will refer to a patient in the training set as patient i, where $\{i = 1...154\}$. The mean number of T&T observations in the training set was 5.3 samples per patient. There were a total of 872 samples acquired from the 176 patients in the training set.

5.3   Challenge

The low sampling rate of the data (every 4 hours) poses a challenge. It means that there are, on average, 5.3 samples per patient in the normal-recovery group. In previous work [9], it was shown that a population-based model of normality may be constructed using the data in this training set. However such a model does not take into account any uncertainty in the modelling process that may occur due to the small mean sample size of 5.3 samples per patient (taken from the last day of patient observation). [11] used a similar population-based approach, where the vital-sign data in the training set were collected continuously at a sampling rate of one sample every 20 seconds. 18,000 hours of data were collected from a total of 333 patients, with a total of 2×10^6 samples acquired. This gives an average of 54 hours of data per patient, and an average of 9,720 samples per patient. Thus the resulting pdf obtained from the training set could be expected to be an accurate representation of the distribution for each patient. In comparison, the small number of samples per patient in the CALMS-2 dataset means that a population-based approach is therefore no longer suitable, motivating our proposed Bayesian method for patient-based modelling.

6   Methodology and Results

Here we first describe our approach for assessing the performance of the proposed model in the absence of explicit labelling of episodes of deterioration in the vital-sign data, and later present results obtained using this approach. Traditionally, a classification task requires the availability of class labels. If a classifier estimates an "abnormal" event correctly, it is deemed to be a true positive (*TP*) case, and a false negative

(*FN*) case otherwise. Similarly, a correctly classified "normal" event is considered to be a true negative (*TN*) case, and a false positive (*FP*) case otherwise. The performance of the classifier is assessed using two metrics: its sensitivity $= \frac{TP}{TP+FN}$, and its specificity $= \frac{TN}{TN+FP}$. Explicit labelling of adverse events could be carried out by clinical experts who review vital-sign recordings and annotate the recording retrospectively. However, labelling by clinical experts is far from being in common practice, and for large datasets such as the one used in this work, where a patient's vital-sign recording can be > 48 hours on average, and where there are 200 sets of vital-sign recordings, this is not feasible.

Another approach is to use outcome-based labels, such as ICU readmission, death, or discharge. However, in this latter case it is difficult to define an "event" based solely on the outcome. For instance, which period of a patient's vital-sign data should be considered "abnormal" if the patient was ultimately admitted to the ICU under emergency conditions? Abnormality is a patient-specific concept: one patient can have a sudden onset of vital sign abnormality, while another may have a more gradually developing abnormality in their vital signs.

One solution is to define escalation on a per-sample basis, i.e. if any vital-sign sample generates an alarm, it is considered as an escalation. Here there may be multiple escalations for a single patient. A more clinically-sound approach is to consider escalations on a per-patient basis. If, at any point during a vital-sign recording of a patient, an alarm is generated, then the patient is considered to have had a positive event. Thus only one escalation may occur per patient. It might be argued that in the clinical setting, it is only the first alarm that counts; i.e., one alarm is sufficient to indicate that the patient is unwell. However in this case there is a risk of mis-detecting transients due to nurse transcription error as escalations.

There is therefore no ideal solution. As mentioned previously, the traditional metrics of sensitivity and specificity are not suitable for use with our dataset. Therefore we we define the following metrics in order to assess model performance.

6.1   Model Assessment

1. Per-patient assessment. Is an alarm generated during the last 24 hours before an event (or before discharge for the normal patient)? r_1 is defined to be the percentage of patients for whom at least one alarm was generated during the last 24 hours. It is expected that the better system will result in a low value of r_1 for the normal-recovery group, and a high value of r_1 for the adverse-event group.
2. Per-sample assessment. How often does the model generate an alarm for a patient in the last 24 hours? r_2 is defined to be the percentage of a patient's vital-sign data whose corresponding novelty score is above the threshold T in the last 24 hours. Often vital signs, and therefore the corresponding novelty score, will exhibit oscillatory behaviour, even for a normal-recovery patient. If the abnormality is variability-related then we expect an adverse-event patient to have a higher value of r_2 than a normal-recovery patient.

6.2   Results

In the absence of clinically labelled episodes of deterioration, models were assessed using the approach described above. Figure 3 shows the performance of the proposed model when applied to the test set. The population-based model was also tested, the results of which are shown in Figure 4. From Figure 3(a) it may be seen that as the threshold T is raised, r_1 decreases for both normal-recovery and adverse-event groups. This is as expected – with a higher value of the threshold T, more test samples from a patient are considered to be "normal". At $T = 9$, for example, over 94% of the patients in the adverse-event group generate an alarm in the last 24 hours before an event.

However at the same threshold $T = 9$, nearly 40% of the patients in the "normal-recovery group also generate an alarm. This suggests that while at $T = 9$ the proposed method is performing well at detecting "true" deterioration in patients with an adverse event, it is also detecting "false" deterioration in 40% of the patients with no adverse event. However as the threshold is raised the performance of the model improves. At $T = 14$, an alarm is generated in the last 24 hours for 79% of the patients with an

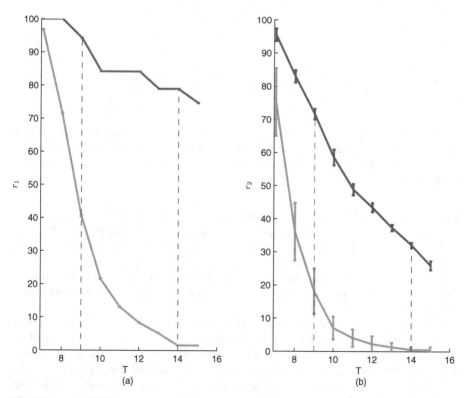

Fig. 3. (a) r_1 and (b) r_2 for the proposed patient-based model, over a range of thresholds T. The average performance for the normal-recovery group, and for the adverse-event group, is shown in green and red, respectively. T = 9 and T = 14 are indicated by dashed lines.

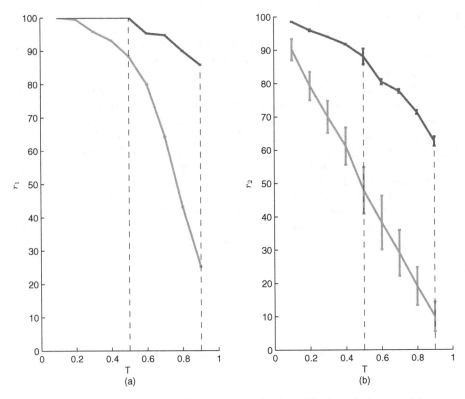

Fig. 4. (a) r_1 and (b) r_2 for the reference population-based Parzen windows model, over a range of thresholds T . The average performance for the normal-recovery group, and for the adverse-event group, is shown in green and red, respectively. T = 0.5 and T = 0.9 are indicated by dashed lines.

adverse event, while it is generated for only 2% of the patients with normal recovery. Additionally, it may be seen from Figure 3(b) that at T = 14, an average of 32% of the vital-sign observations for an adverse-event patient generate an alarm in the last 24 hours before an adverse event, while only 0.5% of the observations of a normal-recovery patient generate an alarm in the last 24 hours before discharge. In comparison, at T = 9, 18% of the total observations of a patient in the normal-recovery group generate an alarm.

A Parzen windows model, as described in Section 4, was also applied to the test set. The threshold range for this method is different from that of the proposed method so it is not possible to compare the results directly. However, at its highest threshold of T = 0.9, the model detects an adverse-event in 86% adverse-event patients, and in 25% normal-recovery patients. Thus while both methods perform well at detecting escalations in the adverse-event patients, the population-based method mis-detects escalations in a maximum of 25% of the normal-recovery patients, compared to a maximum of only 2% with the proposed patient-based method.

7   Discussion and Conclusions

We presented a patient-based model for detection of deterioration in multivariate vital-sign data. The proposed automated method was designed to cope with uncertainty incurred in the modelling process due to low sampling rate of T&T data in a principled manner. It was shown that the model is able to detect deterioration in the T&T vital-sign observations in the 24 hours before an adverse event in 79% patients. The model was also shown to result in 23% fewer mis-detections in normal patients than the reference method.

Although the method described in this paper is a patient-based model, it is not patient-specific – ideally, a patient monitoring system should be able to monitor deviations from population-based norms, as well be able to re-calibrate to monitor any patient-specific departures from the population-based norms. In future work we propose a full Bayesian model averaging approach which considers other parametric forms, and the extension of the proposed model to a fully patient-specific approach.

Acknowledgments. This work was supported by the National Institute for Health Research (NIHR) Biomedical Research Centre Programme, Oxford. The work of S. Khalid was supported by the Rhodes Trust and the Qualcomm Trust. The work of D. Clifton was supported by the Wellcome Trust and Engineering and Physical Sciences Research Council (EPSRC) under Grant WT088877/Z/09/Z.

References

1. Buist, M., Jarmolowski, E., Burton, P., Bernard, S., Waxman, B., Anderson, J.: Recognising clinical instability in hospital patients before cardiac arrest or unplanned admission to intensive care. A pilot study in a tertiary-care hospital. The Medical Journal of Australia 171(1), 22–25 (1999)
2. Sharpley, J., Holden, J.: Introducing an early warning scoring system in a district general hospital. Nursing in Critical Care 9(3), 98–103 (2004)
3. Franklin, C., Mathew, J.: Developing strategies to prevent in-hospital cardiac arrest: analysing responses of physicians and nurses in the hours before the event. Critical Care Medicine 22(2), 244–247 (1994)
4. NCEPOD. An acute problem? A report of the National Confidentiality Enquiry into Patient Outcomes and Death (NCEPOD), NCEPOD, London (2005)
5. Centre for Clinical Practice. Nice Guidelines: Acutely Ill patients in hospital. Technical report, National Institute of Clinical Excellence (2007)
6. Duckitt, R., Buxton-Thomas, R., Walker, J., Cheek, E., Bewick, V., Venn, R., Forni, L.: Worthing physiological scoring system: derivation and validation of a physiological early-warning system for medical admissions. An observational, population-based single-centre study. British Journal of Anaesthesia 98(6), 769–774 (2007)
7. Gardner-Thorpe, J., Love, N., Wrightson, J., Walsh, S., Keeling, N.: The value of Modified Early Warning Score (MEWS) in surgical in-patients: a prospective observational study. Annals of the Royal College of Surgeons of England 88(6), 571–575 (2006)
8. Markou, M., Singh: Novelty detection: a review—part 1: statistical approaches. Signal Processing 83(12), 2481–2497 (2003)

9. Pimentel, M., Clifton, D., Clifton, L., Watkinson, P., Tarassenko, L.: Modelling Physiological Deterioration in Post-operative Patient Vital-Sign Data. Medical & Biological Engineering & Computing (in press), doi: 10.1007/s11517-013-1059-0 [PDF]

10. Hravnak, M., Edwards, L., Clontz, A., Valenta, C., Devita, M., Pinsky, M.: Defining the incidence of cardiorespiratory instability in patients in step-down units using an electronic integrated monitoring system. Archives of Internal Medicine 168(12), 1300–1308 (2008)

11. Tarassenko, L., Hann, A., Patterson, B., Davidson, K., Barber, V.: BioSign TM: Multi-parameter monitoring for early warning of patient deterioration. Medical Applications of Signal Processing, pp. 71–76 (2005)

12. Mackay, D.: Information Theory, Inference, and Learning Algorithms (2003)

13. Duda, R., Hart, P., Stork, D.: Pattern Classification, 2nd edn., p. 654. Wiley-Interscience (2000)

14. Clifton, D.: Novelty Detection with Extreme Value Theory in Jet Engine Vibration Data. PhD Thesis. University of Oxford (2009)

15. Murphy, K.: Machine Learning A Probabilistic Perspective. The MIT Press (2012)

16. Bishop, C.: Pattern Recognition and Machine Learning (Information Science and Statistics). Springer (2007)

17. Hoeting, J., Madigan, D., Raftery, A., Volinsky, C.: Bayesian model averaging: a tutorial. Statistical Science, 382–401 (1999)

18. Clifford, G., Clifton, D.: Wireless Technology in Disease State Management and Medicine. Annual Review of Medicine 63, 479–492 (2010/2012)

19. Khalid, S., Clifton, D., Clifton, L., Tarassenko, L.: A Two-Class Approach to the Detection of Physiological Deterioration in Patient Vital Signs, with Clinical Label Refinement. IEEE Transactions on Information Technology in Biomedicine 16(6), 1231–1238 (2012)

Performance of Early Warning Scoring Systems to Detect Patient Deterioration in the Emergency Department

Mauro D. Santos, David A. Clifton, and Lionel Tarassenko

Institute of Biomedical Engineering, Department of Engineering Science,
University of Oxford, United Kingdom
{mauro.santos,david.clifton,lionel.tarassenko}@eng.ox.ac.uk

Abstract. Acute hospital wards in the UK are required to use Early Warning Scoring (EWS) systems to monitor patients' vital-signs. These are often paper-based, and involve the use of heuristics to score the vital signs which are measured every 2-4 hours by nursing staff. If these scores exceed pre-defined thresholds, the patient is deemed to be at risk of deterioration. In this paper we compare the performance of EWS systems, that use different approaches to score abnormal vital-signs, to identify acutely-ill patients, while attending the Emergency Department (ED). We incorporate the use of data acquired from bed-side monitors into the EWS system, thereby offering the possibility of performing patient observations automatically, between manual observations.

Keywords: Emergency Department, Early Warning Scoring System, Receiver Operator Characteristic Analysis.

1 Introduction

The ED is often one of the busiest wards in the hospital due to unscheduled admissions, diverse patient clinical conditions, and the requirement to diagnose, provide initial treatment, and discharge 98% of the patients within 4 hours within the UK NHS [1]. In these conditions, patient deterioration may be missed between clinical observations. Vital signs are often monitored using paper-based Track and Trigger (T&T) charts, where an alert is generated if the combined scores of heart rate (HR), respiration rate (RR), oxygen saturation (SpO_2), systolic blood pressure (Sys BP), temperature (Temp), and Glasgow Coma Scale (GCS) is higher than a predefined threshold. T&T charts use Early Warning Scoring (EWS) systems to score vital-signs and although a wide variety of EWS systems have been proposed, there is no clear evidence for their validity, reliability, utility, or performance [2,3]. Continuous monitoring systems such as bed-side monitors are also present in some areas of the ED and can identify, during the intervals between the intermittent nurse observations, patients who will require escalation of care in the ED. However, studies have shown that these systems suffer from a high rate of false alerts, such that they are often ignored [4].

J. Gibbons and W. MacCaull (Eds.): FHIES 2013, LNCS 8315, pp. 159–169, 2014.
© Springer-Verlag Berlin Heidelberg 2014

1.1 Patient Care in the Emergency Department

Depending on the triage result the patient is sent to one of three areas in the ED[1]: "Minors" , "Majors" , or the "Resuscitation room" (Resus). The Minors area admits patients who do not require immediate treatment, and whose condition is deemed to be of low severity. The Majors area accommodates adult patients that have a high likelihood of needing further treatment in the hospital, and Resus includes patients with life-threatening illnesses or injury.

The frequency of the clinical observations taken by nurses is dependent on the area of the ED to which the patient has been admitted and on the patient's condition. Patients from Majors and Resus will typically also be continuously monitored, being connected to bed-side monitors.

2   Methods

2.1 Dataset

We used a dataset obtained from 3039 patients (age > 15 years), from an observational study that occurred in 2012, in the Majors area of the ED of the John Radcliffe Hospital, Oxford (Figure 1). A total of 6812 clinical observations, comprising the vital signs previously mentioned, were collected from ED T&T paper charts. About 6325 hours of continuous vital-sign data comprising HR, RR, and SpO_2 were obtained, sampled approximately every 30 seconds, and BP sampled every 30 minutes, from bed-side monitors. Patients are observed by nursing staff every hour in the Majors area if the vital signs are normal, and at 30- and 15-minute intervals when the EWS is greater than or equal to 3. Nurses report to the hospital's Electronic Patient Record (EPR) System the times the patients moved between different ED clinical areas. The times of patients moving from the Majors to the Resus area were collected from this system. All data was anonymised with study numbers.

2.2 Early Warning Scoring Systems

One single-parameter EWS and three multi-parameter EWS systems are used in the retrospective analysis of the dataset:

1. The single-parameter EWS is called Medical Emergency Team (MET, Table 2) calling criteria [5], which is used to call a Medical Emergency Team when there are gross changes in a single vital sign or a sudden fall in the level of consciousness. It was implemented with the assumption that the physiological processes underlying catastrophic deterioration, such as cardiopulmonary arrest, are identifiable and treatable 6 to 8 hours before the condition occurs [5,6]. This system has the advantage of being easy for clinical staff to follow.

---

[1] This set of ED areas exists in the John Radcliffe Hospital, Oxford, equivalents to which may be found in most UK hospitals.

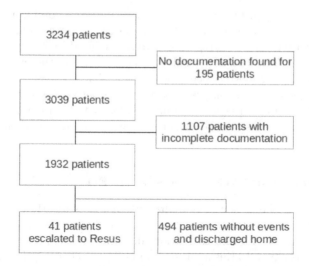

Fig. 1. Consort Diagram with the total amount of patients attending the ED Majors area between April 23rd and June 10th, 2012, and number of patients with and without escalation events used to study the performance of EWS in identifying physiological deterioration.

2. The modified EWS (MEWS, Table 3) [7] is a multi-parameter system where abnormal vital-signs (HR, RR, SpO$_2$, Sys BP, Temp, and GCS) are scored as 0, 1, 2 or 3 according to their level of abnormality. If one of the individual scores is 3 or if the aggregated score is greater than or equal to 3, 4 or 5 (see below) the patient is considered to be at risk of deteriorating and a clinical review is requested. In our analysis, we test an aggregated score of 3 or 4 for MEWS to trigger an alert. Also the abnormal thresholds previously described were assigned to vital-signs according to expert opinion from doctors working at the John Radcliffe ED [8].
3. The centile-based EWS, (CEWS, Table 4) [9] has scores assigned to the vital signs depending on their centile value in a distribution computed from 64,622 h of vital sign data. We also perform the analysis with alerting thresholds of 3 and 4 for the aggregated score for CEWS.
4. The National EWS (NEWS, Table 5) [10] where the scores are optimised for predicting 24-hour mortality. It uses scores of 3 and 5 for the single and multi-parameter alerting criteria, respectively. This system uses an additional parameter: the presence of supplemental oxygen provided to the patient, which adds 2 points to the total score.

2.3   Application of EWS to Bed-Side Monitor Data

In this paper we use the EWS systems to score physiological abnormality both on the intermittent vital signs collected by nurses (i.e. the clinical observations), as well as the continuous vital-sign data collected by bed-side monitors. EWS systems were created primarily to manage the patient's condition using intermittent observations. Applying an EWS to continuous data requires a different methodology to trigger an alert, since artefacts caused by body movement or probe disconnection could easily result in a false alert. We therefore use a "persistence criterion": an alert is deemed to begin if a physiological abnormality (EWS above alerting threshold) is scored for 4 minutes in a 5-minute window, and is deemed to end if less than 1 minute of physiological abnormality exists in a 3-minute window. This criterion has been applied in other patient monitoring studies [11].

2.4   Performance of EWS Systems in the ED

This paper follows the patient-based analysis formulated in [12]. From the 3039 patients, we focus on "stable" and "unstable" (or "event") patients that presented both complete clinical observations documentation and bed-side monitor data (continuous data). In this analysis, "stable" patients comprise patients that did not move to Resus, and who were discharged home at the end of their stay in the Majors area (494 patients). 65 patients needed to be removed due to incomplete timestamps documentation. "event" patients include patients that were escalated from Majors to Resus, due to physiological abnormality during their stay in the ED, including neurological abnormality (41 patients). Inaccuracies may exist in reporting this data in the EPR, therefore only escalations happening 30 minutes after the patient arrival to the ED were considered. Earlier escalations times could have already been planned at patient arrival (for example for patients coming in an ambulance).

The remaining patients, that had both clinical observations and continuous data, but were admitted elsewhere in the hospital, were removed from this analysis. These patients may have had other escalations that did not require them to move to Resus. The analysis was subsequently carried out on a total of 494 patients, with a total of 1519 observations sets and about 1318 hours of continuous bed-side monitor data.

True Positives (TP) are defined as the "event" patients for whom moving to Resus was detected successfully by an abnormal period scored by the EWS systems. False Negatives (FN) are "event" patients that were not detected because no abnormal periods were identified by the EWS system under consideration. We define a TP to have occurred if the alert is generated within an interval t before the first escalation and 10 min after the escalation (because the times of escalation to Resus are not precise). For this study, the performance of the systems is evaluated when the interval $t = 1$ hour.

A True Negative (TN) is considered to be a "stable" patient for whom there were no alerts generated and finally a False Positive (FP) is a "stable" patient for whom at least one alert was generated. One of the effects of the use of this methodology is the fact that the specificity (defined as being $\frac{TN}{FP+TN}$) will be the same in all cases since the TN and FP do not depend on time t.

The performance of the EWS systems as a tool to detect patient deterioration in "event" patients is analysed for five different patient monitoring cases: (a) using nurses' intermittent clinical observations data only; (b) using bed-side monitor continuous data only; (c) using bed-side monitor continuous data with the persistence criterion (as explained in section 2.3); (d) using clinical observations and continuous data; and (e) using clinical observations and continuous data with the persistence criteria. Cases (a), (c) and (e) try to simulate three possible scenarios of patient monitoring in an ED. Cases (b) and (c) allow the effect of the persistence criterion on alert generation on continuous data to be studied. The accuracy ($ACC = \frac{TP+TN}{TP+TN+FP+FN}$) and the Matthews correlation coefficient (MCC) were used to study the performance. The MCC is a balanced measure of quality of binary classifications, which can be used even if the classes are of very different sizes [2].

3   Results

The median time to escalation to the Resus area for the "event" patients considered in this paper was 1.8 hours (range is 38 min to 9 hours, Figure 2). Patient that were escalated to the Resus area within the first 30 min were assumed to be escalated at arrival. In this paper we are interested in reviewing the use of EWS in patients that escalated after arrival.

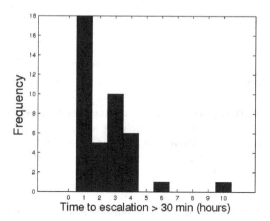

Fig. 2. a) Distribution of time from patients arrival to the ED Majors area to their escalation to the Resus areas. The escalations that happened within 30 min of the patient arrival to the ED were removed. The mean and median times to escalation for a total of 41 patients are 2.4 hours and 1.8 hours respectively (range is from 38 min to 9 hours).

---

[2] $MCC = \frac{TP*TN - FP*FN}{\sqrt{(TP+FP)(TP+FN)(TN+FP)(TN+FN)}}$. The MCC returns a value between -1 and 1. 1 represents a perfect prediction, 0 no better than random prediction and -1 indicates total disagreement between prediction and observation.

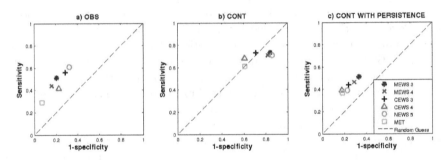

Fig. 3. Performance of EWS systems when considering patients escalated to Resus after arrival for three monitoring cases, and two different aggregated score thresholds for MEWS and CEWS. When appropriate, the aggregated score threshold used is presented next to the EWS system in the legend.

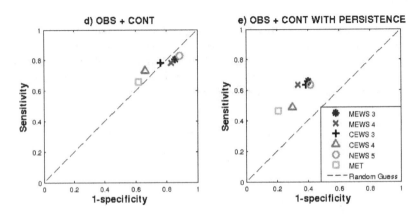

Fig. 4. Performance of EWS systems when considering patients escalated to Resus after arrival for the ideal patient monitoring cases, with and without persistence criterion on the continuous data and two different aggregated score thresholds for MEWS and CEWS. When appropriate, the aggregated score threshold used is presented next to the EWS system in the legend.

Table 1. Results of performance of EWS systems to identify physiological deterioration within 1 hour of the escalation to Resus. Results are sorted by accuracy (ACC).

EWS System	TP	TN	SE (%)	SP (%)	ACC (%)	MCC
MET	19	390	46	79	76	0.16
CEWS 4	20	345	49	70	68	0.107
MEWS 4	26	328	63	66	66	0.165
CEWS 3	26	303	63	61	61	0.134
MEWS 3	27	295	66	60	60	0.138
NEWS 5	26	289	63	59	59	0.118
Total	41	494	-	-	-	-

Figure 3 shows the performance results for detecting physiological abnormality, using the EWS systems previously described, within 1 hour of the escalation time, when only using either the clinical observations or the continuous data. These are shown in a Receiver Operator Characteristic (ROC) plot. The system with best accuracy and MCC was MET when using the clinical observations (ACC=88% and MCC=0.21, Table 6). When only using clinical observations MEWS shows the next best performance, but when using continuous data CEWS shows higher accuracy then MEWS, but lower MCC. The best performing systems present high specificity (70 to 80%) but low sensitivity (30 to 50 %). The use of continuous data without the persistence criterion generates many false alerts, contributing for a lower accuracy.

Figure 4 shows the performance of EWS systems when using both clinical observations and continuous data, and consequently the combination of their alerting criteria. Case (d), with no persistence criterion for the continuous data presents a low accuracy ($<$50%). The ideal patient monitoring case should use the persistence criterion on continuous data, and although this presents a lower sensitivity, the accuracy is indeed improved because it generates much less false alerts. These results are shown in Table 6 for case (e). The system with highest accuracy for the ideal patient monitoring scenario was MET (76%) followed by CEWS, with an aggregate score threshold of 4, and the worst accuracy is observed for NEWS (59%).

When taking the MCC into account, MET (MCC=0.16) is followed by MEWS instead, CEWS scoring the lowest MCC with an aggregated score of 4 (M=0.107), but scoring higher than NEWS when using and aggregated score of 3.

4   Discussion

We start by noting that some noise may be present in the selected dataset, due to the nature of the work in the ED. It may happen that some patients from Majors should have gone to the Resus area, but because there was no space in this area, they remained in the same area to be treated. Patients that escalated to the Resus areas within 30 min could fall in this category. Furthermore, the group of patients without Resus escalations may contain numerous examples of abnormality, and therefore contribute to the total number of FP.

A period of t=1 hour before the escalation was selected due to the fact that in clinical practise, doctors are required to review the patient within 1 hour of the EWS alert. This was a first approach to include this clinical response delay into our analysis.

Applying EWS systems to the continuous data identified more patients with physiological abnormality within 1 hour of being escalated than when using only manually observed data. Although the use of the persistence criterion increased the accuracy, it decreased the sensitivity: 46% in the cases of the system with best accuracy in the ideal patient monitoring scenario, case (e). Increasing the aggregated score alerting threshold also improved the accuracy of the systems (but not the MCC in the case of CEWS). The final results are shown in Table 6 in the appendices.

There are a number of challenges in calibrating these systems. It is interesting to observe that MET showed a better accuracy and MCC than the multi-parameter EWS in the ideal monitoring scenario (e). Both MET and MEWS perform better when clinical observations are used, and CEWS performs better when using continuous data, in particular when the persistence criteria is not present because it has smoother transitions between the abnormal thresholds. This may indicate that these systems are tuned to the data sources used to built them, since CEWS was derived from a large dataset of bed-side monitor data.

Finally, NEWS, which is also an evidence-based system, optimized to predict patient mortality in 24 hours, presented the lowest accuracy in identifying physiological deterioration in patients requiring to move to Resus, when using both clinical observations and continuous data.

5 Conclusion

Our patient-based analysis has allowed us to evaluate the performance of different EWS systems in identifying patients who needed to be escalated to the Resus area to avoid further deterioration, while attending the ED. In this analysis, when using both clinical observations and continuous data (with a persistence criterion) an expert based system, MET, showed the best overall accuracy, although it presented low sensitivity, followed by an evidence-based system derived from vital-signs distributions (CEWS), while an evidence-based system optimized to predict patient mortality in 24 hours (NEWS) presented the lowest accuracy.

6 Future Work

We are currently undertaking a 3-stage observational study [8]. In each stage, data from 3000 patients will be captured for 2-month periods. In this trial we will test how introducing a system that calculates the EWS electronically, on hand-held devices, and a data fusion system that analyses bed-side monitor data [11], will influence short-term mortality and hospital length of stay. Other secondary outcomes such as escalation to the Resus area (used in this analysis) and admission to the Intensive Care Unit, will also be collected.

The current vital-sign scoring systems do not take the dynamical changes of the vital signs into account, and generating clinically useful alerts from abnormal trends within the heterogeneous population attending an ED requires a large amount of validated clinical data. We intend to demonstrate the importance of introducing trend analysis and prior information into the vital-sign scoring models.

The response of clinical staff may also play an important role in how these decision support systems should be delivered. For instance, the escalation pathway used in our current EWS system requires that a doctor should review a patient within 1 hour of the EWS alert. We aim to introduce this information into our analysis to better calibrate the electronic decision support systems.

Acknowledgements. This work was supported by the NIHR Biomedical Research Centre Programme, Oxford. Mauro Santos, would like to acknowledge the support of the RCUK Digital Economy Programme grant number EP/G036861/1 (Oxford Centre for Doctoral Training in Healthcare Innovation). David A. Clifton was supported by the Centre of Excellence in Personalised Healthcare funded by the Wellcome Trust and EPSRC under grant number WT 088877/Z/09/Z.

References

1. NICE: Acutely ill patients in hospital, CG50 (2007), http://www.nice.org.uk/
2. Gao, H., McDonnell, A., Harrison, D.A., Moore, T., Adam, S., Daly, K., Esmonde, L., Goldhill, D.R., Parry, G.J., Rashidian, A., Subbe, C.P., Harvey, S.: Systematic review and evaluation of physiological track and trigger warning systems for identifying at-risk patients on the ward. Intensive Care Medicine 33(4), 667–679 (2007)
3. Kyriacos, U., Jelsma, J., Jordan, S.: Monitoring vital signs using early warning scoring systems: a review of the literature. Journal of Nursing Management 19(3), 311–330 (2011)
4. Tsien, C.L., Fackler, J.C.: Poor prognosis for existing monitors in the intensive care unit. Critical Care Medicine 25(4), 614–619 (1997)
5. DeVita, M., Braithwaite, R., Mahidhara, R., Stuart, S., Foraida, M., Simmons, R.: Use of medical emergency team responses to reduce hospital cardiopulmonary arrests. Quality & Safety in Health Care 13(4), 251–254 (2004)
6. Etter, R., Ludwig, R., Lersch, F., Takala, J., Merz, T.: Early prognostic value of the medical emergency team calling criteria in patients admitted to intensive care from the emergency department. Critical Care Medicine 36(3), 775–781 (2008)
7. Subbe, C.P., Kruger, M., Rutherford, P., Gemmel, L.: Validation of a modified early warning score in medical admissions. QJM: Monthly Journal of the Association of Physicians 94(10), 521–526 (2001)
8. Clifton, D.A., Wong, D., Fleming, S., Wilson, S.J., Way, R., Pullinger, R., Tarassenko, L.: Novelty detection for identifying deterioration in emergency department patients. In: Yin, H., Wang, W., Rayward-Smith, V. (eds.) IDEAL 2011. LNCS, vol. 6936, pp. 220–227. Springer, Heidelberg (2011)
9. Tarassenko, L., Clifton, D.A., Pinsky, M.R., Hravnak, M.T., Woods, J.R., Watkinson, P.J.: Centile-based early warning scores derived from statistical distributions of vital signs. Resuscitation 82(8), 1013–1018 (2011)
10. RCP London: National early warning score (NEWS): standardising the assessment of acute-illness severity in the NHS - report of a working party (2012)
11. Tarassenko, L., Hann, A., Young, D.: Integrated monitoring and analysis for early warning of patient deterioration. British Journal of Anaesthesia 97(1), 64–68 (2006)
12. Clifton, D., Wong, D., Clifton, L., Wilson, S., Way, R., Pullinger, R., Tarassenko, L.: A large-scale clinical validation of an integrated monitoring system in the emergency department. IEEE Journal of Biomedical and Health Informatics 17(4), 835–842 (2013)

Appendix: EWS Systems Criteria

Table 2. Single-channel Medical Emergency Team (MET) abnormal vital-signs criteria [5]. Only the parameters that are used in the analysis are shown in this table.

	Lower Limit	Upper Limit
HR (bpm)	40	140
RR (rpm)	8	36
Sys BP (mmHg)	80	200
Dia BP (mmHg)	-	110
SpO$_2$ (%)	80	-
Temp (°C)	-	-
GCS	13 or decrease in GCS $\geq$ 2	-

Table 3. MEWS system, used in the ED of John Radcliffe Hospital until 2010 [8].

Score:	3	2	1	0	1	2	3
HR (bpm)		$\leq$ 40	41 - 50	51 - 100	101 - 110	111 - 129	$\geq$ 130
RR (rpm)	$\leq$ 8			9 - 18	19 - 24	25 - 29	$\geq$ 30
SpO$_2$ (%)	$\leq$ 92			$\geq$ 93			
Sys BP (mmHg)	$\leq$ 90	91 - 99		100 - 179			$\geq$ 180
Temp (°C)		$\leq$ 35		35.1 - 39.9			$\geq$ 38
GCS	$\leq$ 12	13	14	15			

Table 4. CEWS system [9], currently used in the ED of the John Radcliffe Hospital.

Score:	3	2	1	0	1	2	3
HR (bpm)	$\leq$ 42	43 - 49	50 - 53	54 - 104	105 - 112	113 - 127	$\geq$ 128
RR (rpm)	$\leq$ 7	8 - 10	11 - 13	14 - 25	26 - 28	29 - 33	$\geq$ 34
SpO$_2$ (%)	$\leq$ 84	85 - 90	91 - 93	$\geq$ 94			
Sys BP (mmHg)	$\leq$ 85	86 - 96	97 - 101	102 - 154	155 - 164	165 - 184	$\geq$ 185
Temp (°C)	$\leq$ 35.4		35.5 - 36.9	36.1 - 37.3	37.4 - 38.3		$\geq$ 38.4
GCS	$\leq$ 13		14	15			

Table 5. NEWS system [10]. * The conversion used between GCS and AVPU is: GCS 15 = A; GCS 14 = V; GCS 13 - 9 = P; GCS $\leq$ 8 = U. Since V, P, U are considered score 3 in NEWS, a GCS equal or lower to 14 is used in score 3.

Score:	3	2	1	0	1	2	3
HR (bpm)	≤ 40		41 - 50	51 - 90	91 - 110	111 - 130	≥ 131
RR (rpm)	≤ 8		9 - 11	12 - 20		21 - 24	≥ 25
SpO$_2$ (%)	≤ 91	92 - 93	94 - 95	≥ 96			
Sys BP (mmHg)	≤ 90	91 - 100	101 - 110	111 - 219			≥ 220
Temp (°C)	≤ 35		35.1 - 36.0	36.1 - 38.0	38.1 - 39.0	≥ 39.1	
GCS*	≤ 14			15			
Supplemental O$_2$						Yes	

Table 6. Results of performance of EWS systems to identify deterioration in a window of 1 hour before the escalation (sorted by ACC).The abnormal threshold for the aggregated score is shown next to the system's name. CONT' - the persistence criterion was used in these cases.

Case	EWS System	TP	TN	SS	SP	ACC	MCC
OBS	MET	12.0	459.0	29.3	92.9	88.0	0.21
OBS	MEWS 4	18.0	416.0	43.9	84.2	81.1	0.19
CONT'	CEWS 4	16.0	407.0	39.0	82.4	79.1	0.14
CONT'	MET	15.0	405.0	36.6	82.0	78.5	0.12
OBS	MEWS 3	21.0	392.0	51.2	79.4	77.2	0.19
OBS + CONT'	MET	19.0	390.0	46.3	78.9	76.4	0.16
OBS	CEWS 4	17.0	382.0	41.5	77.3	74.6	0.12
CONT'	NEWS 5	16.0	382.0	39.0	77.3	74.4	0.1
CONT'	CEWS 3	18.0	377.0	43.9	76.3	73.8	0.12
OBS	CEWS 3	23.0	352.0	56.1	71.3	70.1	0.16
CONT'	MEWS 4	19.0	351.0	46.3	71.1	69.2	0.1
OBS + CONT'	CEWS 4	20.0	345.0	48.8	69.8	68.2	0.11
OBS	NEWS 5	25.0	334.0	61.0	67.6	67.1	0.16
OBS + CONT'	MEWS 4	26.0	328.0	63.4	66.4	66.2	0.17
CONT'	MEWS 3	21.0	330.0	51.2	66.8	65.6	0.1
OBS + CONT'	CEWS 3	26.0	303.0	63.4	61.3	61.5	0.13
OBS + CONT'	MEWS 3	27.0	295.0	65.9	59.7	60.2	0.14
OBS + CONT'	NEWS 5	26.0	289.0	63.4	58.5	58.9	0.12
CONT	CEWS 4	28.0	194.0	68.3	39.3	41.5	0.04
CONT	MET	25.0	194.0	61.0	39.3	40.9	0
OBS + CONT	MET	27.0	188.0	65.9	38.1	40.2	0.02
OBS + CONT	CEWS 4	30.0	166.0	73.2	33.6	36.6	0.04
CONT	CEWS 3	30.0	143.0	73.2	28.9	32.3	0.01
OBS + CONT	CEWS 3	32.0	117.0	78.0	23.7	27.9	0.01
CONT	MEWS 4	29.0	89.0	70.7	18.0	22.1	-0.08
OBS + CONT	MEWS 4	32.0	83.0	78.0	16.8	21.5	-0.04
CONT	MEWS 3	30.0	78.0	73.2	15.8	20.2	-0.08
OBS + CONT	MEWS 3	33.0	70.0	80.5	14.2	19.3	-0.04
CONT	NEWS 5	29.0	70.0	70.7	14.2	18.5	-0.11
OBS + CONT	NEWS 5	34.0	56.0	82.9	11.3	16.8	-0.05
Total	-	41	494	-	-	-	-

Early Fault Detection Using Design Models for Collision Prevention in Medical Equipment*

Arjan J. Mooij[1], Jozef Hooman[1,2], and Rob Albers[3]

[1] Embedded Systems Innovation (ESI) by TNO, P.O. Box 513, 5600 MB Eindhoven,
The Netherlands
{arjan.mooij,jozef.hooman}@tno.nl
[2] Computing Science Department, Radboud University Nijmegen, The Netherlands
[3] Philips Healthcare, Best, The Netherlands
r.albers@philips.com

Abstract. In the medical domain there is a tension between the requested speed of innovation and the time needed to deliver a certifiable system. To ensure the required safety, usually a long test and integration phase is needed. To shorten this phase and to avoid late bug fixing, the aim is to detect faults (if any) much earlier in the development process. This can be achieved by combining a number of model-based techniques such as (1) architecture validation by simulating executable models, (2) development of a Domain-Specific Language (DSL) to combine precision with higher levels of abstraction, and (3) transformations from DSLs to analysis models for performance evaluation and formal verification. We illustrate such techniques using an industrial study project on a new architecture for movement control including collision prevention.

1 Introduction

In the medical domain there is a tension between the requested speed of innovation and the time needed to deliver a certifiable system. To ensure the required safety, usually a long test and integration phase is needed. The problem is that often faults are found in this late phase of the development process.

In industrial development processes, the first formal artefacts are usually at the level of implementation code (or close to it), whereas the architecture and design phases are based on informal documents; see Fig. 1(a). Faults are often detected during or after developing such formal artefacts. However, the detected faults do not only include implementation faults, but also faults that were introduced in the requirements, architecture and design phases [19]. For example, during test and integration it may turn out that the requirements are incomplete, or that a design cannot fulfil the requirements. Such faults are often costly to repair in such a late phase.

The aim of our work is to detect such faults (if any) much earlier in the development process, thus reducing late bug fixing in the test and integration phase,

---

* This research was supported by the Dutch national program COMMIT and carried out as part of the Allegio project.

J. Gibbons and W. MacCaull (Eds.): FHIES 2013, LNCS 8315, pp. 170–187, 2014.

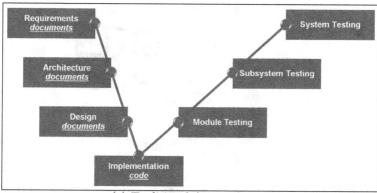

(a) Traditional Approach

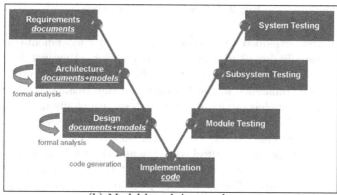

(b) Model-based Approach

Fig. 1. Development Processes and Phases

and hence increasing the rate of innovation. To this end, we combine a number of model-based techniques, which introduce formality in earlier development phases; see Fig. 1(b). We emphasize high-level design models and their potential for early analysis.

We have applied these techniques while participating in an industrial study project at Philips Healthcare, in the context of interventional X-ray systems; see Fig. 2. Such systems are used for minimally-invasive surgery, where X-ray images guide the surgeon during an operation. These systems consist of one or two so-called C-arms, each carrying an X-ray generator and a detector. During the treatment, the C-arms, the detectors, and the patient table may move to obtain optimal projections for the images.

Physical safety of these systems includes avoiding any collisions between these heavy moving objects and the humans, such as patient and medical staff. The study project has focused on redesigning the software components for movement control, which includes functionality for collision detection and prevention.

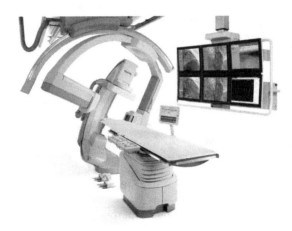

Fig. 2. Interventional X-Ray system

We have first developed a reference architecture for movement control. Architectures are usually described using informal drawings. However, it is difficult to use such drawings to decide whether the architecture will really work in practice. To obtain more confidence in the feasibility of the architecture, we have used high-level formal models, which can be analysed using simulation and domain visualization. By limiting the amount of detail in such models, the required effort remains acceptable. In our experience, such models trigger more detailed discussions about the architectural concepts and their interactions.

Afterwards we have designed the component that is responsible for collision prevention. The main challenges were to identify the main reasoning concepts, and to represent the rules for collision prevention in a concise, precise and readable way, such that they can be inspected and analysed easily. To stay close to the requirements formulation, we have developed a Domain-Specific Language (DSL) that is targeted at the type of rules we want to express. We have generated code from these DSL models, and evaluated it on the physical hardware. In addition we have analysed these models by defining transformations to and from several analysis tools. As the collision prevention component is a safety-critical real-time component, we have evaluated the required execution time and we have verified some formal correctness properties.

Overview In Sect. 2 we address the description and analysis of the proposed reference architecture. In Sect. 3 we focus on the design and analysis of the collision prevention component. In Sect. 4 we discuss related work. Finally, in Sect. 5 we draw some conclusions and sketch further work.

2   Reference Architecture for Movement Control

In this section we focus on the architecture phase from Fig. 1(b), where the aim was to develop a reference architecture for movement control. An architecture provides a high-level view of a specific system, whereas a reference architecture

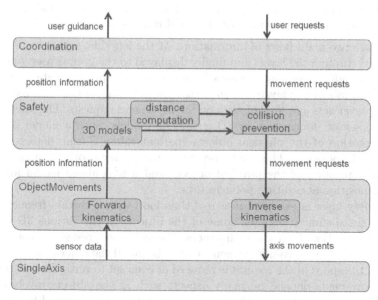

Fig. 3. Reference Architecture for Movement Control

provides a high-level view of a family of systems (or a product line). Architectures are developed in an early development phase, where the goal is to decompose the functionality in layers and components, and to identify the interfaces.

Traditionally (reference) architectures are described using various informal drawings that are easy to make and modify. However, once the developers start to reach an agreement on such informal drawings, it is still very difficult to decide whether the architecture will really work in practice. Often the only way to decide this is to start implementing it.

To gain more confidence in the feasibility of the architecture, we investigate the use of formal modelling and analysis. In this development phase, where there are many uncertainties and fast experimentation with variations is needed, it is inappropriate to make a detailed formal model of the complete system. It would be too time consuming, both to design and to modify the model, and it would require too many details. In a later phase, it may be useful to model and analyse some safety-critical components in detail. In this section we discuss the potential for high-level formal modelling and analysis in the architecture phase.

2.1 Reference Architecture for Movement Control

Fig. 3 contains a simplified description of the reference architecture for movement control that was proposed in this study project and that uses a layered approach [8]. It consists of four layers:

- *Coordination*: interaction with the user about movements and procedures;
- *Safety*: restriction of movement requests in order to prevent collisions;

- *ObjectMovements*: translation of complex movements to individual axes;
- *SingleAxis*: interaction with the physical motors and sensors.

There are two main flows of information. At the left side, sensor readings are propagated through the layers and finally displayed to the user as user guidance. At the right side, movement requests from the user are propagated to motors.

The interfaces of the layers are such that the safety layer can be removed; so the safety layer acts as a kind of filter on the movement requests. The safety layer stores the sensor information in 3D geometric models. Such a model contains a representation of the physical objects (patient table, C-arm, detector, etc.) and their 3D position. The safety layer contains, among others, a model for the current position of the physical objects and a look-ahead model for their expected position at a future point in time.

The safety layer is executed in a real-time loop with a certain frequency. In this loop the distances between some of the objects in the various 3D models are computed. Based on these distances, the collision prevention component determines whether a given movement request is safe. If the request might lead to collisions, the speed of the request is reduced or even set to zero. The restrictions on the movements depend on many aspects such as the objects involved, the accelerations and positions of the objects, the reaction time needed to influence movements and the required brake distances. Look-ahead models are needed to take response times and brake distances into account.

2.2   Required Functionality for Movement Control

The architecture phase has also been used to increase the insight in the functionality that needs to be redesigned. In this type of systems there is always a tension between safety and usability. On the one hand no dangerous situation may be introduced, but on the other hand the physician wants to have maximum freedom in controlling the system to obtain optimal projections for the images. Moreover, users expect a very predictable system.

The existing system has evolved over many years, starting as a simple X-ray system for diagnosis, and later on extended with functionality for interventional X-ray, 3D scans, and hybrid operating rooms. In particular the latter leads to new requirements and interfaces for additional external equipment. There have also been several modifications and extensions on request of medical users. To achieve a consistent user experience within the product family, both regular design decisions and late modifications may become requirements that restrict the design of future systems. These trends have introduced a number of incidental complexities and intricate dependencies between pieces of functionality.

To be able to develop a new reference architecture where components have clear responsibilities and clean interfaces, it was essential to challenge the need for complex functionality and to identify the real underlying requirements. By discussions with domain specialists, the requirements have been simplified significantly, eliminating some notorious complexities and disentangling pieces of functionality. We expect that these simplifications will reduce the potential for faults in further development phases.

2.3   High-level, Formal Modelling

Before starting the implementation, we would like to validate the architecture
in order to reduce risks. For instance, to gain confidence that several typical
scenarios can really be implemented effectively, and to investigate how the architectural choices impact the system as the user would experience it. To keep
the workload manageable, it is crucial to focus on critical scenarios that have a
high impact on the system. In this application, we have considered some manual joystick movements and a few medical procedures that involve moving the
C-arm according to a special trajectory.

To perform such validation, we have added some formality to the informal
drawings such that we obtain executable models. In this development phase
we only make high-level models that abstract from many of the details. We
have used very simplistic models of the hardware (motors and sensors); detailed
models with continuous behaviour and differential equations are far outside our
scope. Making such models triggers many questions to the developers about
their exact ideas. By clarifying these issues in an early development phase, costly
misunderstandings and repairs later on can be avoided.

To model the relevant scenarios, we have used a language called POOSL (Parallel Object-Oriented Specification Language, [31]), which has a formal semantics
defined in terms of a timed probabilistic labelled transition systems. POOSL uses
two types of building blocks: cluster (with a blue border) and process (with a
black border). Clusters can contain again clusters and processes, and thus they
can be used to model hierarchical system structures. Processes focus on individual behaviours and are specified using a textual object-oriented process algebra.
Each block has an external interface consisting of ports (drawn near its border)
that can be used for synchronous one-to-one message communication; that is, a
message can be communicated when a pair of a sender and a receiver are both
ready for communication.

Fig. 4(a) shows the graphical representation of our POOSL model in the
SHESim tool [14]. All the blocks in this diagram are clusters. In particular in
the bottom left corner there are four clusters for the architectural layers from
Fig. 3. The other blocks are clusters that expose the external interfaces of the
architecture to other validation tools as we need in the next section. In turn,
Fig. 4(b) shows the graphical representation of one of the clusters. All the blocks
in this diagram are processes. Processes themselves are specified textually. Most
of our processes follow the structure of a state machine.

Note that in this development phase we do not aim at formal verification.
The emphasis is on rapid prototyping of architectural concepts in a powerful
modelling language. Formal verification would impose additional restrictions on
the models and would require further abstractions from many relevant data
aspects, such as 3D position information and movement requests.

It is not easy to show that later implementations of the architecture are a formal refinement of our architectural model. Our high-level models do not cover
all scenarios, they typically ignore detailed timing issues, and they can use simplified external interfaces. Hence, at best we can expect this refinement only

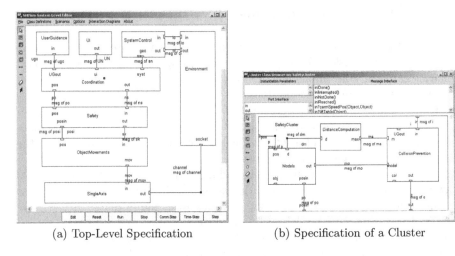

(a) Top-Level Specification   (b) Specification of a Cluster

Fig. 4. Executable Model in POOSL

for restricted scenarios, and with additional conversions to make the interfaces homogeneous; see also [19]. In this study project we have not tried to show any formal refinement between different models. Still the analysis of individual design models gives useful results.

2.4   Interactive Simulation and Domain Visualization

To validate the modelled behaviour, we use interactive simulation. In our experience, it is important to relate the architectural model to the user-perceived system behaviour. That is, not only consider internal software aspects, but also include their impact on the full system. This includes user interactions and external system behaviour such as physical movements and X-ray. To achieve this, we combine simulation with domain visualizations [24,19].

Fig. 5 shows the combination of simulation and two types of domain visualization. In the middle there is a simulator for the architectural model, which focuses on the system's functionality. At the left side there is a Java GUI that simulates user interfaces such as joysticks, that displays user guidance messages, and that can inject special simulated events such as faults or collisions. At the right side there is a 3D model of the physical hardware that is modelled using the 3D modelling and game engine Blender [7]. It shows the physical state of the system, and it can be used to trigger X-ray requests via the pedals.

For example, by clicking on the picture of the joysticks, the user can trigger events that start a movement or select a certain medical procedure that involves movements. These events are sent to the simulator of the architecture. The architectural model then determines whether certain user guidance messages have to be generated; in this case an event is send to the Java GUI. The architectural model might also trigger certain movements; in this case events are send to Blender. The communication between these tools uses sockets (see also [24,19]).

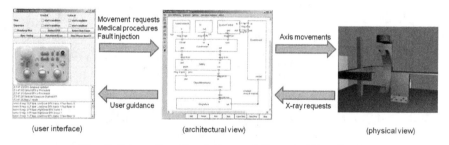

(user interface)   (architectural view)   (physical view)

Fig. 5. Interactive Simulation and Domain Visualization

The combination of interactive simulation and domain visualization helps to see the impact of design decisions on the system as a whole. Moreover, it turns out to trigger again a lot of discussion, although there was common agreement on the earlier informal drawings. Certain implications, omissions or faults can be seen more quickly using an interactive simulation, in particular in combination with a realistic domain visualization. This applies to the validation of both the architectural concepts and the component interfaces.

Validation includes checking the completeness of the interfaces, the information that is available in each component, and whether the components can together collect enough information for making the right decisions. This concerns, for instance, sensor data and decisions where to store movement trajectories. By formally modelling different choices, the developers can really experience the consequences of different architectural decisions.

The analysis is particularly interesting when it comes to feature interaction. Because we have a single executable model for multiple scenarios, interferences can be identified early. For instance, in our model we had to make very explicit which manual movements are allowed during certain medical procedures. Moreover, the possibility to inject faults makes it easy to experiment with, for instance, graceful degradation strategies.

For the simulation we have used the SHESim tool [14] that includes an interactive simulator for POOSL. It can show interaction diagrams with the flow of messages between parts of the model. Moreover, during simulation the internal state of the model can be inspected. In our experience these facilities give insight in the model, and also help in debugging the models, in a way that is more convenient than debugging prototype implementations in some traditional programming language.

2.5 Results

The applied modelling and simulation approach focuses on rapid prototyping of the proposed reference architecture. In particular we have connected the reference architecture with the user-perceived system behaviour. This approach has triggered more discussions among the developers during the architecture phase, in which it is relatively easy to experiment with different alternatives. Thus we have gained confidence in the feasibility of the proposed architecture.

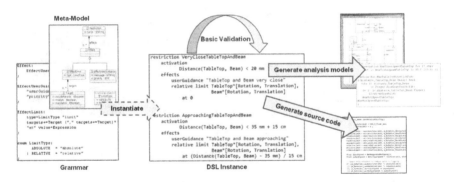

Fig. 6. Domain-Specific Language and Transformations

The proposed architecture has finally been implemented as a prototype, which has been evaluated on the physical hardware.

3   Design for Collision Prevention

In this section we focus on the design phase from Fig. 1(b), and consider the collision prevention component from Fig. 3. Collision prevention is based on rules that describe in which situations the movement requests have to be restricted. Although there are basic rules about required minimal distances between objects (for example, between C-arm and table), there are many exceptions for special procedures or situations. In addition there are detailed slowdown patterns that describe how to restrict the movement requests in a safe and comfortable way. Moreover, the set of rules varies depending on the product configuration.

An important goal of the redesign is to simplify the collision prevention component, and to support further modifications of the collision prevention rules. To represent the rules in a concise, precise and readable way, we aim to capture the rules at a high level of abstraction, close to the requirements formulation. To this end, we have developed a Domain-Specific Language (DSL).

Fig. 6 summarizes our work in relation to this DSL. At the left side, there is a fragment of the developed meta-model and grammar for this DSL. These are not specific for a single system, but they can be used for a family of similar systems (for example, a product line). In the middle of Fig. 6, there is a fragment of a DSL instance, which is specific for a single system. Based on such a DSL instance we generate source code for an implementation, and we generate analysis models for early validation of the rules.

3.1   Domain-Specific Language for Collision Prevention

The development of a Domain-Specific Language (DSL, [13,33]) includes a meta-model and a grammar; see Fig. 6. The meta-model (abstract syntax) identifies the essential concepts that we need for modelling the collision prevention rules, and the relations between these concepts; see the snapshot in Figure 7(a). The

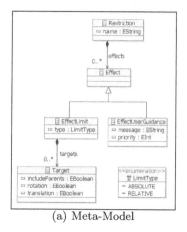

```
Effect:
    EffectUserGuidance | EffectLimit
;

EffectUserGuidance:
    "userGuidance" message=STRING
    "priority" priority=INT_LITERAL
;

EffectLimit:
    type=LimitType "limit"
    targets+=Target ("," targets+=Target)*
    "at" value=Expression
;

enum LimitType:
    ABSOLUTE   = "absolute"
    | RELATIVE  = "relative"
;
```

(a) Meta-Model   (b) Grammar

Fig. 7. DSL Snapshots

grammar (concrete syntax) defines the textual language used for describing instances of the language; see the snapshot in Figure 7(b).

Fig. 8 contains a snapshot of an instance of the language. It starts with a specification of the available 3D geometric models (as mentioned in Section 2.1), including the geometric objects they contain. The collision prevention rules themselves are specified in terms of restrictions. For each restriction there are criteria that specify when the restriction is active. The effects of an active restriction can include user guidance and speed limits on the movements. Moreover, there are several mechanisms to specify how to deal with hysteresis effects of the sensors and processing latencies in the system, but these are not shown in this snapshot.

As mentioned in [25], DSLs trade generality for expressiveness in a limited domain, leading to improved ease of use compared to general-purpose languages. We aim that also non-programmers are able to use our language. As an example, we have used measurement units for numbers instead of data types; confusion about measurement units is a known source of faults.

The development of this DSL has been an iterative process. We have started with a small set of language concepts, which were clearly essential for basic collision prevention rules. Afterwards we have analysed more challenging rules, thus gradually identifying some extra language concepts, which we have added to the DSL. More details of this process are described in [26]; special emphasis is given to gaining industrial confidence for the use of DSLs.

We have defined the DSL using Xtext [2], which is based on the Eclipse Modelling Framework (EMF, [30]). Based on the grammar, an Eclipse-based editor, parser and meta-model are generated automatically. Also convenient starting points are provided for defining validation and code generation.

Clearly the definition of a DSL for modelling collision prevention rules requires some additional effort. To make sure that these efforts pay off, DSLs should mainly be considered when several instances (or modifications over time) are to be expected, which is the case for the collision prevention rules.

```
// --- Context Declarations -------
object Table
object CArm
object Detector


model Actuals          predefined
model LookAhead        userdependent

// --- Restrictions -------
restriction ApproachingTableAndCArm
  activation
    Distance[Actuals](Table, CArm) < 35 mm + 15 cm
  effect
    absolute limit CArm[Rotation]
      at ((Distance[Actuals](Table, CArm) - 35 mm) / 15 cm) * 10 dgps


restriction ApproachingTableAndDetector
  activation
    Distance[LookAhead](Table, Detector) < 35 mm + 15 cm
 && Distance[LookAhead](Table, Detector) <
                              Distance[Actuals](Table, Detector)
  effect
    relative limit Detector[Translation]
      at ((Distance[LookAhead](Table, Detector) - 35 mm) / 15 cm)
```

Fig. 8. Snapshot of a DSL Instance

Moreover, it is important to have a clear understanding of the semantics of the modelling language. In the context of DSLs, the code generator often defines the semantics. In [21] we give a mathematical semantics of some key concepts in our DSL. Furthermore we have chosen the syntax of the DSL in such a way that most of the language elements are practically self-explanatory; there are only a few features whose semantics requires a more detailed explanation.

3.2   Generation of Source Code

For the generation of source code in Fig. 6, we have developed a custom code generator (using Xtend [1]) that transforms the high-level concepts from our DSL into executable code. By means of some glue code, we have integrated the generated code with existing systems.

The generated code can be used in various ways. First of all, the code generation gives semantics to the concepts in the meta-model and grammar of the DSL. When developing the DSL, we use the generated code to evaluate whether we have correctly captured all essential concepts. Next, we use the code generation for testing whether a specific set of rules has been modelled correctly, by running the generated code on the physical hardware. Finally, the code generation can be used for generating production code and then it adds immediate value to the modelling efforts [16].

3.3   Basic Validation and Generation of Analysis Models

A high-level description in terms of a DSL has a lot of potential for analysis, even before generating any source code for implementation in a general-purpose language. When applied to implementation code, many analysis techniques would require the prior use of abstraction techniques. DSLs facilitate analysis by providing a domain-specific abstraction that naturally fits the problem domain.

Fig. 6 shows two types of analysis. We have started with some basic validation on the DSL instance. This includes, for instance, type checking and checks that certain relations are acyclic. Clearly such checks are limited and there is a need for more analysis before code generation and time-consuming system tests. As the collision prevention component is a safety-critical real-time component, we have considered two types of analysis: performance evaluation of the required execution times and formal verification of some correctness properties.

In selecting analysis tools, we have used two criteria [21]. The first one is that no user interaction should be required, as the idea is to hide the analysis tools from the user of the DSL. This means that the analysis models have to be generated from the DSL instance, and the analysis results have to be translated back to the DSL level. Ideally, the results are showed as warnings and errors in the DSL editor.

The second criterion is that analysis results should be available in a short amount of time, such that the analysis can be run after any modifications of the DSL instance, such as changing or adding rules. Basic validation of DSL instances is performed whilst typing. The other types of analysis are more time consuming, and hence we do not intend to perform them whilst typing. We aim for an analysis time of at most a few minutes (say a short coffee break).

Performance Analysis. The collision prevention component is part of a real-time control loop that executes with a certain frequency; see Sect. 2.1. Hence it is important that the collision prevention component can execute within the period of the real-time loop. The performance analysis aims to predict quickly how much execution time is needed based on the description in the DSL instance; any other scheduling issues are not considered.

Fig. 9 gives an overview of the approach as described in [6]. In the top-left corner we start with a DSL instance. To meet our criteria for the analysis tools (fully automated, and time efficient), we create a POOSL model and analyse it using the high-speed simulation tool Rotalumis [14]. The POOSL model is generated using a model transformation (in Xtend [1]) from the DSL instance. In addition, in the top-right corner, we collect performance profiles of basic operations. These are added to the POOSL model. Finally, in the bottom-left corner the statistical results are depicted, consisting of expected execution times and their likelihood.

As the collision prevention acts as a safety layer, one may expect that we are only interested in worst-case scenarios. However, we have performed a statistical analysis instead, as a worst-case analysis would assume the extremely unlikely case that all functionality under-performs at the same time. Focusing on the worst-case only may thus result in serious over-dimensioning of the system, which, in turn, increases its costs. Moreover, the safety layer is not the only means to ensure safety; for example, the lower layers in the architecture from Fig. 3 contain various collision detection mechanisms.

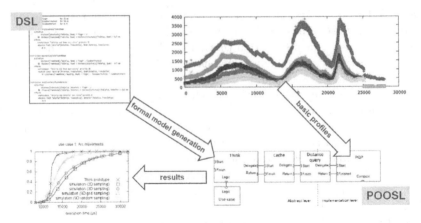

Fig. 9. Performance Analysis using the DSL

The most time-consuming basic operations are the distance computations between objects in the geometric models. The required *amount* of distance computations is basically determined by the instance of the DSL, which specifies which distances are relevant for the specified set of rules. However, the generated implementation code uses conditional and lazy evaluation. That is, depending on the positions of objects, some distances may not need to be computed.

The required *time* for a single distance computation depends on the used package for distance computations. In [6] we have considered distance computations on the basis of the Proximity Query Package (PQP, [23]), which is used in the context of robotics [9]. The execution times in PQP vary depending on the shapes of the objects and their relative geometric position. For each pair of objects, we have profiled the execution time for distance computations.

In the POOSL performance model we abstract from the geometric positions of the objects, and perform random sampling from the basic performance profiles. In addition we use probabilities to model the conditional and lazy evaluation. By simulating the performance model, we obtain a statistical indication of the expected execution times. In [6] these times are compared with measurements based on the generated implementation code.

Formal Verification. The collision prevention component is part of the safety layer; see Fig. 3. The formal verification aims to check quickly whether the following types of correctness properties hold for the DSL instance:

- well-defined expressions: checks whether there cannot be any "division by zero" or "exponentiation resulting in a complex number".
- ranges: checks whether the specified speed limits come from a proper range of values; for example, whether they are non-negative in all situations.
- safety: checks various properties such as that if two objects are close to each other and still approaching, then their speeds are restricted.
- deadlock: checks whether there is no position of the objects such that no further movements are possible.

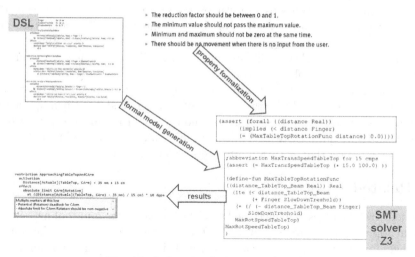

Fig. 10. Safety Analysis using the DSL

Fig. 10 gives an overview of this approach as described in [21]. In the top-left corner we start with a DSL instance. To meet our criteria for the analysis tools (fully automated, and time efficient), we create a Satisfiability Modulo Theories (SMT, [3]) model and analyse it using the SMT-solver Z3 [12]. The SMT model is generated using a model transformation (in Xtend [1]) from the DSL instance. In addition, in the top-right corner, we formulate the properties, and also formalize them in an SMT model. The combination of these models is analysed by the SMT-solver. For any failed property, an automated debugging procedure identifies a place in the DSL instance that contributes to the failure. At this place the results are displayed in the Eclipse-based editor for the DSL.

To make the formal verification feasible, we have applied several abstractions. First of all, we abstract from the acceleration characteristics of the physical objects. Similarly, we abstract from timing aspects of the system, such as the latency between sensing and acting in the real-time control loop of the safety layer. Moreover, we do not consider the physical shapes of the objects; basically we consider completely independent object positions and distances between objects.

Using these abstractions, the experiments in [21] show that fast analysis and user feedback is feasible for realistic instances of the DSL. For the correctness properties mentioned above, the applied abstractions may result in false positives. Moreover, for the deadlock check it may also result in false negatives. Nevertheless, also the deadlock check is useful as it can detect certain typical mistakes in the collision prevention rules.

3.4 Results

The development of this DSL has triggered many discussions about the collision prevention rules. By making the rules more explicit, we continuously had to decide what is really essential, and what is just an implementation detail.

The initial expectation was that there would be a lot of variability in the rules. However, the combined study of the movement control architecture and the collision prevention design has shown that a lot of the variability can be isolated. In further work we will consider whether DSLs can play a useful role in the design of these isolated parts.

Using language development frameworks like Xtext/Xtend, DSL instances can easily be transformed to various types of analysis models. When applied to implementation code, many analysis techniques would require the prior use of abstraction techniques. Instead, DSLs facilitate analysis by providing a domain-specific abstraction that naturally fits the problem domain.

4   Related Work

To model architectures, we have used the POOSL language and tooling, but the general approach is not restricted to POOSL. An overview of many other formal languages for describing architectures is provided by [17]. Our focus is on how to apply such languages and methods effectively in industrial practice. A particular challenge identified in [17] is scalability, which we address by making high-level models that omit many details and focus on parts of the functionality.

For example, we could also consider architecture description languages such as the SAE Architecture Analysis and Design Language (AADL, [29]) standard. However, at the moment that we decided to use POOSL, the AADL tools were still too much under development without convenient simulation possibilities. We could also have used MatLab, but we prefer a light-weight tool specializing in discrete event systems. In particular we focus on specification and not on implementation or verification. The goal here is to keep the models simple, in order to facilitate rapid experimentation.

In the context of the architectural validation, the goal is not to generate code out of the POOSL models, in contrast to formal methods such as VDMTools [11], Atelier B [10], SCADE Suite [15], and ASD:Suite [32]. The last tool has also been used at Philips Healthcare [20,19,27]. The goal of our architectural validation is rapid prototyping of the architectural concepts, in such a way that alternatives can easily be explored, and changes can be made quickly.

It is interesting to compare such formal methods approaches with the DSL approach. Both approaches aim for models at a higher abstraction level than implementation code, and aim to generate implementation code from these models. The code generators for formal methods approaches are usually generic and predefined (based on a formal semantics), and hence the modelling cannot abstract a lot from the implementation level. Typically the formal methods models are a kind of state machines. As the code generators for DSLs are custom, higher-level and domain-specific abstractions are feasible. Finally, the formal methods approaches focus on formal verification using sophisticated model checkers. To bring similar benefits to the DSL approach, we have introduced the transformations to various types of analysis models.

The architecture models from [22] are similar to our POOSL models. Their analysis, however, focuses on validating the requirements by observing external behaviour, whereas in our analysis we focus equally on how this behaviour is established internally.

The BIP (Behavior, Interaction, Priority; [5]) framework as described in [28] uses a similar structure as our DSL approach. However, we use a DSL whereas BIP is more a general-purpose language somewhat comparable to POOSL.

In earlier work [18] we have translated UML models into the formats of several existing validation tools like model checkers and theorem provers. Also the work on design space exploration from [4] has a similar flavour as our transformations to analysis models. Also there the goal is to create a specification at a convenient abstraction level, and then provide transformations to and from various analysis tools. In both cases the transformations hide all the low-level encodings.

5   Conclusions and Further Work

We have participated in an industrial study project for redesigning the collision prevention components of interventional X-ray systems. In this context, we have demonstrated various model-based techniques that allow for fault detection in early development phases. Thus we have gained confidence in the feasibility of the proposed redesign. Finally a prototype implementation has been delivered, which has been evaluated on the physical hardware.

The architecture analysis has led to more discussions before going into the design and implementation phases. The DSL approach has led to simple descriptions of collision prevention rules, from which a prototype implementation is generated. In our experience, the Xtext/Xtend tools enable the quick development of languages and their transformations. Our analysis techniques for DSL instances show potential, but they became available to late during the study project to have a significant impact.

An important challenge for all the analysis techniques described here is to find a good balance between the level of detail and the potential for analysis. In general, modelling in more detail is more time consuming, but it can enable more extensive analysis. Note that more detail can also significantly increase the time needed for the analysis. This is a serious issue, as we aim for quick feedback in early development phases (when many details are still unknown).

The composition of the study team has also contributed to its success. First of all it contains young people with fresh ideas. Secondly, it contains people with a lot of experience and domain expertise, which was important to avoid too many iterations of erroneous attempts. Finally it contains developers that made prototype implementations of new ideas using the existing code base; this includes both the new product features and the use of new development techniques like DSLs.

Further Work. Architectural POOSL models are currently used to validate proposed architectural changes of other parts of the system. It requires more experimentation to define clear guidelines on how to handle with the tension between level of detail and analysis power. In particular we would like to support a notion of refinement on a series of models from requirements via architecture to design.

To make sure that analysis results on the DSL are relevant for the generated code, we need to establish that the code generators and model transformations are consistent. We are currently investigating an approach where we first define a formal semantics for the DSL, and then analyse which properties of the DSL are maintained by the code generators and model transformations. A particular challenge is to do this in such a way that it can be applied in industrial practice in a cost effective way.

Finally we are improving the usability aspects of the POOSL tools. This includes the use of DSL technology for developing an Eclipse-based editor. In particular we are adding all kinds of validation checks while editing the POOSL models, in order to support early fault detection.

Acknowledgements. The authors like to thank Freek van den Berg and Sarmen Keshishzadeh for their work on analysis models for our DSL, and for providing relevant screenshots. The authors also like to thank Hans Driessen and Jan Stevens for their active participation in this study project.

References

1. Xtend. version 2.3 (2012), http://www.eclipse.org/xtend/
2. Xtext. version 2.3 (2012), http://www.eclipse.org/Xtext/
3. Barrett, C., Sebastiani, R., Seshia, S., Tinelli, C.: Satisfiability Modulo Theories. Handbook of Satisfiability 185, 825–885 (2009)
4. Basten, T., Hendriks, M., Trcka, N., Somers, L., Geilen, M., Yang, Y., Igna, G., de Smet, S., Voorhoeve, M., van der Aalst, W., Corporaal, H., Vaandrager, F.: Model-driven design-space exploration for software-intensive embedded systems. In: Model-Based Design of Adaptive Embedded Systems. Springer (2013)
5. Basu, A., Bozga, M., Sifakis, J.: Modeling heterogeneous real-time components in BIP. In: Proceedings of SEFM 2006, pp. 3–12. IEEE Computer Society (2006)
6. van den Berg, F., Remke, A., Mooij, A., Haverkort, B.: Performance evaluation for collision prevention based on a domain specific language. In: Balsamo, M.S., Knottenbelt, W.J., Marin, A. (eds.) EPEW 2013. LNCS, vol. 8168, pp. 276–287. Springer, Heidelberg (2013)
7. Blender, http://www.blender.org/
8. Brooks, R.: A robust layered control system for a mobile robot. IEEE J. Robot. Autom. 2(1), 14–23 (1986)
9. Carpin, S., Mirolo, C., Pagello, E.: A performance comparison of three algorithms for proximity queries relative to convex polyhedra. In: Proceedings of ICRA 2006, pp. 3023–3028 (2006)
10. ClearSy: Atelier B, http://www.atelierb.eu/en/
11. CSK Systems Corporation: VDMTools, http://www.vdmtools.jp/en/
12. de Moura, L., Bjørner, N.S.: Z3: An efficient SMT solver. In: Ramakrishnan, C.R., Rehof, J. (eds.) TACAS 2008. LNCS, vol. 4963, pp. 337–340. Springer, Heidelberg (2008)
13. van Deursen, A., Klint, P., Visser, J.: Domain-specific languages: an annotated bibliography. SIGPLAN Notices 35(6), 26–36 (2000)
14. Eindhoven University of Technology: Software/Hardware Engineering (SHE) - Parallel Object-Oriented Specification Language (POOSL), http://www.es.ele.tue.nl/poosl/
15. Esterel Technologies: SCADE Suite, http://www.esterel-technologies.com/products/scade-suite/

16. Fitzgerald, J.S., Larsen, P.G.: Balancing insight and effort: The industrial uptake of formal methods. In: Jones, C.B., Liu, Z., Woodcock, J. (eds.) Formal Methods and Hybrid Real-Time Systems. LNCS, vol. 4700, pp. 237–254. Springer, Heidelberg (2007)

17. Garlan, D.: Formal modeling and analysis of software architecture: Components, connectors, and events. In: Bernardo, M., Inverardi, P. (eds.) SFM 2003. LNCS, vol. 2804, pp. 1–24. Springer, Heidelberg (2003)

18. Graf, S., Hooman, J.: Correct development of embedded systems. In: Oquendo, F., Warboys, B.C., Morrison, R. (eds.) EWSA 2004. LNCS, vol. 3047, pp. 241–249. Springer, Heidelberg (2004)

19. Hooman, J., Mooij, A.J., van Wezep, H.: Early fault detection in industry using models at various abstraction levels. In: Derrick, J., Gnesi, S., Latella, D., Treharne, H. (eds.) IFM 2012. LNCS, vol. 7321, pp. 268–282. Springer, Heidelberg (2012)

20. Hooman, J., Huis in 't Veld, R., Schuts, M.: Experiences with a compositional model checker in the healthcare domain. In: Liu, Z., Wassyng, A. (eds.) FHIES 2011. LNCS, vol. 7151, pp. 93–110. Springer, Heidelberg (2012)

21. Keshishzadeh, S., Mooij, A.J., Mousavi, M.R.: Early fault detection in DSLs using SMT solving and automated debugging. In: Hierons, R.M., Merayo, M.G., Bravetti, M. (eds.) SEFM 2013. LNCS, vol. 8137, pp. 182–196. Springer, Heidelberg (2013)

22. Kramer, J., Magee, J., Uchitel, S.: Software architecture modeling & analysis: A rigorous approach. In: Bernardo, M., Inverardi, P. (eds.) SFM 2003. LNCS, vol. 2804, pp. 44–51. Springer, Heidelberg (2003)

23. Larsen, E., Gottschalk, S., Lin, M., Manocha, D.: Fast distance queries with rectangular swept sphere volumes. In: Proceedings of ICRA 2000, vol. 4, pp. 3719–3726 (2000)

24. Li, L., Hooman, J., Voeten, J.: Connecting technical and non-technical views of system architectures. In: Proceedings of CPSCom 2010, pp. 592–599 (December 2010)

25. Mernik, M., Heering, J., Sloane, A.M.: When and how to develop domain-specific languages. ACM Computing Surveys 37(4), 316–344 (2005)

26. Mooij, A.J., Hooman, J., Albers, R.: Gaining industrial confidence for the introduction of domain-specific languages. In: Proceedings of COMPSAC workshops, IEESD 2013, pp. 662–667. IEEE (2013)

27. Osaiweran, A., Schuts, M., Hooman, J., Wesselius, J.H.: Incorporating formal techniques into industrial practice: an experience report. In: Proceedings of FESCA 2013. ENTCS, vol. 295 (2013)

28. Poulhiès, M., Pulou, J., Rippert, C., Sifakis, J.: A methodology and supporting tools for the development of component-based embedded systems. In: Kordon, F., Sokolsky, O. (eds.) Monterey Workshop 2006. LNCS, vol. 4888, pp. 75–96. Springer, Heidelberg (2007)

29. SAE International: Architecture Analysis & Design Language (AADL). SAE Standard AS5506B (September 2012)

30. Steinberg, D., Budinsky, F., Paternostro, M., Merks, E.: Eclipse Modeling Framework. Pearson Education (2008)

31. Theelen, B.D., Florescu, O., Geilen, M., Huang, J., van der Putten, P.H.A., Voeten, J.: Software/hardware engineering with the Parallel Object-Oriented Specification Language. In: Proceedings of MEMOCODE 2007, pp. 139–148. IEEE (2007)

32. Verum Software Technologies: ASD:Suite, http://www.verum.com/

33. Voelter, M.: DSL Engineering, Version 1.0 (2013), http://dslbook.org

OR.NET: Safe Interconnection of Medical Devices

(Position Paper)

Franziska Kühn[1,2] and Martin Leucker[1]

[1] Institute for Software Engineering and Programming Languages
University of Lübeck
[2] Graduate School for Computing in Medicine and Life Science
University of Lübeck

Abstract. This position paper gives an overview on the OR.NET project which focuses on the dynamic and safe interconnection of medical devices in an operating room. A brief overview of the legal situation for the approval of medical devices is given to highlight today's limitations of the dynamic interconnection of safety critical devices in hospitals. A collection of methods equipped with a methodology is presented and discussed, which is intended to replace current integration tests at runtime.

1 Introduction

Nowadays in Europe the interconnection of medical devices in an operating room is almost always limited to devices from a single manufacturer or the clinic operator assumes the role of a manufacturer. This is partially due to technical restrictions but especially due to the legal requirements needed in the medical domain. These legal requirements impose that a complete system-of-systems has been successfully tested and certified before its use in an operating room.

Especially for clinic operators this situation limits the technological and economical benefits that could be obtained by the interconnection of medical devices from different vendors. The OR.NET project[1] focuses on the safe, secure and dynamic interconnection of medical devices from different manufacturers in an operating room. The project is funded by the German federal ministry of education and research (BMBF) and includes nearly 50 project partners, ranging over medical device manufacturers, clinic operators, standardization organizations and universities. A main project objective is the *standardized interoperability* for medical devices. More specifically, the goal is to build future medical devices with interoperable capabilities, to facilitate their simple integration.

There exist many descriptions of interoperability [1]. The *Association for the Advancement of Medical Instrumentation* defines interoperability as follows [1]: *"Medical device interoperability is the ability of medical devices, clinical systems, or their components to communicate with each other in order to safely fulfill an*

---

[1] `www.ornet.org`

J. Gibbons and W. MacCaull (Eds.): FHIES 2013, LNCS 8315, pp. 188–198, 2014.

intended purpose." This definition focuses on safety as well as intended purpose, which agrees well with our intention. From a technical perspective, though, the definition is imprecise. Regarding interoperability, one can distinguish different levels (e.g. described in [2,1,3,4]). While there exist different definitions of levels of interoperability, most of them share the following classifications. Basic interoperability is achieved at the level of *connectivity*, i.e. devices are able to exchange unstructured data. The level of *integratability* is reached when the devices agree on common data formats. Full interoperability is achieved, when the devices expose their state and behavior at least partially. From our point of view full interoperability should be supported in context of the OR.NET project.

We distinguish core and additional functionality. As core functionality we consider e.g. a microscope or a dissector, where one system implements all functionality required for a certain intended use. While functionalities might be distributed over several subsystems, the system has been designed as a whole. E.g. a dissector consists mainly of a hand-piece and a control unit. Additional functionality only provides better usability and overview in order to relieve staff, e.g. that the information of the dissector can be displayed on the monitor of a microscope, thereby providing the surgeon with a better overview. We consider mainly settings, where core functionalities are provided by single devices and interconnection of devices is employed only to provide additional functionality. In contrast, Hatcliff et al. [5] and the MD PnP project[2] focus on distributing core functionality and consider not primarily the critical area of the operating room.

The project goal is that the clinic operators have the freedom to choose medical devices from different manufacturers fulfilling the intended use. Furthermore it should be possible to connect the devices safely in a plug-and-play-manner. If a device fails (also during surgery), it must be possible to exchange it dynamically by one having the capabilities to fulfill the same intended use. Moreover, the particular combination of devices must not require a dedicated certification and must not require the clinic operator to take over the role of a manufacturer.

It is not possible that all combinations of medical devices (of all manufacturers and all releases) are tested before connection resulting that medical devices are possibly connected together, but have not worked together before and tested a priori. Because safety in the medical domain has high priority, our goal is to compensate the safety risks induced by the missing integration and system test.

In the following section we give a short overview of today's legal situation for approval of medical devices in Germany and highlight the resulting current limitations of their dynamic interconnection. In Section 3 we present a collection of methods equipped with a methodology which is intended to replace the missing integration test at runtime. In Section 4 we conclude with a discussion about the outcome and the further challenges related to the safety of medical devices in the context of the dynamic interconnection.

---

[2] www.mdpnp.org

2   Legal Situation and Limitations of Interconnection

The objective of the so called *New Approach*[3] is the elimination of technical restrictions to European trade and thereby to facilitate open exchange of goods within the European Union. So far more than 20 European directives were adopted, including directives for medical devices. It is mandatory for all European member states to implement the European directives into national law.

The European directives 93/42/EEC (Medical Device Directive) [6], 98/79/EC (In-vitro Diagnostic Directive) [7] and 90/385/EEC (Active implantable medical devices directive) [8] are the basis for medical devices, whereby the last two are more specific than the first one. The German implementation of the three European directives for medical devices, supplemented by regulations, is the Medical Devices Act (in German: *Medizingproduktegesetz*, MPG).

The Medical Device Directive demands the following requirements [9]: consideration of quality aspects, execution of risk management, consideration for software life cycle processes and proof of usability. Before bringing a product on the market, medical device manufacturers have to verify in a conformity assessment procedure that their products fulfill the essential requirements of the corresponding directives – guaranteeing that their products are safe and effective.

Harmonized norms are a support for manufacturers to fulfill the essential requirements of the European directives. The most important harmonized norms to fulfill the requirements are EN ISO 13485 [10], EN ISO 14971 [11], EN 62304 [12], EN 62366 [13] and EN 60601-1-6 [14].

By law, before bringing a product on the market, the manufacturers have to guarantee that their devices are safe and effective. This includes the validation and verification of the entire system (including an integration and system test) and defining appropriate risk control measurements for possible safety risks. This must also be done by the manufacturer when interconnecting medical devices, considering the interconnection as one system.

When a clinic operator interconnects medical devices which were not certified as a system-of-systems before, he becomes a manufacturer and is taking the responsibilities. Though norm IEC 80001-1 [15] may support him when integrating medical devices in IT-networks, the operator does in general not have the abilities (e.g. staff, skills and medical devices information) to perform an appropriate risk management. Therefore, besides developing techniques for the standardized interoperability of different devices, a main objective of the OR.NET project is to develop a technical as well as a legal framework for the safe interconnection of medical devices. The goal is to allow the individual certification of devices and to release the clinic operator from the burden of taking legal responsibilities.

3   Proposal of Methods and Methodologies for a Safe Interconnection

In this section, we elaborate on the quest of checking the compatibility of systems after deployment in the special setting of medical devices. Technically, we

---

[3] http://www.newapproach.org

propose a two layered approach that intends to guarantee that the interconnected devices perform correctly, even without a comprehensive integration test.

The Need for Deferred Integration Testing. Connecting devices that have been developed and tested individually but have not been tested together means that no integration test has been performed. As outlined in the previous section, such an integration test is by law either required from the vendor or the hospital itself. In the presence of different vendors only the operator could take over this job.

Therefore, we propose that systems that are intended for interconnection by the operator are designed to provide a thorough support for an integration test to be performed after delivery. We formulate our first main thesis:

T1 *Systems have to be designed in such a way that they perform an integration test when connected to each other.*

At this stage, one may also take the position that any interface like human interfaces and also network interfaces have to be considered within the risk analysis of medical devices. One may argue that the carefully carried out risk analysis and the intensive testing of each device individually does not require any further integration testing, neither by the manufacturer nor by the operator. We do not consider this position adequate, neither from a technical nor a legal point of view. During development it may not be foreseen every scenario a device is used for later. Moreover when testing systems implicit assumptions of the system behavior are often made and thus important test cases are possibly skipped.

Let us stress that following our first thesis has a significant draw back compared to the integration testing by the vendor. The testing functionality is part of the system and may as such be faulty and insufficient for finding problems in the interconnection of devices. However, we think that the testing functionality as well as the interfaces as outlined below provide a high level of confidence that integrated system test may perform correctly.

Performing Deferred Integration Testing. Clearly, thorough integration testing as done by the manufacturer would be desirable when connecting devices also from different vendors. Such a test requires both a decent knowledge about the individual functionality as well as the combined functionality of the systems. In general such combined functionality may not be foreseen completely when developing each device individually unless we are faced with an a priori precisely defined interconnection. In general, we have to distinguish two different scenarios:

1. An official (industry) standard defines precisely the intended interconnection as well as the intended functionality.
2. Proprietary defined features of the connection of devices are used to obtain a single system resulting in a partially unknown behavior.

In the first case, it seems possible that a correct and complete test case, presumably provided by the standardization body, is used to test the interconnection of the systems. Such a test might be carried out by the operator whenever individual systems are combined. However, profound integration testing is partly manual and time consuming, thus, it is only feasible when no flexible, say daily recombination of systems, is necessary.

In the second case, the existence of suitable test cases does not seem to be plausible for different reasons. First, such tests require some knowledge about the combined functionality of the systems, which may be not be foreseen completely when developing each device individually. Moreover, one manufacturer of a system might not be willing to provide a test suite making sure that his devices work also with those from competitors. In addition, the connection possibilities may change quickly from revision to revision of the corresponding devices, following the enhanced functionality of each device.

To provide support for the interconnection especially in the second case, we suggest the following approach, which is a well-known approach in computer science and consists of three steps.

1. Define precisely the interface intended for connectivity.
2. Check compatibility of interfaces whenever connecting two devices.
3. Check each device for conformance with its interface specification.

In the following we discuss the advantages of this approach and how to realize the individual steps.

The Need for Interface Definitions. A precise interface definition has many advantages. It is helpful to make sure that the manufacturer has himself a precise understanding of the intended system's connection functionality. It is typically also necessary for the manufacturer's risk analysis of the device to be carried out for getting the machine certified. In our setting, it may be used, as explained in the next sections, as a basis for checking compatibility of interconnected devices as well as that each device adheres to its specified interface.

Many different forms of interface definitions are known in computer science. UML's component diagrams, for example, specify for each component the methods including parameter types that it provides. With Henzinger's and de Alfaro's interface automata [16], also the intended behavior of a component may be specified precisely, at least on the level of a finite automaton.

In our setting, we aim for a formalism that has a rich expressiveness but at the same time allows for certain analysis techniques. A promising approach presented recently is given in [17]. We consider a formal interface specification to include at least the methods which are delivered by the medical devices, but also the external methods which are necessary to fulfill a functionality. Furthermore we consider the specification to include the parameters and return values of the methods (including datatypes and the intended ranges) and their pre- and postconditions as well as some form of the behavior of the component. In addition qualities as for example the probability of failure and maximum latency time as well as safety and liveness properties of the medical devices (especially those properties which can be affected by the interconnection) should be included.

A favorable approach given in [18] allows to describe the behavior of medical devices by a modal specification language. Furthermore it partially allows to verify safety and liveness properties based on a device model. Session types [19] allow to specify the allowed sequences of messages, expressing an interaction protocol between components. Suitable logics, for example linear temporal logic [20] (LTL) or timed linear time logic [21] can be used to describe safety and liveness properties of the individual components and for quality aspects.

Another axis to distinguish interfaces is by means of their level of dynamics. In traditional programming languages, there is a fixed interface when calling functions. In service oriented architectures, on the other hand, interfaces come with a lot of variability and a so-called service request broker takes care of the connection from so-called service users and corresponding service providers. For example is it possible that the interfaces of two medical devices do not have syntactically the same methods, but actually the devices provide same services. Thus, the relationship between the syntactic interfaces of the semantically compatible components have to be inferred automatically.

Checking Compatibility of Interfaces. When connecting two devices, the compatibility of their interfaces should be checked. We suggest that only if their interfaces are compatible, the devices continue any operation, following the idea that a new system is created via the interconnection of the two individual ones.

We use the term compatible here in a broad sense that has to be made precise depending on the notion of interface. In Java, for example, an interface is a set of method signatures. In this setting, compatibility means that a class is implementing the interface by providing methods for each method signature in the interface.

As mentioned before we aim for more specific interface specifications comprising pre- and post- conditions, information on the expected behavior, quality aspects and safety and liveness properties. Compatibility then becomes less obvious to define. For example is it necessary to determine whether a service provider is delivering the methods a service user is needing and whether the delivered values have the expected types and fits in the estimated range. Likewise it has to be determined whether the service user is calling the functionality of a service provider correctly, for example whether the service user calls an external method with the correct number and types of parameters. In general, every kind of input parameter has to be exactly or more specific than expected and every kind of output parameter has to be more general.

Defining compatibility of two behavioral specifications is even more involved. All the behavior expected by one system has to be provided by the other system and vice versa. Corresponding work in the field of interface automata, session types and the work described in [18] might be of help here, yet precise definitions for our setup are to be defined. In general, interfaces may only be compatible on a small part of the respective services. It may be helpful to define levels of compatibility of two systems provided that each system can cooperate with the other one in terms of different cooperation levels.

We presume that checking compatibility usually boils down to some satisfiability problem in a suitable logic, following the idea that two specifications are compatible iff there is no entity provided by one system that cannot be consumed by the other. Moreover, we presume that checking compatibility of behavioral interface specifications can be checked by automata theoretic techniques. It remains to be active research to work out the details. In general, we require that

T2 *Interface specification languages have to be designed such that checking compatibility is decidable.*

Checking Conformance with Interfaces. Following the rule of separation of concerns, checking correctness of the combined system is divided into checking compatibility of interfaces and conformance to interfaces. We mean by conformance that a system adheres to all the constraints in the interface specification.

As the first part is required to be decidable and most interesting properties are undecidable, we cannot expect that checking conformance with an interface specification is in general decidable. As such, there are two possibilities to check conformance. Either before delivery of the complete system using, for example, theorem provers, or, dynamically at runtime of the respective system.

It is important to understand that checking conformance is to be done by both systems. These systems are in general developed by different manufacturers and the systems cannot trust each other. Thus, checking conformance before delivery of the system is not enough. The system should be checked and delivered with a proof of conformance. The latter can be easily checked by the other system to make sure that the connecting part is indeed working correctly. We presume that concepts of proof carrying code can be used for this scenario.

As a different approach we suggest to use runtime verification [22] techniques to monitor at runtime the interface compliance of the medical devices, whereby the monitors are automatically generated by for example the pre- and postconditions as well as safety and liveness properties of the interface specification. Furthermore, this approach allows to detect misbehavior at runtime and enables to react if problems occur. If an abstract model of the medical devices exists we presume that techniques as described in [23,24] can be used to detect the satisfaction or violation of LTL formulae even before it actually occurs. Furthermore, as described in [23] it is also detected when the runtime behavior of a component does not agree with the specified behavior of the abstract model, which is highly important when an abstract model is the basis for other verification techniques.

As described in a previous section it may be possible that the interfaces (or parts of it) are semantically but not syntactically the same. Ontologies [25] can be used to define concepts of application domain and the semantics meaning of interfaces of components. Given such an ontology the relationship between syntactic interfaces of semantically compatible components might be inferred automatically. The goal is to synthesize a mediator [26], performing syntactic transformation between interfaces.

4   Discussion

An important question is whether medical devices can just be interconnected if there exist a precisely defined standard for an interconnection scenario or whether it is possible to interconnect medical devices if there just exist proprietary defined features of the interconnection. In general medical devices should be interconnected to fulfill an intended purpose.

An advantage of precisely defined standards for interconnection scenarios is the possibility to provide reference implementations for the systems of an interconnection scenario. These implementations may be useful for manufacturers to evaluate that a system can be used in an interconnection scenario and also be helpful to support the risk management process and for system tests. Additionally, precisely defined interface specification can be delivered by the standardization bodies as well as comprehensive test cases. This may be helpful to ensure that the systems are build to be able to work in certain interconnection scenarios.

Nevertheless, in our opinion it will limit the dynamic as it will take a long time for standardizing interconnection scenarios. Additionally it will be difficult (especially by the struggle for market share) that all manufacturers agree on such precisely defined functionality and implement a standardized interface. Especially without the possibility of manufacturer-specific device capabilities.

Especially when proprietary features of interconnection are defined the check of compatibility between the devices is inevitable. There are several possibilities when checking the compatibility of interfaces: during the initial start-up of a medical device, during the preparation of the surgery, dynamically when connecting the medical devices together.

When devices should be installed in a hospital an initial start-up is necessary, which includes for example a training session for future users. We presume that also an initial start-up for interconnected devices is useful, for example to train the users and to define which users are allowed to use the functionality of interconnected devices (it may be possible that a user is allowed to use one medical device of an interconnection, but not the other – is the user then allowed to use the interconnected functionality?). Furthermore it is possibly time-consuming to check the compatibility and if it is determined that the interfaces of devices are not compatible during the preparation of the surgery (or when connecting the devices during operation) it may be problematic for the upcoming (or running respectively) surgery. Also it may prevent a dynamic exchange of medical devices during surgery when we assume that it is time-consuming or incompatibilities might not be detected in advance. Nevertheless at runtime (whenever devices are connected) it has to be checked whether all devices are available and already checked to be compatible. This check has to be repetitive, for example when a device fails (or a device is added), preventing that an interconnection functionality can be fulfilled (or facilitating to fulfill an interconnection scenario respectively).

When connecting devices together several problems can occur. For example is it possible that a device does not adhere to its interface specification, the network connection breaks down, resulting in unavailability of medical devices, safety or liveness properties are violated and the runtime behavior of a medical device does not comply with the specified behavior of an abstract device model.

We suppose that devices of an interconnection have a work-alone mode. The work-alone mode is not useful for all interconnection scenarios, but especially when the goal of an interconnection is to provide better usability or overview only. In the work-alone mode a device should be able to provide its basic functionality without relying on other devices. When a problem is observed (injuring the functionality of the interconnected devices) the involved medical devices should fall into work-alone mode, thereby maintaining all required functionality to continue e.g. an ongoing medical procedure.

Particularly for that a classification of failures, relating to the possible consequences would presumably be helpful. For example when detecting that the observed behavior of a system does not comply with the behavior of a specified device model, additionally installed and then activated runtime verification techniques can be helpful checking the functionality that was checked statically related to the model. When one device is for example unavailable in an interconnection it could be tried to identify the cause automatically and tried to be recovered. For those scenarios also runtime reflection [27] techniques can help to trigger adequate recover measures. It requires further investigation to define when it is useful to recover a system and when to continue or interrupt an interconnection.

Especially when interconnecting many different components, it is possibly necessary to monitor at runtime safety and liveness properties not only in pairwise fashion. We suppose that also runtime verification techniques can be used allowing the consideration of properties which involve several distributed components. Assuming that a central component (monitoring the distributed medical devices) is used for this purpose (placed inbetween the devices) latency of exchanged data or observed events may pose various challenges. For example is it possible that the order of the observed sequences of events/messages is not the order that actually occurs. Above all a suitable logic (especially logics which also take data into account) and a time or synchronization model is required. A major challenge is the consideration of a monitor which is distributed on the several components (for example when a central component is not possible).

We suppose that automated verification techniques help to increase the safety of interconnected medical devices. Therefore a comprehensive interface specification (done by the manufacturer or if, standardized, by the standardization organization) is necessary, facilitating verification techniques, both carried out statically and also at runtime. We also assume that those verification techniques are suitable for risk control measurements. To relieve an operator from the responsibilities when dynamically connecting devices, the corresponding norms should be changed to require the outlined interface specification and verification approaches as mandatory for the device manufacturers.

To this end, also a classification of failures would be useful to define adequate risk control measurements and for the triggering actions when a problem is observed. Such a classification is for example described in [28], but should go down to each method of a device instead of components. It would also be helpful to define cooperation levels. This means for example that a high critical function cannot be used by another device without the use of additional risk control measurements.

Altogether, it remains a challenge to provide the technical and legal means for a safe interconnection of medical devices.

References

1. Association for the Advancement of Medical Instrumentation: Medical Device Interoperability (AAMI MDI/March 30, 2013) (2013)
2. Turnitsa, C.D.: Extending the Levels of Conceptual Interoperability Model. In: Proceedings IEEE 2005 Summer Computer Simulation Conference, IEEE CSP (2005)
3. C4ISR Architecture Working Group: Levels of Information Systems Interoperability, LISI (1998)
4. National Committee on Vital and Health Statistics (NCVHS): Report on Uniform Data Standards for Patient Medical Record Information (2000)
5. Hatcliff, J., King, A.L., Lee, I., Macdonald, A., Fernando, A., Robkin, M., Vasserman, E.Y., Weininger, S., Goldman, J.M.: Rationale and architecture principles for medical application platforms. In: IEEE ICCPS, pp. 3–12 (2012)
6. Council Directive 93/42/EEC of 14 June 1993 concerning medical devices. OJ L 169 (July 12, 1993)
7. Directive 98/79/EC of the European Parliament and of the Council of 27 Oct 1998 on in vitro diagnostic medical devices. OJ L 331 (July 12,1998)
8. Council Directive 90/385/EEC of 20 June 1990 on the approximation of the laws of the Member States relating to active implantable medical devices. OJ No L 189 (July 20, 1990)
9. Johner, C., Hölzer-Klüpfel, M., Wittorf, S.: Basiswissen Medizinische Software: Aus- und Weiterbildung zum Certified Professional for Medical Software. Dpunkt (2011)
10. Medical devices - Quality management systems - Requirements for regulatory purposes (EN ISO 13485:2003)
11. Medical devices - Application of risk management to medical devices (ISO 14971) (2007), Corrected version (January 10, 2007)
12. Medical device software - Software life-cycle processes (IEC 62304) (2006)
13. Medical devices - Application of usability engineering to medical devices (IEC 62366) (2007)
14. Medical electrical equipment – Part 1-6: General requirements for basic safety and essential performance - Collateral standard: Usability (IEC 60601-1-6) (2010)
15. Application of risk management for IT-networks incorporating medical devices - Part 1: Roles, responsibilities and activities (IEC 80001-1) (2010)
16. de Alfaro, L., Henzinger, T.A.: Interface automata. In: ESEC / SIGSOFT FSE, pp. 109–120. ACM (2001)
17. Masson, B., Hélouët, L., Benveniste, A.: Compatibility between DAXML Schemas (March 2011)
18. King, A.L., Feng, L., Sokolsky, O., Lee, I.: A modal specification approach for on-demand medical systems. In: Preproceedings of FHIES (2013)
19. Takeuchi, K., Honda, K., Kubo, M.: An interaction-based language and its typing system. In: Halatsis, C., Philokyprou, G., Maritsas, D., Theodoridis, S. (eds.) PARLE 1994. LNCS, vol. 817, pp. 398–413. Springer, Heidelberg (1994)

20. Pnueli, A.: The temporal logic of programs. In: Proceedings of the 18th IEEE Symposium on the Foundations of Computer Science (FOCS 1977), pp. 46–57. IEEE (1977)
21. Raskin, J.F.: Logics, Automata and Classical theories for Deciding Real Time. Thèse de doctorat, FUNDP, Namur, Belgium (June 1999)
22. Leucker, M., Schallhart, C.: A brief account of runtime verification. JLAP 78(5), 293–303 (2009)
23. Kühn, F.: Pink states for runtime verification. Master's thesis, Univ. of Lübeck (2013)
24. Leucker, M.: Sliding between model checking and runtime verification. In: Qadeer, S., Tasiran, S. (eds.) RV 2012. LNCS, vol. 7687, pp. 82–87. Springer, Heidelberg (2013)
25. Gruber, T.R.: A translation approach to portable ontology specifications. Knowledge Acquisition 5, 199–220 (1993)
26. Bennaceur, A., Chilton, C., Isberner, M., Jonsson, B.: Automated mediator synthesis: Combining behavioural and ontological reasoning. In: Hierons, R.M., Merayo, M.G., Bravetti, M. (eds.) SEFM 2013. LNCS, vol. 8137, pp. 274–288. Springer, Heidelberg (2013)
27. Leucker, M.: Checking and enforcing safety: Runtime verification and runtime reflection. ERCIM News 2008(75) (2008)
28. Vasserman, E.Y., Venkatasubramanian, K.K., Sokolsky, O., Lee, I.: Security and interoperable-medical-device systems, part 2: Failures, consequences, and classification. IEEE Security & Privacy 10(6), 70–73 (2012)

A Modal Specification Approach for On-Demand Medical Systems*

Andrew L. King, Lu Feng**, Oleg Sokolsky, and Insup Lee

Department of Computer & Information Science, University of Pennsylvania
{kingand,lufeng,sokolsky,lee}@cis.upenn.edu

Abstract. The on-demand approach, where systems are assembled from components by lay users, has seen success in the consumer electronics industry. Currently, there is growing demand for on-demand capabilities in medical systems so caregivers can create larger medical systems from smaller medical devices. Unlike consumer electronics, medical systems pose challenges for the on-demand approach due to attributes such as device complexity, device variability and safety requirements. In this paper, we propose a formal specification language for on-demand (medical) systems. Our approach is based on the formalism of Modal I/O Automata, which allows system designers to express complex device requirements and can be used to reason about safety and liveness properties of on-demand medical systems directly from their specifications. We illustrate the applicability of our approach through a case study of a closed-loop patient controlled analgesia system.

1 Introduction

An on-demand system is any system assembled by a lay user out of components that have not been previously tested together. An example on-demand system is a home entertainment system: A typical home theater is composed of speakers, an audio/visual receiver, a content source (such as a DVD player or streaming video device), and television. Assembly of these on-demand systems is facilitated by a 'plug-and-play' capability in the components themselves; in theory each component conforms to a well defined standard (*e.g.,* USB, HDMI, Bluetooth) which then ensures that the components properly compose to form a functioning system. The standards typically define a small set of rigid component classes. For example, the USB standard defines around 20 classes for different component types such as mass storage (external hard drives), human interface device (keyboards and mice), audio, and video. The feature sets for each class are fixed (and relatively simple).

---

* Research is supported in part by NSF grants CNS-1035715 and IIS-1231547.

** Lu Feng is supported by James S. McDonnell Foundation 21st Century Science Initiative - Postdoctoral Program in Complexity Science/Complex Systems - Fellowship Award.

J. Gibbons and W. MacCaull (Eds.): FHIES 2013, LNCS 8315, pp. 199–216, 2014.

Recently, there has been interest in on-demand medical systems where health care workers can assemble larger medical systems out of smaller medical devices at the bedside in order to provide better therapy for their patients [25]. These on-demand systems would be used to provide better physiologic alarms (by combining data streams from multiple medical devices) and closed loop control (using physiologic sensors to drive actuators). While there is demand from the medical community, critical care medical systems have two major attributes which pose engineering challenges for the on-demand approach.

First, medical devices tend to be more **complex**. Unlike consumer electronics, critical care medical devices are very complex and variable, even among devices designed for a similar purpose (*e.g.,* infusion pumps). Often, this complexity and variability is the result of different ways device manufacturers have chosen to mitigate certain safety hazards. The complexity and variability means it is difficult to capture the range of behavior of a single device class in a standard similar to USB where the features and behavior of each class are fully enumerated beforehand. Second, on-demand medical systems serve a **safety critical** purpose; if the composite system malfunctions or is implemented incorrectly injury or death could result. Traditional safety critical systems such as aircraft, nuclear power plants and standalone medical devices are evaluated for safety before they are delivered to the user. The state of the art in safety assesment is to consider the completely assembled system as a whole. In on-demand medical systems this would not be possible because each system instance may be assembled by combining devices that have never been tested together. There must be some mechanism in place to analyze the behavior of *all* instantiations of a on-demand system in order to ensure that any instantiation only exhibits safe behavior.

There have been a number of high-level proposals for how to achieve safe on-demand medical systems [20,11,25,5]. These proposals all involve separating system functionality between *interoperable* componenets: *coordination applications* (apps), medical devices, and a Medical Application Platform (MAP). In these proposals, each type of system component would be regulated, certified, and then obtained by the health-care organization separately [12]. We now provide a brief overview of the role and use of each system component type.

Apps are software programs that provide the coordination algorithm for a specific clinical scenario (*i.e.,* smart alarms, closed-loop control of devices, *etc.*). In addition to executable code, these apps contain *device requirements* declarations: a formal model of the medical devices they need to operate correctly. These apps would be validated and verified against their requirements specification before they are marketed. Symmetrically, the interoperable medical devices carry a self-descriptive model, known as a *capabilities* specification. Each medical device would be certified that it conforms to its specification before it is marketed and sold to end users.

The MAP provides a trusted base: It executes the coordination apps and facilitates the assembly of the on-demand system. When a user connects a medical device to the network, that medical device will transmit its capabilities specification to the MAP. Likewise, when a user attempts to launch an app, the MAP analyzes the app's requirements specification and the connected devices' capabilities specifications. If the devices do not have the required capabilities, the MAP will prevent the app from running and notify the user. This functionality is critical to the assembly of on-demand medical systems because it is the foundation for any safety or effectiveness claim; in theory only systems which exhibit the behavior captured by the app (and its associated requirements specification) will be instantiated. This enables various stakeholders (*e.g.,* app developers and regulatory agencies) to verify and validate the behavior of all possible instantiations of an on-demand system by checking the behavior of the application against its requirements specification.

Finally, each of these components would implement an *interoperability standard*. The standard would specify allowed network transport protocols, how medical and system information is encoded on the network, provide a basic means to establish an interconnection between components, and expose logical interfaces for the transmission of data or commands. Current interoperability standards, such as IEEE-11073 POC [16], IEEE-11073 PHD [9,8] and Health Level 7 (HL7) [10] focus mainly on *data* interoperability (*i.e.,* they provide a mechanism for the exchange of data). Notably absent in current standards is the ability to address the reactive behavior of various medical systems. This means that current standards are largely unsuitable for interoperable medical systems where multiple devices are coordinating to provide autonomous delivery of care.

Our ability to reason about an on-demand medical system *a priori* (*i.e.,* before it is instantiated) depends on how the app requirements and device capabilities are specified. There are three major goals that must be met by a suitable specification language:

G1 The language must enable us to automatically relate app device requirements specifications to device capabilities specifications: properties which must hold for apps composed with their requirements specification must hold for any ad hoc system where the app is composed with compatible devices.

G2 The language must enable app developers to explicitly specify variability in required device behavior: if all safety properties are satisfied with a highly variable device requirements specification it means the app is compatible with a larger set of medical devices.

G3 The language must be expressive enough to specify arbitrarily complex and reactive behavior.

In this paper, we propose a modal specification language for on-demand systems which addresses **G1**, **G2** and **G3**. This formalism could be layered onto existing standards to enable the specification of device behavior. Syntactically, it is a simple, state-based language inspired by Alur and Henzinger's *Reactive Modules* formalism [1]. Semantically, each module defined in the language is equivalent to a modal I/O automaton (MIOA) [24], a formalism that extends labeled transitions systems with a may/must modality on transitions and an input/output/internal distinction on action labels.

MIOAs are well suited for reasoning about on-demand systems for the following reasons. First, the may/must distinction of transitions is useful for specifying the behavioral variability of devices: must transitions denote required behavior and may transitions represent allowed behavior. Thus, we can use MIOAs to reason about all possible instantiations of an on-demand system based on the specification. Second, we show that the *weak modal refinement* relation of MIOAs preserves both *safety* (nothing bad happens) and *liveness* (something good eventually happens) properties. The guarantee of safety and liveness properties are essential for on-demand medical systems, *e.g.,*

- "the patient's SpO$_2$ level should never be lower than 95" (safety)
- "the laser must be completely deactivated to allow the flow of the oxygen concentrate from the ventilator" (liveness)

Third, the compositionality of MIOAs allows us to easily verify the behavior of component-based on-demand systems by verifying their specifications. For example, if we find a medical device that refines an app's requirements specification, then we can claim that the system created by composing the app with that device will satisfy all safety and liveness properties satisfied by the composition of that app and its requirements specification.

We have prototyped our approach using the MIO Workbench tool [6] and the PRISM model checker [22], and applied it to a few case studies. In this paper, we report on the application of our approach to the case study of a closed loop patient controlled analgesia system.

The rest of this paper is organized as follows: in Section 2 we describe one possible application of on-demand medical systems as a motivating example. In Section 3 we describe our proposed specification language and the underlying MIOA semantics. Section 4 contains a case study where we apply language to specify an on-demand medical system and then verify properties of that system. We conclude the paper, discuss current weaknesses of the approach, and propose directions for future work in Section 5.

2   Motivating Example

In this section we describe Patient Controlled Analgesia (PCA), the hazards of PCA, and how a closed-loop system could be used to mitigate those hazards. The purpose of the example itself is twofold. First it illustrates how the functionality of the closed-loop system can be divided between an app and medical devices. Second, it allows us to show variability among the same class of medical device and how that variability can affect the safety of an on-demand system.

After trauma (*e.g.,* invasive surgery) patients convalescing in an ICU are often placed on PCA therapy for pain management. During PCA therapy, patients are attached to an infusion pump loaded with a painkiller (*e.g.,* an opiod). When the patient desires additional pain-relief, they press a trigger which causes the pump to deliver a bolus of medication. While PCA lets patients manage their own pain-levels effectively [15] it also creates an opportunity for overdose. Opiod

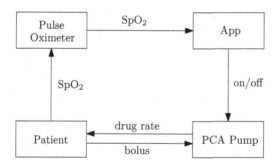

Fig. 1. A closed-loop PCA system

overdose can result in respiratory depression, which in turn can result in injury or death [17,27,13]. One possible way to mitigate the hazard posed by PCA is to 'close the loop': analyze data from sensors attached to the patient in real-time to determine if the patient is nearing respiratory distress and, if so, disable the pump [26,19].

As shown in Figure 1, the system consists of four components: a pulse oximeter, an app, a PCA infusion pump and a patient. The system operates in a closed-loop fashion: the pulse oximeter keeps monitoring the patient's SpO_2 value (measure of blood oxygenation), and the app controls the PCA pump based on the SpO_2 value read from the pulse oximeter (the app would stop the pump if the detected SpO_2 value is lower than 95). When the PCA pump is turned on, it delivers drug to the patient with a normal infusion rate pre-programmed by the caregiver; however, if it receives a bolus request from the patient, then a higher drug dose will be supplied, unless the pump is stopped by the app.

This application has one main safety property: the infusion rate of the pump should always be 0 (*i.e.,* the pump is off) whenever the patient has an SpO_2 below a certain threshold (*e.g.,* $SpO_2 < 95$). The satisfaction of this property depends on both the algorithm implemented by the app and the behavior of the PCA pump the app is managing. Figure 2 illustrates the behavior of three different types of PCA pumps as state machines. Figure 2a represents a simple infusion pump that infuses while it receives the *on* signal. Technically speaking, the pump of Figure 2a is not a PCA pump because it doesn't provide any mechanism for the patient to request a bolus. Figure 2b represents a PCA pump that will infuse at a rate of 1 while it receives the *on* signal and it will infuse at a rate of 2 when the patient requests a bolus, even if it is receiving the *off.* Finally, Figure 2c represents an even more complex PCA pump. This pump will autonomously disable itself under a number of conditions in order to mitigate several hazards associated with infusion pumps [4]. For example, if the pump detects air bubbles in the infusion line, it will halt infusion and raise an alarm in order to prevent an air-embolism.

So, which pump should we choose to use? If we plug any of these three pumps into the system, will the patient's safety be guaranteed? And is there an easy way to verify the effectiveness of the PCA system? These questions will be answered

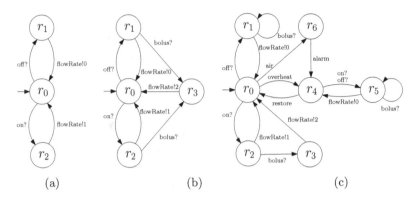

Fig. 2. MIOAs for three different PCA pump devices

in Section 4 by applying our modal specification approach, which is explained in the next section.

3   A Specification Language for On-Demand Systems

In this section, we propose a simple, state-based specification language for describing the requirements of on-demand systems. This language can be applied, for example, by app developers to specify the desirable behavior of compatible medical devices. The language is based on Alur and Henzinger's *Reactive Modules* formalism [1], with the extension of transition modality (*i.e.*, distinguishing *must* and *may* transitions). We first define the syntax of our proposed language in Section 3.1, and then give its semantics in Section 3.2.

3.1   Syntax

We define each component of an on-demand system as a module M, which is a tuple $((in_M, out_M, int_M), var_M, (must_M, may_M))$ where (in_M, out_M, int_M) is the signature of M representing sets of *input*, *output* and *internal* actions, var_M is a set of state variables, and $(must_M, may_M)$ are sets of *must* and *may* transitions.

A module communicates with the external environment via input and output actions in the CSP style [14]; that is, an input (resp. output) action, denoted by $c?v$ (resp. $c!v$), enables the module to receive (resp. send) message v over a named channel c. The message v, which for example can be an expression about some previous inputs or a valuation of some local variable of the module, must be typed. Sometimes, message v is omitted from an input/output action, denoted by $c?$ or $c!$, with the interpretation that there is only a single possible message can be transmitted through channel c. The set of internal actions int_M, representing internal events of module M, are not observable to the external environment.

```
module M₁

    input: a?integer[0..1], b?;
    output: c!;
    internal: τ;

    s : [0..3] init 0;

    [a?v]  (s = 0)  ──must──▸  (s' = 1);
    [c!]   (s = 2)  ──must──▸  (s' = 3);
    [τ]    (s = 3)  ──must──▸  (s' = 3);

    [τ]    (s = 0)  ──may──▸   (s' = 2);
    [b?]   (s = 1)  ──may──▸   (s' = 3);

endmodule
```

Fig. 3. An example module specification

The variable set var_M defines the local state space of module M. A state variable $s \in var_M$ can be either a Boolean value, or an integer within a predefined finite range. We suppose that each variable s has an initial value $\bar{s}$.

The behavior of module M is defined by the set of must/may transitions $(must_M, may_M)$. Each transition $t \in must_M \cup may_M$ takes the form (a, g, m, u), comprising an action label a, a guard g, a modality label m and an update u. The action $a \in in_M \cup out_M \cup int_M$ can be either an input/output action synchronizing with the external environment, or an internal event occurring within the module. The guard g is a predicate over the state variables var_M, determining if transition t is enabled. The modality label $m \in \{must, may\}$ indicates if the transition is required (*i.e.*, must occur) in all implementations or if it is allowed (*i.e.*, may occur) in any implementation. The update u describes the effect of transition t on state variables; more specifically, $u = (s'_1 = expr_1) \wedge \cdots (s'_n = expr_n)$ where s'_i denotes the updated value of state variable $s_i \in var_M$, and $expr_i$ is an expression in terms of the state variables.

Example 1. Figure 3 shows an example module M_1 described in our proposed specification language. The description is split into four parts, defining actions, state variables, as well as must and may transitions of the module. The module M_1 has two input actions: "a?**integer[1..2]**" that receives a integer value within the range $\{1, 2\}$ via channel "a", and "b?" that receives an input via channel "b" (the message is omitted). The module may send an output through action "c!", and has a single internal action τ.

We also see that M_1 has a single interger-valued variable s with the range $\{0, \ldots, 3\}$ and an initial value 0. There are four transitions in M_1. Each transition $t = (a, g, m, u)$ is written in a line "$[a]\ g \xrightarrow{m} u;$". For example, line "$[a?v]\ (s = 0) \xrightarrow{must} (s' = 1);$" represents a "must" transition with action "a?v", guard $(s = 0)$ and update $(s' = 1)$.

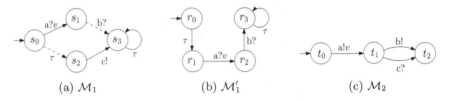

Fig. 4. Three example MIOAs

3.2   Semantics

The semantics of our specification language is based on Modal I/O Automata [24] which in turn are extensions of Modal Transition Systems [23]. A modal I/O automaton (MIOA) can be considered as a (nondeterministic) state transition system with an input/output/internal distinction on action labels and a must/may distinction on its transition relations.

Definition 1 (MIOA). *A modal I/O automaton P is a tuple $(S_P, \bar{s}_P, in_P, out_P, int_P, \rightarrow_{\Box P}, \rightarrow_{\Diamond P})$ where S_P is a finite set of states, $\bar{s}_P \in S_P$ is an initial state, in_P, out_P and int_P are disjoint sets of input, output and internal actions, $\rightarrow_{\Box P} \subseteq S_P \times act_P \times S_P$ is the must transition relation describing required behavior, and $\rightarrow_{\Diamond P} \subseteq S_P \times act_P \times S_P$ is the may transition relation describing allowed behavior $(act_P = in_P \cup out_P \cup int_P)$.*

The mapping from a module $M = ((in_M, out_M, int_M), var_M, (must_M, may_M))$ described in our proposed specification language to a MIOA P is straightforward. We define the state space S_P of P to be the set of all valuations of the state variables in var_M. The initial state $\bar{s}_P$ is given by the initial values of variables in var_M. The action sets $in_P = in_M$, $out_P = out_M$, and $int_P = int_M$. And each transition $t \in must_M$ (resp. $t \in may_M$) maps to a transition $p \xrightarrow{a}_{\Box P} p'$ (resp. $p \xrightarrow{a}_{\Diamond P} p'$) in P, where p and p' are states given by the guard and update of t, respectively.

Example 2. The module M_1 described in Figure 3 maps to the MIOA $\mathcal{M}_1$ shown in Figure 4a. There are four states $\{s_0, s_1, s_2, s_3\}$ in $\mathcal{M}_1$, each of which maps to a valuation of variable $s = i$ for $i \in \{0, \dots, 3\}$ in M_1. The initial state of $\mathcal{M}_1$ is s_0, indicated by an incoming arrow in Figure 4a. The must transitions are drawn in solid arrows, while the may transitions are drawn in dashed arrows.

In this paper, we consider only *syntactically consistent* MIOA where $\rightarrow_{\Box P} \subseteq \rightarrow_{\Diamond P}$, i.e., every required transition is also allowed. If the must and may transition relations of a MIOA P coincide, denoted $\rightarrow_{\Box P} = \rightarrow_{\Diamond P}$, then we call P an *implementation*. An abstract MIOA with nonempty must and may transition relations specifies a set of concrete implementations: a must transition asks that any legal implementation must include that transition, while a may transition indicates that implementations are allowed (but not required) to have that transition. Formally, the relation between an abstract specification MIOA and a concrete implementation MIOA is captured by *refinements*. There are many different types of refinement relations between MIOAs [24,7]. In our setting, we adopt the *weak modal refinement* relation [7], which ensures that the observable behavior of an implementation (*e.g.*, actual medical device) refines the specification (*e.g.*, app requirements).

We need the notion of *weak transitions* to reason about the observable behavior of MIOAs. Given an input/output action a of a MIOA P, there exists a weak must transition between states p and p', denoted by $p \ (\xrightarrow{a}_{\Box P})^* \ p'$, iff there exist a pair of states $p_1, p_2 \in S_P$ such that $p \ (\xrightarrow{\tau}_{\Box P})^* \ p_1 \xrightarrow{a}_{\Box P} p_2 \ (\xrightarrow{\tau}_{\Box P})^* p'$, where τ denotes any arbitrary internal action and $p \ (\xrightarrow{\tau}_{\Box P})^* \ p_1$ represents finitely many (zero or more) transitions from p to p_1 labelled with internal actions. The notion of weak may transitions $p \ (\xrightarrow{a}_{\Diamond P})^* \ p'$ can be defined analogously.

Definition 2 (Weak Modal Refinement). *Given two MIOAs P and Q with $in_P = in_Q$ and $out_P = out_Q$, a relation $R \subseteq S_P \times S_Q$ is called a weak modal refinement for P and Q iff for all $(p, q) \in R$ and $a \in act_P \cup act_Q$ it holds that:*

- *if $q \xrightarrow{a}_{\Box Q} q'$ then there exists $p' \in S_P$ such that $p \ (\xrightarrow{\hat{a}}_{\Box P})^* \ p'$ and $(p', q') \in R$,*
- *if $p \xrightarrow{a}_{\Diamond P} p'$ then there exists $q' \in S_Q$ such that $q \ (\xrightarrow{\hat{a}}_{\Diamond Q})^* \ q'$ and $(p', q') \in R$,*

where $(\xrightarrow{\hat{a}}_{\Box P})^* = (\xrightarrow{a}_{\Box P})^*$ if $a \in int_P \cup out_P$, and $(\xrightarrow{\hat{a}}_{\Box P})^* = (\xrightarrow{\tau}_{\Box P})^*$ otherwise. If there exists a refinement relation R such that $(\bar{s}_P, \bar{s}_Q) \in R$, then we claim that P weakly modally refines Q, denoted by $P \leq_m^* Q$.

The weak modal refinement relation defined above allows implementations to contain different (*i.e.*, unspecified) internal behavior as long as the internal behavior does not prevent the implementation from performing required external behavior. The refinement also prevents implementations from performing 'extra' external behavior as long as the extra behavior is specified in the signature of the specification. It does allow implementations to introduce new external behavior if that behavior is an action-label not specified in the specification; in this case, the transitions labled with that action are treated as τ transitions.

Example 3. The MIOA $\mathcal{M}_1'$ shown in Figure 4b weakly modally refines the MIOA $\mathcal{M}_1$ shown in Figure 4a, under relation $R = \{(r_0, s_0), (r_1, s_0), (r_2, s_1),$ $(r_3, s_3)\}$. Note that the required transition $s_2 \xrightarrow{c!}_{\Box} s_3$ in $\mathcal{M}_1$ does not have a mapping in $\mathcal{M}_1'$, because $\mathcal{M}_1'$ does not contain a refinement of the allowed transition $s_0 \xrightarrow{\tau}_{\Diamond} s_2$ in $\mathcal{M}_1$ such that no refinement of state s_2 is reachable in $\mathcal{M}_1'$.

Recall that, in our proposed specification language, a module (medical device) can comminucate with the external environment via sending/receiving messages. We now introduce a binary *composition* operator [24] to reason about the message passing. We say that two MIOAs P_1 and P_2 are *composable* iff the overlapping of their actions only occur on complementary types, *i.e.*, $(in_1 \cup int_1) \cap (in_2 \cup int_2) = \emptyset$ and $(out_1 \cup int_1) \cap (out_2 \cup int_2) = \emptyset$.

Definition 3 (Composition). *The composition of two composeable MIOAs P_1 and P_2 is given by a MIOA $P_1 \otimes P_2 = (S, \bar{s}, in, out, int, \rightarrow_\Box, \rightarrow_\Diamond)$, where the state*

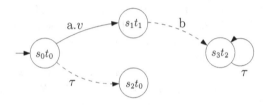

Fig. 5. A MIOA composition $\mathcal{M}_1 \otimes \mathcal{M}_2$.

space $S = S_1 \times S_2$, the initial state $\bar{s} = (\bar{s}_1, \bar{s}_2)$, in $= (in_1 \backslash out_2) \cup (in_2 \backslash out_1)$, out $= (out_1 \backslash in_2) \cup (out_2 \backslash in_1)$, int $= int_1 \cup int_2 \cup (in_1 \cap out_2) \cup (in_2 \cap out_1)$, and the transition relations are given by the following rules (for $\gamma \in \{\Box, \Diamond\}$):

$$\frac{p_1 \xrightarrow{a!}_\gamma p_1' \quad p_2 \xrightarrow{a?}_\gamma p_2'}{p_1 \otimes p_2 \xrightarrow{a}_\gamma p_1' \otimes p_2'} \quad \frac{p_1 \xrightarrow{a?}_\gamma p_1' \quad p_2 \xrightarrow{a!}_\gamma p_2'}{p_1 \otimes p_2 \xrightarrow{a}_\gamma p_1' \otimes p_2'}$$

$$\frac{p_1 \xrightarrow{a}_\gamma p_1' \quad a \notin act_2}{p_1 \otimes p_2 \xrightarrow{a}_\gamma p_1' \otimes p_2} \quad \frac{a \notin act_1 \quad p_2 \xrightarrow{a}_\gamma p_2'}{p_1 \otimes p_2 \xrightarrow{a}_\gamma p_1 \otimes p_2'}$$

Example 4. Figure 5 shows the composition of two MIOAs $\mathcal{M}_1$ (Figure 4a) and $\mathcal{M}_2$ (Figure 4c). $\mathcal{M}_1$ expects an input action "a?v" in state s_0 while $\mathcal{M}_2$ sends an output action "a!v" in state t_0, these two transitions are composed into a transition $s_0 t_0 \xrightarrow{a.v}_\Box s_1 t_1$ in $\mathcal{M}_1 \otimes \mathcal{M}_2$. Similarly, the may transition $s_1 \xrightarrow{b?}_\Diamond s_3$ in $\mathcal{M}_1$ composes with the must transition $t_1 \xrightarrow{b?}_\Box t_2$ in $\mathcal{M}_1$, resulting in a may transition $s_1 t_1 \xrightarrow{b}_\Diamond s_3 t_2$ in the product. Since τ is an internal action of $\mathcal{M}_1$, the τ-labelled transitions of $\mathcal{M}_1$ compose with atomic transitions (self-loops) of $\mathcal{M}_2$, see for example, $s_0 t_0 \xrightarrow{\tau}_\Diamond s_2 t_0$. Note that $s_2 t_0$ is a deadlock state.

A motivation of our work is to design a specification language that makes verifying properties of medical devices easy. In particular, we are interested in two kinds of properties: *safety* (something bad will never happen) and *liveness* (something good will eventually happen). Formally, a safety property ϕ_{safe} is defined as a liner-time property over a set of actions such that any infinite word w where ϕ_{safe} does not hold contains a bad prefix (*i.e.*, a finite prefix w' where the bad thing has happened); a liveness property ϕ_{live} (over a set of actions) is an linear-time property such that each finite word can be extended to an infinite word that satisfies ϕ_{live}.

Given a MIOA P and a safety or liveness property ϕ over act_P, we define two satisfaction relations:

- $P \models_\Box \phi$, under-approximates "all refinements of P satisfy ϕ";
- $P \models_\Diamond \phi$, over-approximates "some refinement of P satisfies ϕ".

To verify property ϕ on P, we need to prove that $P \models_\Box \phi$ is true; and to refute property ϕ, we need to establish that $P \models_\Box \neg\phi$ holds.

We prove that weak modal refinement preserves the verification of safety and liveness properties as follows.

Lemma 1. *Let P and Q be two MIOAs such that $P \leq_m^* Q$. Given a safety property ϕ_{safe} over actions $in_P \cup out_P$, if $Q \models_\Box \phi_{safe}$, then $P \models_\Box \phi_{safe}$.*

Proof. For the sake of contradiction, suppose $Q \models_\Box \phi_{safe}$ and $P \not\models_\Box \phi_{safe}$. The latter means that there may exist some path ρ in P containing a bad prefix. For simplicity, assume that the bad behavior is represented by a single word a. We have a path $\rho = p_0 \rightarrow \cdots \rightarrow p_{n-1} \xrightarrow{a}_{\Diamond P} p_n$. Based on $P \leq_m^* Q$ and Definition 2, there exists a pair of states q and q' in Q such that $(p_{n-1}, q) \in R$, $(p_n, q') \in R$ and $q (\xrightarrow{\tau}_{\Diamond Q})^* q_{i-1} \xrightarrow{a}_{\Diamond Q} q_i (\xrightarrow{\tau}_{\Diamond Q})^* q'$. Therefore, there may exist a path in Q containing the bad word a, which is a contradiction with $Q \models_\Box \phi_{safe}$. $\quad\square$

Lemma 2. *Let P and Q be two MIOAs such that $P \leq_m^* Q$. Given a liveness property ϕ_{live} over actions $in_P \cup out_P$, if $Q \models_\Box \phi_{live}$, then $P \models_\Box \phi_{live}$.*

Proof. Since $Q \models_\Box \phi_{live}$, every (infinite) path in Q must eventually reach the good condition. For simplicity, assume that the good condition is represented by a single word a. Then, there must exists a pair of states q_{n-1} and q_n in any (infinite) path ρ of Q such that $\rho = q_0 \rightarrow \cdots \rightarrow q_{n-1} \xrightarrow{a}_{\Box Q} q_n \rightarrow \cdots$. Based on $P \leq_m^* Q$ and Definition 2, for each pair of q_{n-1} and q_n, there must exists a pair of corresponding states p, p' in P such that $(p, q_{n-1}) \in R$, $(p', q_n) \in R$ and $p (\xrightarrow{\tau}_{\Box P})^* p_{i-1} \xrightarrow{a}_{\Box P} p_i (\xrightarrow{\tau}_{\Box P})^* p'$. Therefore, every infinite path in P must eventually reach the good condition, so that we have $P \models_\Box \phi_{live}$. $\quad\square$

Another nice feature about weak modal refinement is the following compositionality result:

Theorem 1 (Compositionality [2]). *Let P_1, P_1' and P_2 be MIOAs (P_1 and Q are composable). If $P_1' \leq_m^* P_1$, then $P_1' \otimes P_2 \leq_m^* P_1 \otimes P_2$.*

Based on the above theorem and Lemmas 1 and 2, we can verify safety and liveness properties on medical devices without composing the (large) complete systems. For example, let P_1 be the specification for some medical device, P_1' be an implementation of the actual device, P_2 be the external environment (*e.g.*, app, patient) and ϕ be the desirable safety or liveness property. When designing the specification, the app developers make sure that $P_1 \otimes P_2 \models_\Box \phi$. We only need to check whether the device P_1' weakly modally refines the specification P_1. If $P_1' \leq_m^* P_1$ holds, then we can claim that $P_1' \otimes P_2 \models_\Box \phi$ without actually verifying the composed system $P_1' \otimes P_2$.

4   Case Study

Now we apply our proposed specification approach to analyze the closed-loop PCA example from Section 2. We model each system component (*i.e.*, app, patient, Pulse Oximeter and PCA pump) as a MIOA. To answer the question that, from the three PCA pumps shown in Figure 2, which one should we choose

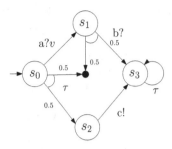

Fig. 6. Translation of the MIOA in Figure 4a for PRISM

to use, we use the MIO Workbench tool [6] to check weather the MIOA of a pump weakly modally refines the MIOA of the pump specification. If the refinement relation holds, then the pump is good in the sense that the PCA system should be able to guarantee the required safety property; otherwise, the pump is not safe to use.

To demonstrate that our approach can help to preserve system properties, we also use the (probabilistic) model checker PRISM [22] to verify the required safety property of composed PCA systems because of PRISM's relative maturity and ease of use. PRISM does not actually support the verification of MIOAs. We instead translate MIOAs as probabilistic automata (PAs): each must transition becomes a transition with probability 1 and each may transition becomes a transition with probability 0.5 [1]. For example, Figure 6 shows the probabilistic translation of the MIOA in Figure 4a; the may transition from s_0 to s_2 now becomes a transition with probability 0.5 (the black dot is the sink state). If PRISM verifies that certain property is *true* with probability 1, then the property "must" be satisfied by the on-demand medical system; and if the verification result is a real value p such that $0 < p < 1$, then the system "may" satisfy the property.[2]

4.1   Modelling

Figure 7 shows the detailed model for the pulse oximeter, which is a two-state modal I/O automaton synchronizing with the patient model via a must transition labelled with the input action "toSensor?SpO_2" and then immediately sending the data to the app via another must transition with the output action "toApp!SpO_2". Note that, in both actions, $SpO_2 \in [0, 100]$ is an integer value transmitted over the input/output channel.

---

[1] To make probabilistic distributions full, we complement each may transition with a transition (with probability 0.5) to a sink state; however, the verification result would exclude all the paths leading to the sink state.

[2] While an evaluation of scalability is beyond the scope of this paper, PRISM implements a number of efficient model-checking algorithms for probabilistic systems and can scale to models with at least 10^7 states.

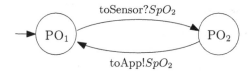

Fig. 7. MIOA for the pulse oximeter

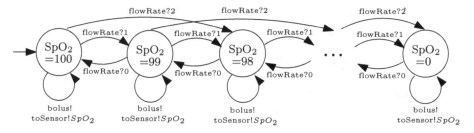

Fig. 8. MIOA for the patient dynamics

We adopt a simple patient model which only considers the patient's discrete SpO_2 measurements.[3] As shown in Figure 8, each state of the MIOA for the patient model represents a single SpO_2 value, ranging from 0 to 100. With an initial value of 100, the patient's SpO_2 measurement decreases by 1 or 2 upon receiving drug from the PCA pump at a normal infusion rate ("flowRate?1") or a bolus rate ("flowRate?2"), respectively. On the other hand, the SpO_2 value increases by 1 if the PCA pump stops ("flowRate?0"), modeling the restoration of the patient's vital sign as the drug concentration reduces. At any point, the patient has the option of pressing the button to request one more dose from the PCA pump (denoted by the output action "bolus!"). The patient's SpO_2 level is constantly monitored by the pulse oximeter via synchronizing over "toSensor!SpO_2".

The behavior of the control app is illustrated in Figure 9 using our proposed specification language[4]. The app has an input action "toApp?" carrying integer values SpO_2 sent by the pulse oximeter, and two output actions "on!" and "off!" which control the PCA pump. There are two state variables a and v. Initially we assume $a = 0$ and $v = 100$. If an input action "toApp?SpO_2" is detected, the app updates a as 1 and sets v with the received SpO_2 value. If $v > 95$, meaning that the patient's vitals are not endangered, then the app outputs an "on!" signal to the PCA pump for allowing drug delivery; otherwise, an "off!" signal is sent to stop the PCA pump.

Figure 10a describes the specification for the PCA pump, which should be provided by the app developers, and Figure 10b shows the corresponding MIOA. Under this specification, if the pump is enabled by the "on?" command from the

---

[3] See [26] for an example of how continuous patient dynamics can be related to a discrete model.

[4] The corresponding MIOA has more than 200 states and thus is too large to be drawn here.

```
module app

input: toApp?integer[0..100];
output: on!, off!;

a : [0..1] init 0;
v : [0..100] init 100;

[toApp?SpO₂] (a = 0)                    ──must──→ (a' = 1) ∧ (v' = SpO₂);
[on!]        (a = 1) ∧ (v > 95) ──must──→ (a' = 0);
[off!]       (a = 1) ∧ (v ≤ 95) ──must──→ (a' = 0);

endmodule
```

Fig. 9. App that controls the PCA pump

```
module pumpSpec

input: on?, off?, bolus?;
output: flowRate!integer[0..2];
internal: τ;

s : [0..5] init 0;

[off?]       (s = 0) ──must──→ (s' = 1);
[on?]        (s = 0) ──must──→ (s' = 2);
[on?]        (s = 4) ──must──→ (s' = 5);
[off?]       (s = 4) ──must──→ (s' = 5);
[flowRate!0] (s = 1) ──must──→ (s' = 0);
[flowRate!0] (s = 5) ──must──→ (s' = 4);
[flowRate!1] (s = 2) ──must──→ (s' = 0);
[flowRate!2] (s = 3) ──must──→ (s' = 0);

[bolus?]     (s = 1) ──may──→ (s' = 1);
[bolus?]     (s = 2) ──may──→ (s' = 3);
[bolus?]     (s = 5) ──may──→ (s' = 5);
[tau]        (s = 0) ──may──→ (s' = 4);
[tau]        (s = 4) ──may──→ (s' = 0);

endmodule
```

(a)   (b)

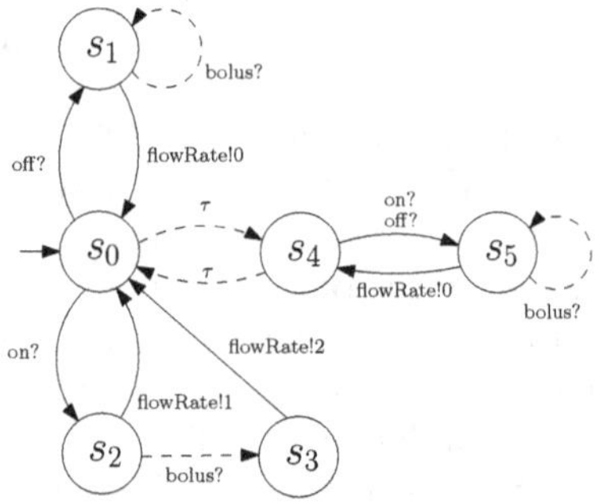

Fig. 10. The PCA pump specification and its corresponding MIOA

app, then it can deliver drug to the patient at a normal infusion rate "flowRate!1"; however, if it is disabled by the "off?" command, then no drug will be delivered ("flowRate!0"). Some pump may allow receiving "bolus?" request from the patient, which are described as "may" transitions in the specification (dashed lines in Figure 10b). To avoid the overdose of drug, the "bolus?" request is only effective (i.e., the pump delivers drug at a higher rate "flowRate!2") when the pump is enabled by the app. A pump may shut itself down due to various reasons and may also restore from the shutdown; the specification allow these behavior by describing them "may" transitions labelled with an internal action τ. When a pump is shutdown, it would not respond to any command from the app/patient and no drug will be delivered.

4.2   Analysis

Figure 2 shows three PCA pump devices with different functionality. Device (a) has the basic functions of receiving commands from the app and delivering drug to the patient accordingly. Device (b) has the additional function of adjusting the drug infusion rate based on patients' bolus requests. Device (c) is the most sophisticated equipment: apart from the functions of receiving app commands (bolus requests) and delivering drug, it can detect air bubbles in the infusion line and issue alarm, and also protect itself from overheating; if any of these hazards is detected, the pump will shutdown automatically until the device is restored.

Our experiments indicate that devices (a) and (c) meet the specification requirements, because their corresponding MIOAs (Figures 2a and 2c) are both weak refinements of the specification's MIOA (Figure 10b). However, device (b) does not meet the specification: the path

$$r_0 \xrightarrow{\text{off?}} r_1 \xrightarrow{\text{bolus?}} r_3 \xrightarrow{\text{flowRate!2}} r_0$$

in the device's MIOA (Figure 2b) does not have a mapping (allowed path) in the specification's MIOA.

We verified the safety property "patient's SpO_2 level should always be above 94" on the PCA systems composed using these three devices. It is not surprising to find that both systems of devices (a) and (c) satisfy the safety property, but the system of device (b) violates the property. The violation is due to the fact that device (b) always admits patients' bolus request even if the app has issued the "off" command.

5   Conclusion and Discussion

In this paper we have described an approach to specify on-demand systems and applied that approach to an example application from the medical domain. This approach uses a specification language with the semantics of MIOA. We showed that weak modal refinement can be used to check the compatibility between app requirements and device capabilites by proving that weak modal refinement preserves both safety and liveness properties. This enables medical systems developers to express complex medical device behavioral requirements, explicitly specify allowed variability and reason about the behavior of on-demand systems *a priori*.

While we provided a case study as a proof-of-concept for the approach, there are many open questions concerning the engineering, safety and application of on-demand medical systems in a critical care setting. First we note that there are several areas where our proposed specification language and associated semantics would need to be extended to make the approach more applicable to real medical systems. For example, the action labels in our language are only tagged with simple data-types. Often, medical device actions relate directly to an interaction with the physical world (*e.g.,* an infusion pump *infusing* a drug). It would be useful if action labels could also be tagged with *physical* types which would denote the physical interaction of the action. Furthermore, our approach only supports reasoning about discrete time systems. Real medical devices exhibit continuous time behavior, and the ability to capture real-time behavior is critical if we want to apply our approach to real medical systems. For example, the on-demand medical systems described in [3,26,18] all rely on 'timeout' behavior in the medical devices to guarantee system safety in the presence of inter-device communications failures. Additionally, many medical devices exhibit continuous behavior in terms of their interactions with the patient. For example, infusion pumps deliver drugs continuously according to 'trumpet' curves [28]. It is not known to what fidelity a specification will need to capture device behavior: Is continuous time plus discrete behavior enough, or is a fully hybrid specification required? The answer to this question will likely depend on the types of on-demand systems clinicians will want to employee.

Second, the approach described in this paper requires that medical devices comply with their specifications. In theory this seems reasonable, but in practice it may not be possible to have total confidence in a device's compliance with its specification. For example, a device may be non-compliant due to an uncaught systematic defect (*i.e.,* a design or implementation error), uncaught manufacturing errors, or unaccounted for environmental interference (*e.g.,* artifical light interfering with a physiologic sensor). Should the specification approach be extended to capture the possibility of these errors? If so, what types of errors and faults should be captured in the specification versus left to other risk management mechanisms?

Finally, medical devices can interact with each other indirectly through the patient (*e.g.,* a pulse-oximeter attached to a patient on supplementary oxygen will sometimes give abnormally high readings). Should on-demand systems check for these types of interactions automatically? Or should we rely on the medical caregiver to determine which combinations of medical devices are appropriate to use in a given situation? The answer is not clear; though at first it may appear that automatic interaction checking could improve the safety of the system, in practice doing thisis very difficult due to the fact we currently lack a detailed understanding of human physiology. This in turn can result in overly conservative or sensitive checks. For example, modern computerized physician order entry (CPOE) systems automatically check if a doctor prescribes drugs that *may* interact adversely. In many cases hospitals have worked with vendors to disable these checks because these checks are too conservative (*i.e.,* generate an overwhelming number of alerts) and the caregivers are competent enough to know how the drugs will interact and whether or not the risk is justified for a particular patient [21]. The answer to this question will depend on the complexity of on-demand medical systems, our level of understanding of patient physiology, and the fidelity of care those system are intended to deliver.

References

1. Alur, R., Henzinger, T.A.: Reactive modules. Formal Methods in System Design 15(1), 7–48 (1999)
2. Antonik, A., Huth, M., Larsen, K.G., Nyman, U., Wasowski, A.: 20 years of modal and mixed specifications. European Association for Theoretical Computer Science. Bulletin (95) (2008)
3. Arney, D., Goldman, J.M., Whitehead, S.F., Lee, I.: Synchronizing an x-ray and anesthesia machine ventilator: A medical device interoperability case study (2009)
4. Arney, D., Jetley, R., Jones, P., Lee, I., Sokolsky, O.: Formal methods based development of a pca infusion pump reference model: Generic infusion pump (gip) project. In: Joint Workshop on High Confidence Medical Devices, Software, and Systems and Medical Device Plug-and-Play Interoperability, HCMDSS-MDPnP, pp. 23–33. IEEE (2007)
5. Medical devices and medical systems - essential safety requirements for equipment comprising the patient-centric integrated clinical environment (ice), http://enterprise.astm.org/filtrexx40.cgi?+REDLINE_PAGES/F2761.htm
6. Bauer, S.S., Mayer, P., Legay, A.: Mio workbench: A tool for compositional design with modal input/output interfaces. In: Bultan, T., Hsiung, P.-A. (eds.) ATVA 2011. LNCS, vol. 6996, pp. 418–421. Springer, Heidelberg (2011)
7. Bauer, S.S., Mayer, P., Schroeder, A., Hennicker, R.: On weak modal compatibility, refinement, and the MIO workbench. In: Esparza, J., Majumdar, R. (eds.) TACAS 2010. LNCS, vol. 6015, pp. 175–189. Springer, Heidelberg (2010)
8. Carroll, R., Cnossen, R., Schnell, M., Simons, D.: Continua: An interoperable personal healthcare ecosystem. IEEE Pervasive Computing 6(4), 90–94 (2007)
9. Clarke, M., Bogia, D., Hassing, K., Steubesand, L., Chan, T., Ayyagari, D.: Developing a standard for personal health devices based on 11073. In: 29th Annual International Conference of the IEEE Engineering in Medicine and Biology Society, EMBS 2007, pp. 6174–6176 (2007)
10. Dolin, R.H., Alschuler, L., Boyer, S., Beebe, C., Behlen, F.M., Biron, P.V., Shvo, A.S.: Hl7 clinical document architecture, release 2. Journal of the American Medical Informatics Association 13(1), 30–39 (2006)
11. Hatcliff, J., King, A., Lee, I., Macdonald, A., Fernando, A., Robkin, M., Vasserman, E., Weininger, S., Goldman, J.M.: Rationale and architecture principles for medical application platforms. In: IEEE/ACM Third International Conference on Cyber-Physical Systems, ICCPS 2012, pp. 3–12. IEEE Computer Society, Washington, DC (2012), http://dx.doi.org/10.1109/ICCPS.2012.9
12. Hatcliff, J., Vasserman, E., Weininger, S., Goldman, J.: An overview of regulatory and trust issues for the integrated clinical environment. In: Proceedings of HCMDSS 2011 (2011)
13. Hicks, R.W., Sikirica, V., Nelson, W., Schein, J.R., Cousins, D.D.: Medication errors involving patient-controlled analgesia. American Journal of Health-System Pharmacy 65(5), 429–440 (2008)
14. Hoare, C.A.R.: Communicating sequential processes. Prentice-Hall, Inc., Upper Saddle River (1985)
15. Hudcova, J., McNicol, E., Quah, C., Lau, J., Carr, D.B.: Patient controlled intravenous opioid analgesia versus conventional opioid analgesia for postoperative pain control: A quantitative systematic review. Acute Pain 7(3), 115–132 (2005)
16. Iso/ieee 11073 committee, http://standards.ieee.org/findstds/standard/11073-10103-2012.html

17. Joint Commission: Sentinel event alert issue 33: Patient controlled analgesia by proxy (December 2004),
    http://www.jointcommission.org/sentinelevents/sentineleventalert/
18. Kim, C., Sun, M., Mohan, S., Yun, H., Sha, L., Abdelzaher, T.F.: A framework for the safe interoperability of medical devices in the presence of network failures. In: Proceedings of the 1st ACM/IEEE International Conference on Cyber-Physical Systems, pp. 149–158. ACM (2010)
19. King, A., Arney, D., Lee, I., Sokolsky, O., Hatcliff, J., Procter, S.: Prototyping closed loop physiologic control with the medical device coordination framework. In: Proceedings of the 2010 ICSE Workshop on Software Engineering in Health Care, pp. 1–11. ACM (2010)
20. King, A., Procter, S., Andresen, D., Hatcliff, J., Warren, S., Spees, W., Jetley, R., Jones, P., Weininger, S.: An open test bed for medical device integration and coordination. In: Proceedings of the 31st International Conference on Software Engineering (2009)
21. Kuperman, G.J., Bobb, A., Payne, T.H., Avery, A.J., Gandhi, T.K., Burns, G., Classen, D.C., Bates, D.W.: Medication-related clinical decision support in computerized provider order entry systems: A review. Journal of the American Medical Informatics Association 14(1), 29–40 (2007),
    http://www.sciencedirect.com/science/article/pii/S106750270600209X
22. Kwiatkowska, M., Norman, G., Parker, D.: PRISM 4.0: Verification of probabilistic real-time systems. In: Gopalakrishnan, G., Qadeer, S. (eds.) CAV 2011. LNCS, vol. 6806, pp. 585–591. Springer, Heidelberg (2011)
23. Larsen, K.G., Thomsen, B.: A modal process logic. In: Proceedings of the Third Annual Symposium on Logic in Computer Science, LICS 1988, pp. 203–210 (1988)
24. Larsen, K.G., Nyman, U., Wąsowski, A.: Modal I/O automata for interface and product line theories. In: De Nicola, R. (ed.) ESOP 2007. LNCS, vol. 4421, pp. 64–79. Springer, Heidelberg (2007)
25. Medical device "plug-and-play" interoperability program (2008),
    http://mdpnp.org/
26. Pajic, M., Mangharam, R., Sokolsky, O., Arney, D., Goldman, J., Lee, I.: Model-driven safety analysis of closed-loop medical systems. IEEE Transactions on Industrial Informatics (2013)
27. Paul, J.E., sawhney, M., Beattie, W.S., McLean, R.F.: Critical incidents amongst 10033 acute pain patients. Canadian Journal of Anesthesiology 51, A22 (2004)
28. Voss, G.I., Butterfield, R.D.: 27.1 performance criteria for intravenous infusion devices. Clinical Engineering, 415 (2003)

Towards Formal Safety Analysis in Feature-Oriented Product Line Development

Sara Bessling and Michaela Huhn

Department of Informatics, Clausthal University of Technology
Clausthal-Zellerfeld, Germany
{sara.bessling,michaela.huhn}@tu-clausthal.de

Abstract. Feature-orientation has proven beneficial in the development of software product lines. We investigate formal safety analysis and verification for product lines of software-intensive embedded systems. We show how to uniformly augment a feature-oriented, model-based design approach with the specification of safety requirements, failure models and fault injection. Therefore we analyze system hazards and identify the causes, i.e. failures and inadequate control systematically.

As features are the main concept of functional decomposition in the product line approach, features also direct the safety analysis and the specification of system-level safety requirements: Safety (design) constraints are allocated to features. Subsequently, the behavior including possible faults is formally modeled. Then formal verification techniques are employed in order to prove that the safety constraints are satisfied and the system level hazards are prevented. We demonstrate our method using SCADE Suite for the model-based product line design of cardiac pacemakers. VIATRA is employed for the model graph transformation generating the individual products. Formal safety analysis is performed by using SCADE Design Verifier. The case study shows that our approach leads to a fine-grained safety analysis and is capable of uncovering unwanted feature interactions.

1 Introduction

Software product line development addresses the engineering of families of similar products by means of systematically sharing development artifacts. In *feature-oriented* approaches to the product line development of software-intensive systems, user-tangible product characteristics - called *features* - that differentiate between the various products or are common to many of them, are used as a first class concept to structure the design. In case of dependable products, safety requirements need to be specified at each design phase and have to be verified to hold for each product. Currently, the use of formal approaches to dependable systems product lines is hampered by (1) rather restrictive product building mechanisms and (2) a lack of support for safety analysis, the specification and finally the verification of product-specific safety constraints that goes along with the design methodology. Both issues limit applicability of formal approaches to dependable systems product lines.

Ex post adding of safety constraints and failure models to a product model can be very costly as it may lead to an additional iteration through design steps when the product model needs to be reinspected and eventually redesigned. Moreover, verifying each

J. Gibbons and W. MacCaull (Eds.): FHIES 2013, LNCS 8315, pp. 217–235, 2014.

single product of a software product line, especially for safety-critical systems, can be very time consuming.

Therefore it looks more promising to extend a feature-oriented design methodology for product lines by an investigation of possible failures and to derive safety constraints feature-wise. As a feature is just a defined part of functionality in comparison to the more complex, complete product, it is easier to define safety constraints and failure models just by feature. However, when combining features to a product we have to consider possible feature interaction and failure propagation which will result in additional system-level safety constraints and failure models.

We already investigated how feature-oriented software product lines can be extended by feature-wise safety constraints in [12]. We showed how single products *and* their associated safety constraints can be derived from a single base model by means of graph transformation. Moreover, we verified the single product models with the SCADE Design Verifier. Here we complement this work by a method for identifying the system-level hazards due to system-theoretic process analysis (STPA) by Leveson [17]. STPA takes a functional view on the system architecture for identifying potentially unsafe behavior which can be naturally extended to our feature-oriented design approach. We apply STPA product-wise, but put an emphasis on the effects of combining features in the product generation and unwanted feature interaction. Errors that have been discovered for single features are reused. The safety analysis results in error models and safety constraints that are associated with the design models. Thus formal verification is now applied to the design models describing the normal behavior as well as to the exceptional behavior in the presence of failures. Unlike to [12], we use VIATRA [28] instead of CVL [11] for the transformation of product models because VIATRA allows for a more fine-grained control on the graph transformation process.

The joint verification of safety requirements and failure models for all products of a product line has been identified as sophisticated in literature by several authors, e.g. [8,23] and specifically for a pacemaker product line by [27]. However, if features are considered a first class concept in product line development, their impact on the safety constraints to hold on the products is evident [5,18]. In our approach we append error models and safety constraints to specific features. We perform a model transformation in which not only features are combined into a new product but also the associated error models and safety constraints are transformed and attached to the new product at the same time. This way it is guaranteed that the building strategies used when combining the design features to a product are uniformly applied to the error models and are properly reflected when formulating the safety constraints.

For demonstrating our approach we use the SCADE development framework for the phases of architectural and functional design. VIATRA is employed to implement the model graph transformation for product generation. The case study on a product line for cardiac pacemakers shows that a transformational approach to product generation can deal with the different kinds of modifications needed for different features. Moreover, the systematic feature-specific fine-grained treatment seems to increase the portion of functionality that is covered by safety analysis, failure modeling and subsequently by safety requirements.

2 Basics

2.1 Feature Models in Product Line Development

Products of product lines are a combination of features. Therefore feature models are used to specify variability. They can already be generated at the problem space level at which the different stakeholders contribute their requirements [24]. A common representation of feature models are tree diagrams in which a hierarchical decomposition of similarities and differences between the single product variants are expressed.

In constructive development phases, the variability specification has to be linked to the artifacts of the solution space. In a model-driven approach to the development of software product lines, the design for variability and the composition of features forming a product have to be framed at the level of architectural and behavioral design models. Azana et al. [3] consider a product generation as a model transformation. A sequence of transformation steps executed on an existing product model lead to a new product model. Each step stands for a modification needed to create or transform into a certain feature. These modifications are described as model deltas or fragments which will be replaced and include a base model, the transformation source, and the target model, the new product. These two models must conform to the same metamodel. Other approaches, which use only a single operator for feature composition, limit the possible the flexibility for product generation whereas transformational approaches offer the possibility to support many different feature-specific adaptations [3,10,11].

2.2 VIATRA

VIATRA [20,21] is the short name of VIsual Automated model TRAnsformations, a meanwhile subproject of eclipse and originally developed by Budapest University of Technology and Economics, OptXware Research and Development LLC and YourKit LLC. VIATRA contains not only a language for model transformations but also a model space to show models and a model transformation engine. The model space contains one or more metamodels as well as at least one model on which the transformations will be done. The single elements of the model space are entities and relations. These two elements are enough to represent a complete model in combination with a metamodel. The transformation language of VIATRA is based on graph patterns as the model itself is understood as graph. A graph pattern is used to search for a specific part of the model. If this part is found, modifications like changing relations or attributes or even removing the part can be executed.

2.3 Dependable System Modeling Using SCADE

The acronym SCADE stands for Safety-Critical Application Development Environment. The main objectives of the SCADE Suite are (1) to support systematic, model-based development of correct software based on formal methods and (2) to cover the whole development process [6]. Its formal semantics is based on a synchronous model of computation. SCADE uses a cycle-based evaluation of events. Events occuring in the same cycle are considered synchronous.

The SCADE Suite is an integrated development environment that covers many development activities of a typical process for safety-critical software: modeling, formal verification using the SAT-based SCADE Design Verifier [1], certified automatic code generation producing readable and traceable C-code, requirements tracing down to model elements and code, simulation and testing on the code level and coverage metrics for the test cases with the Model Test Coverage module. The version 6.3 of the SCADE Suite integrates the SCADE System Designer that allows to specify systems by means of SysML block diagrams. SCADE System Designer offers an integration into the SCADE Suite: The model entities of the System Designer project, i.e. blocks and connectors, are transformed into SCADE blocks and corresponding connections automatically.

In order to model product lines we use SysML blocks which are a concept offered at the architectural layer of SCADE System Designer. The feature modeling and how to build an instance of a product as the synchronous parallel composition of blocks are described in detail in [12]. The product generation process is formalized as model transformation applied on a base model. In difference to [12], we employ VIATRA instead of CVL for the model transformation here, as the underlying graph transformation, the developer of the product line has to implement, is more compact and more controllable in our experience.

2.4 Safety Analysis

Safety analysis is part of the development process of safety-critical systems and aims to identify the hazards and their possible causes. It results in safety requirements and safety design strategies that are capable to eliminate or to mitigate the occurrence of a hazards. Safety analysis techniques like Fault Tree Analysis (FTA) [29] and Failure Modes and Effects Analysis (FMEA) [13] have a long tradition and focus on possible component failures and their consequences. Leveson [17] proposed a new safety analysis approach, called system-theoretic process analysis (STPA), which we will use here. STPA takes unexpected behavior and interactions of components into account in addition to faults.

2.5 Related Work

Design variability in the design space is often realized by associating model fragments to product features. A product is built by using either a minimal model which is augmented by fragments or by a 150% model from which fragments are subtracted, see [2,3] for detailed surveys.

Like us, Liu et al. [18,19] consider a product line of pacemakers as a case study. Their sequential composition is less flexible compared to our synchronous product as they assume that only one feature is currently active. A further difference is that our approach handles the generation of design model and safety constraints uniformly as the safety constraints are bonded to a certain feature.

Different approaches target for formal verification of cardiac pacemakers: High-level models of different pacemakers concerning CSP are given by Tuan, Zheng, and Tho [27]. Their safety properties concern deadlock freedom and upper or lower rate limits. UPPAAL is used by Jee et al. [14,15] to formally develop and verify the software control of pacemakers. As they aim for a product-centric assurance case in [14], a thoughtful combination of methods and results from safety analysis, design and verification is needed. Thus the intended seamless integration of safety analysis, development, and verification is similar to our approach, however, the methods and formalisms applied in [18] and [14] differ from our approach. Furthermore, [14] focuses on a single pacemaker whereas we concentrate on a product line of pacemakers as [18] does. Compared to [18] we take account of a combination of product generation with safety requirements and error models .

3   Towards STPA for Product Lines

As first step we have to identify possible hazards and then we derive safety constraints from the identified hazards. We orientate ourselves on the method of STPA (System-Theoretic Process Analysis) of Leveson [17]. STPA steps due to Leveson are:

1. Define accidents and unacceptable losses. Draw the system boundaries and identify system level hazards. Derive system level safety constraints. Refine the safety constraints in the architectural design phase and allocate them to components. Then design an initial safety control structure.
2. Investigate the safety control structure for "inadequate control that could lead to hazardous states". Four kinds of unsafe software *control actions* (see [17]) are distinguished, namely, (1) a missing or incompletely performed safety *control action*, (2) a *control action* leading to a hazard, (3) a potentially safe, but mistimed *control action*, (4) a *control action* that is applied with wrong parameters.
3. Analyze "how each potentially hazardous *control action* ... could occur" ([17] p. 213). Therefore Leveson recommends to investigate each part of a control loop whether it may contribute to an unsafe action. In case, several controllers operate on the same component or contribute to the same safety constraint, possible conflicts have to be determined. In addition, the degradation of control over time shall be considered. As a mean, the control structure diagram is enhanced by process models which facilitates to identify *causal scenarios*, i.e. the causal factors contributing to a possibly unsafe *control action*.

3.1   STPA-Extension for Product Lines

STPA is an iterative analysis technique: We assume that STPA is applied on each architectural layer and that "components" refer to the building blocks as appropriate at the layer under analysis, i.e. to features at the functional layer and to components at the logical layer. Here we concentrate on safety analysis and verification for the software part of the logical layer of product lines. Thus we assume a system of hardware and software components that respects the constraints induced by the feature-oriented decomposition on the functional layer. Moreover, safety constraints and the control structure diagrams are refined and allocated to the components accordingly.

1. For each product of the product line the coverage, coordination, and consistency of the refined safety constraints allocated to the components has to be checked. The safety control structure is considered product-wise.

2. Each product is analyzed for inadequate control. Thus the additional possibilities for unwanted feature interaction on safety control are:
   - (a) Is a *control action* not provided because it is associated with a feature missing in a specific product or is it suppressed by an additional feature dominating the control loop?
   - (b) May a component, belonging to a specific feature of this product, emit a *control action* that may lead to a hazard?
   - (c1) May a mistimed *control action* occur because the timing depends on the feature selection?
   - (c2) Are *control actions* mistakenly doubled or required ones are suppressed because different features address the same safety constraint?
   - (d) Does the correctness of the parameters of a *control action* depend on a component added or removed in this particular product?
   - (e) Does a required *control action* rely on an active principle that interferes with the active principle used by another feature (even for non-safety-related control)?
3. In step 3 the possible contribution of each part of a control loop to a potentially hazardous *control action* is analyzed. Moreover, in case of dynamic variability, also the mode switches within the system have to be considered.

We adapt the concept of active principles from the engineering sector, see [22]. During the development of new products, the requirement description is transferred into a functional description of the later product. This description is split into smaller partial functional parts. A constructional solution is searched for each functional part based on so-called active principles. These active principles are based on physical, chemical, biological or material effects. When the functional parts are recombined into a product the compatibility of each active principle is examined.

As we do investigate software, we have to identify the active principles for the software part. One active principle is the collective use of one resource. Featuresmay interfere by using the same resource at the same time. The problem is that this may not be clearly recognizable in the control loop. Therefore we have to consider the used resources of the single features in our safety analysis in detail.

The analysis results in a list of scenarios showing potential causes for the identified hazards. In a last step we have to decide, if it is sufficient to derive only safety constraints from our results. Safety constraints lead to a special design in the later product models. Based on them, the model will be designed in such a way that the constraints will stay valid. Further we will add observer nodes for a later verification, in which we want to prove the validity of our safety constraints. If we decide that a cause for a hazard cannot be prevented by a formulated safety constraint, we will formulate an observer constraints. These observer constraints can be seen as warning system. Only if the hazard's cause occurs, they will be valid. These constraints do not influence the model's actual design.

3.2   Error Models and Fault Injection

As a result of the STPA analysis we gain hazards, scenarios of inadequate control actions and their causing errors. Furthermore we can assign these errors to single features.

As next step we have to model these errors and their influence on the system. Errors are modelled as automata which at least consist of two states: an error free state and one for the occurence of an error. Each feature only receives one error model. Thus error models can contain more than two states in case of the assignment of more than one error to a feature. We differentiate between permanent and transient errors.

Errors can be propagated between different error models. For this we introduce propagation events which are sent from one error models to another. The propagation can only occur along already existing connections between features for e.g. communication, data transfer or control flow. This propagation rules are based on the propagation rules of AADL [7]. Further possible ways for propagation are mutual reactions between features or feature decomposition.

Furthermore we need to model the influences of the errors on the system model. For the fault injection, we introduce system modes. This means that a system or a feature can have different behaviours or configurations, each represented by a mode. The error model can send injection events which trigger a mode change in the feature model. This model owns at least one mode for the error free behaviour and further modes for each error impact. So if different errors have the same impact on the system, these errors will trigger a change into the same mode. But we need to follow certain rules when we add error models to a feature. These rules are based on the conservative extension of models proposed by Ortmeier [9].

- The feature model, respectively its error free mode(s), may not be changed.
- The error model has to be added at the top-level of each feature model.
- The error model may not include micro steps.
- Hierarchies and initial states may not be changed.
- When we add modes describing the error impact, we proceed as follows:

  • New modes for error impacts can be added, as well as outgoing transitions from these modes.
  • Conditions of transitions which lead to error modes have to include injection events.
  • Transitions of an active mode which lead to an error mode have to be evaluated first. If more than one transition of an active mode leads to an error mode, all transitions are priorized to guarantee a deterministic behaviour. The priorities are assigned according to the severity of an error. This means that the transition leading to an error mode representing the impact of an error with a high severity, will receive a high priority.

3.3 Implementation of the Approach

In order to derive a specific product model of a product line, we need to perform different steps: After the analysis with STPA, we develop a base product model. A base model is one specific product consisting of its functional features, its associated safety constraints and error models. This base model is modeled in SysML by using the SCADE System Designer. Each feature is modeled as a *part* in the Internal Block Diagram (ibd) of the product model. The safety constraints are as well parts which shall observe if the constraints remain valid, respectively can be falsified, in the later verification.

In comparison to [12] we replaced CVL with VIATRA as it offers a more fine-grained possibility for deriving further product models. The base model is imported into VIATRA to derive further product models. VIATRA transforms the SysML model into a graph representation. The objects of the SysML model and the connections between them are transformed into graph nodes, known as entities. The relations between these nodes are built according to the SysML meta-model. For example, a SysML *part* is a special representation of a block which forms a component of a further block. Therefore VIATRA creates two relations for a part which point in which block this part is included and from which block it is derived. How a SysML model is transformed exactly into a graph representation can be read in [12]. VIATRA offers several possible actions on the graph model like deleting, adding or altering nodes and relations. We use them to derive new product models from our base model. Subsequently we export the new product models from VIATRA into SysML and import them into the SCADE Suite. Next we implement the inner logic to the automatic compiled operators. Further, we have to add explicit error models to our product models. In our case, error models are implemented as state machines.

4   Variability in a Pacemaker Product Line

The heart is a very complex biological system. The single heart beats are triggered by electric impulses which are transmitted over the cardiac conduction system. These impulses trigger the contraction of the cardiac chambers. This conduction system is partitioned into different segments to trigger the contraction of atrium and ventricle in a synchronous order. Failures in this system lead to a misbehavior of the heart. A pacemaker is used to handle this misbehavior. As there are several different points in the system where a single failure can occur, or even several ones in combination, different pacemakers exist to fit the possible failures and the resulting misbehavior.

4.1   The Pacemaker Product Line

Industrial pacemakers are categorized by an international code, the NASPE/BPEG Code [4] which we also use to structure the pacemaker's features as shown in Fig. 1. Its definition enfolds five letters. The first three letters characterize the main functions of a pacemaker as the stimulation of the heart, the sensing of natural heart paces and the response mode to sensing. The letters indicate the heart chambers affected by stimulation or detection, i.e. "V" denotes *ventricular*.

The mandatory functionalities for stimulation, sensing, the sensing response mode and additional functions are classified into feature groups on the first layer. The top-level feature groups are combined by the AND-operator, meaning that a feature from *each* group has to be chosen when building a product. At the second layer, *exactly one* feature is selected from each group according to the the XOR-operator. The "0"-feature (none) does not offer any functionality, but serves as dummy for compliance to the NASPE/BPEG code. Features may not be combined arbitrarily as they depend on each other. The dependencies are depicted as directed edges between the groups in Fig. 1. The labeling indicates the constraint: For instance, "0 $\Rightarrow$ 0" means that selecting the

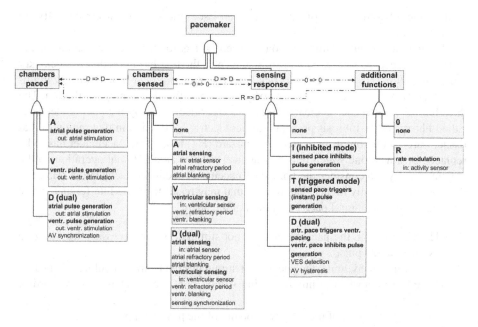

Fig. 1. Feature diagram of pacemaker product line

feature "0" in the feature group *chambers sensed* implies the feature "0" to be selected from the group *sensing response*. For each feature we briefly list its functionality and the timing constraints associated with it in Fig. 1.

For brevity, we will restrict the case study to a subset of possible pacemakers and concentrate on the pacemakers VVI and DDDR. A VVI pacemaker is a variant that stimulates the ventricle, in case no ventricular pace is detected. After a natural pace or a stimulation, two time intervals start, namely the blanking period in which the sensing is switched off and the refractory period in which no stimulation is allowed. In difference, a DDDR pacemaker senses and stimulates both chambers. Moreover, it can detect a ventricular extra-systole (VES), i.e., a natural ventricular pace without a preceding atrial event that needs an exceptional treatment. Furthermore, the DDDR variant comes with a hysteresis functionality changing the length of the AV interval after an atrial pace. The DDDR offers rate modulation of pacing. All behavioral details and an informal specification of the safety requirements originate from an industrial specification document by Boston Scientific [25].

4.2 Safety Analysis of the Pacemaker

In the first step we concentrate on the pacemaker and its interaction beyond its system boundaries. So we consider the pacemaker, the heart and the interaction between them, namely pacing and sensing. We focus on the software control, i.e., hazards, safety constraints, inadequate control actions, and possible errors are only considered if they relate to the software control of a pacemaker, all issues that do not concern the software are neglected.

The first functional requirement on a pacemaker is to stabilize the beating of the heart with respect to frequency and strength. Thus, the first hazard is that a pacemaker fails stimulation (H1). However, artificial pacing in an improper moment is hazardous as well (H2), as it may cause cardiac arrhythmia up to life-threatening fibrillation. The third hazard we consider is cicatrization of the cardiac tissue by the pacing electrode called fibrosis (H3). Fibrosis prevents further electric conduction in that region of that tissue. Early depletion of the battery is a hazard (H4) too, as the pacemaker has to be replaced by a new one which puts the medical risks of an additional operation on the patient. Finally we consider the hazard of pacemaker mediated tachycardia (H5), i.e. a pacing rate critically higher than normal that may result from the interference of the pacemaker and the natural pace generation of the heart.

- H1: Bradycardia, the pacemaker does not stimulate when necessary leading to a insufficient low pulse
- H2: Cardiac arrhythmia, the pacemaker stimulates the heart in a vulnerable phase
- H3: Fibrosis, no forwarding of pacing stimuli due to cicatrization in the cardiac tissue
- H4: Early depletion of the battery, drop out of the power supply
- H5: Pacemaker mediated tachycardia

Table 1. VVI Pacemaker: Unsafe control actions - in case action provided

Control Action	Context	Hazardous?		
		if provided	if provided too early	if provided too late
trigger stimulation	refractory period	H2	H2	H2
trigger stimulation	non-refract. period & no natural pace	-	if frequently H5	-
trigger stimulation	non-refract. period & natural pace	if frequently H3, H4, H5	if frequently H3, H4, H5	if frequently H3, H4, H5
interrupts	refract. period & pm timers synchr. with the heart	if frequently H4	if frequently H4	if frequently H4
interrupts	refract. period & pm timers not synchr. with the heart	H2	H2	H2
interrupts	non-refract. period	-	H5	-
...				

Hazard 4 differs from the others in that it dominates the system design: The requirement is that the battery shall survive for 8 to 10 years. That is only possible when using a processor with sleep modi that run with reduced energy consumption most of the time. Hence the control architecture must be interrupt-driven and the core, the sw-control, is executed only when the interrupt handler signals a timeout for some timing interval or a pace has been sensed.

According to STPA, a functional view on the architecture is provided next in order to investigate the possibilities for inadequate control that may lead to a hazard. We use the four types of unsafe control actions proposed by Leveson [17] and the notion of a *context*, specifying the situation in which a control action is unsafe, introduced by Thomas [26]. Fig. 2 shows the logical architecture of a single chamber pacemaker (one lead only). VVI specifics are contained in the functional blocks, in particular the timers and the sw-control. Table 1 and 2 show a part of the unsafe control actions identified on the logical architecture.The entries for hazards are meant as "'(not) providing this control action *may lead to* H*n*'"..

Table 2. VVI Pacemaker: Unsafe control actions - in case action not provided

Control Action	Context	Hazardous if not provided
trigger stimulation	refractory period	-
trigger stimulation	non-refract. period & no natural pace	H1
trigger stimulation	non-refract. period & natural pace	-
interrupts	refract. period	-
interrupts	non-refract. period	H1
...		

Next, the logical architecture is investigated in order to identify causal factors that may lead to an unsafe action. We again consider the VVI pacemaker (see fig. 2) : The action *trigger stimulation* may be erroneously issued in case the timing parameters of the pacemaker do not fit to the timing of the patient's heart or the interrupt handling activating the sw-control or the pulse generation is deferred e.g. because switching between the processor's sleep modi is mistimed. Other causes may be the lead is dislocated or broken and the natural pace is missed at all or disturbing signals are misinterpreted. The causes for not providing the action *trigger stimulation* may be a hardware defect in the pulse generation circuit itself or depletion of the battery. For the action *interrupts* very similar causes are discovered.

When refining and systematizing the causal scenarios we differentiate between hardware and mechanic errors and causes that relate to the software. Hardware errors like the dislocation of a lead that contribute to an unsafe control action are modeled in an error model that is associated to that hardware component model in the hardware abstraction layer. The software-related causes can be naturally structured along the features: The causes that relate to the pulse generation are associated with the pacing feature., those

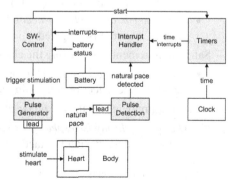

Fig. 2. Logical architecture of a single chamber pacemaker like VVI

that originate from the sensing parts are associated with the sensing feature and so on.

Hardware related errors may be transient or permanent. Furthermore, we distinguish whether some redundancy is provided or not: For instance, in case of a processor failure an additional circuit performs an emergency pace-making. But in case of a dislocated lead the only mean is that abnormal sensor values are logged and read-out when the patient is monitored by a physician.

Software related causes translate to functional safety constraints that must be guaranteed by the software. In general we derive two kinds of safety constraints, namely (1) *if time interval T_X elapses (optional: without a natural pace sensed) than response-specific pacing is triggered* and (2) *if a (natural or artificial) pace is triggered, no action a is performed before time interval T_Y expires*.

As the VVI pacemaker serves as our base model of the product line, STPA is applied purely. How to use the product line extension for STPA we introduced in Sec. 3.1 becomes obvious best when analyzing dual chamber pacemakers. For a dual chamber pacemaker the atrial and ventricular variants of each features cannot be simply added, but the so-called AV-synchronization and hysteresis are introduced in order to harmonize the atrial and ventricular sensing and pacing. An example for the interference of action principles is present in the pacemaker by the possibility of misinterpreting paces generated for one chamber, when sensing the other one. Hence further blanking intervals are introduced in order to avoid sensing in both chambers in the immediate interval when a pace is generated for one of them. Moreover, in the dual response mode ventricular extra-systoles are handled. This additional functionality restricts the interference between the atrial and ventricular pacing features even further in order to mitigate scenarios in which frequent ventricular extra-systoles may lead to H5, (and subordinate to H4 and H3).

In summary we derive the following safety constraints:

- Safety requirements for *Pacing*
  - *At most one pace (PA/PV)* Within the base interval (BI) at most one atrial/ventricular artificial pace occurs[1].
  - *The AV synchrony is respected (PSyn)* An artificial ventricular pace is only triggered if the AV interval (AVI) is expired.
  - *Pacemaker is only active if needed (IR)* The pacemaker sw-control shall only act if an interrupt is triggered.
- Safety requirements for *Sensing* the chambers
  - *Refractory period (SA/SV)* During a refractory period of the atrium/ventricle neither a pace detection nor a stimulation occurs[2].
- Safety requirements for the *Response* on the sensing
  - *The AV synchrony is respected (RSyn)* The period between the atrial and ventricular artificial pacing is exactly AVI.

---

[1] The two safety requirements refer to different outports.

[2] As the atrial and ventricular refractory periods differ, the time interval in the safety requirements have to be adapted accordingly, too.

- *Natural pace inhibits artificial pace (RIA/RIV)* Iff no natural atrial/ ventricular pace is detected within the admissible intervals of the BI, an artificial atrial/ventricular pace is triggered exactly once.
- *AV synchrony and ventricular inhibition (RSynIV)* After an atrial pace a natural ventricular pace is awaited in the interval [0,AVI), in case the natural ventricular pace is missing, at time AVI an artificial ventricular pace is triggered.
- *Response on an ventricular extra-systole (RVES)* If a natural ventricular pace occurs in the interval $[AVI + VRP, BI[^3$ then neither an artificial atrial pace nor an artificial ventricular pace is triggered from this occurrence t_0 on until time $t_0 + BI$.
- *Rate Modulation (RM)* Although in the presence of Rate Modulation the actual BI is always within the limits defined by the Upper (URL) and the Lower Rate Limit (LRL).

4.3   Error Models

The Boston Scientific Product Perfomance Report lists numerous errors for pacemakers in detail. We focus on those that are relevant for the software control and aggregate them into five generic errors that we will model and analyze:

- Undersensing: The pacemaker misses to sense a cardiac pace.
- Oversensing: The pacemaker senses and misinterprets additional signals that do not correspond to a cardiac pace.
- Parameter error: Timing parameters are changed to inappropriate values, e.g. by a storage error.
- Missing pulse generation error: The pulse generation (sporadically) fails, for instance due to transient hardware errors.
- Battery depletion: The battery depletes and consequently the pacemaker stops execution.

Undersensing, oversensing, and missing pulse generation may be a consequence of the dislocation of a lead.

For every error identified, we build an error model in terms of an automaton. An exemplary error model for the ventricular pacing feature is shown in fig. 3. It is a safe-state machine in this case. This model includes two errors: a missing stimulation pace and a battery error. As we already assigned errors to single features, we can now add error models to them. Every error model contains an initial state standing for the error free mode

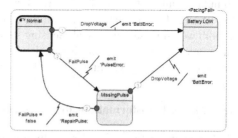

Fig. 3. Exemplary error model

of the feature. For every error, we add then a further state and connecting transitions between this new state and already existing states. In the example, we have a transient

---

[3] VRP is the time interval of the ventricular refractory period.

error for the missing pulse and a permanent error for the low battery voltage. The battery error is also a propagated error, originating from the battery control.

After modeling the error behavior, we have to model the fault injection on the feature model. The feature's error free behavior is integrated into an error free mode. Next, we have to define the impacts of each error on the feature model. In our example, both errors have the same impact: no artificial pace is trig-

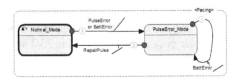

Fig. 4. Fault injection model: ventricular pacing

gered. Thus we need only one error mode. This model is shown in fig. 4, again as safe-state machine. Further we have priorities for every transition. As the battery error has a more severe impact, it has the higher priority.

4.4   The Pacemaker's Base Model and Model Deltas

The VVI pacemaker builds our base model. We chose it, as the VVI is a central pacemaker. It combines features which can be found in more complex dual pacemakers as well as includes features which are part of simple pacemakers like the V00. The V00 pacemaker is characterized by periodic ventricular stimulation after each expiration of the BI and ignores all natural ventricular paces.

The VVI's ibd is depicted in fig. 5. Its architecture consists of the parts `Timers`, `InterruptHandling`, `VVI_Control` and `BatteryControl`. The `Timers` and `BatteryControl` can trigger interrupts in the `InterruptHandling` which triggers the `VVI_Control` to wake up and react to the interrupts sent. The `VVI_Control` consists of different control blocks. In general, the `Control` consists of different control structures depending on the chosen features. This also applies for the `Timers` which also contains a clock and a parameter memory. In case of the VVI the `Timers` consists of timers for base interval (BI), ventricular refractory period (VRP) and the blanking time.

The VRP timer in combination with the control part realizes a deactivation of both stimulation and detection after a natural or artificial pulse. Neither a stimulation nor a forwarding of sensed natural paces of the heart must occur within the refractory period, as both would be safety-critical: Sensing shortly after a pulse may lead to misinterpretation, pacing may cause life-threatening cardiac fibrillation and thus a short blanking period exists at the beginning of the refractory period in which sensing is not possible.

4.5   Model Transformations for Product Generation

Each new product model is derived by transformations on the base model of the VVI. The transformations lead to a transposition of features. This means that features are replaced, added or deleted. In our case features can be also altered leading to a different feature. The features of the group *chambers paced* are an example. The dual feature includes the features atrial and ventricular pulse generation and additional parts to combine these two features.

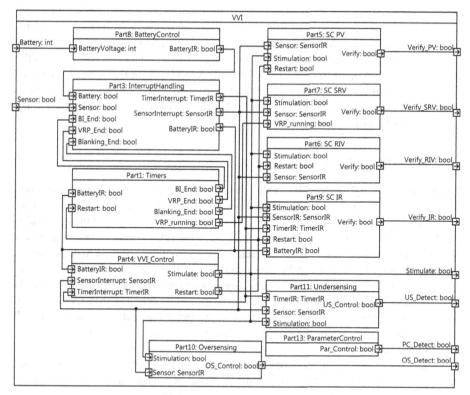

Fig. 5. ibd of VVI pacemaker

The DDD pacemaker design is derived from the VVI base model by essentially doubling all features in the first step. This can be done as the atrial and ventricular related features own a quite similar behavior. So these types of features can be transformed into one another by just minor changes. After these changes, the existing and doubled features are combined leading to dual features. But this can only be done for the feature groups chambers paced and chambers sensed.

For the feature Dual (D) of the group sensing response a new part named VES is introduced that handles extra-ordinary natural pulses of the ventricle. If a VES is sensed, the VES control part triggers a reset of the timer for the atrial TimePulseGeneration and both RefractoryPeriod timers. Moreover, a Hysteresis structure and a PVARP timer are added to the Timers. The PVARP timer is started after an artificial or natural ventricular pace and serves as additional block for the atrial sensor lest no misinterpretation of ventricular signals may occur. For the DDDR pacemaker and its feature rate modulation (R) we assume that rate modulation is based on an activity sensor that measures the ventricular pressure using a piezoelectric crystal and can be incorporated into the pacing lead. The piezoelectric sensor yields a voltage that is used as an input by the SensorControl block for altering the base interval accordingly.

VIATRA is employed for these model transformations. The base model is imported into the VIATRA framework where the model is converted into a graph representation.

Every model element, e.g. parts and connections, are converted into a node of a model graph. These nodes are connected by transitions which are built on behalf of meta information of the model. Model meta information can be information about which part is included in another part or which parts are the ends of a connection. We perform the described transformation from VVI to DDDR by VIATRA scripts. We search for predefined patterns if a model element shall be altered or even deleted. New nodes are built if new elements shall be added into the model. The pattern search is then employed for finding the right spot.

4.6   Verification of Products

When synchronizing the SysML models resulting from the VIATRA transformation with the SCADE Suite the corresponding (bare) operators are generated. For each pacemaker, a SCADE operator is created as well as inner operators for both kinds of blocks, the design and the observers. The SCADE System Designer offers a special interface for importing SysML model files and generates automatically the SCADE operators. Behavioral modeling is done in SCADE manually for the base model and each model delta, i.e. each design operator and each observer node expressing a safety constraint is modeled as prescribed in the functional specification. The operator "SW-Control" (see fig. 2) consists mainly of state machines with the inner logic, the operator "Timers" includes different timers for the single time intervals, a system clock and a storage for the single parameters.

Table 3 shows the verification results. The safety requirements are structured along the feature groups and are described in detail in 4.2 as a result of the safety analysis. An empty field indicates that there is no safety constraint specific to that feature on this product. All safety constraints could be proven. The figures indicate the run-times in seconds of a successful proof by SCADE Design Verifier executed on a Intel Core 2 Duo P9700 2,80 GHz. Most constraints could be verified nearly instantaneously.

Table 3. Verification run-times in seconds

	Chambers Paced		Chambers Sensed		Sensing Response	
	Ventr.	Dual	Ventr.	Dual	Inhibit	Dual
VVI	PV 0 IR 1		SV 9		RIV 0	
DDDR		PA 0 PV 0 PSyn 1 IR 0		SA 0 SV 13		RIA 0 RIV 1 RSynIV 0 RM 0

4.7   Fault Injection and Error Propagation

In addition to the already mentioned safety constraints, we add further observer nodes to our models. Their purpose is to monitor and report if critical errors like oversensing, undersensing or memory errors occur. Memory errors can lead to a change of the pacemaker's parameters like the interval lengths. The pacemaker's design cannot remedy these critical errors, so the observer nodes shall register them and give notice.

We added error models to the pacemaker in combination with a very simple heart model.

– *Undersensing:* If a specific number of stimulated paces occur in a defined interval, under-sensing is reported.
– *Oversensing:* If a specific number of sensed paces occur in a defined interval shortly after the end of the refractory period, oversensing is reported.
– *Parameter:* The time parameters have changed iff the time parameters of in the interval n+1 aren't the same as at interval n.
– *Missing Pulse:* Pulse generation has failed iff an artificial pace shall be generated but no pulse output is observed (at outport of the hardware abstraction of the pulse generator in our model).

In summary, most safety constraints stay valid in case that single errors are tested. Exceptions are the missing pulse error and the depletion of the battery, for which those safety constraints are falsified that request the generation of an artificial pulse. We anticipated these results since even in the presence of error the pacemaker is still working correctly according to its safety constraints. As the oversensing, undersensing and missing pulse error may depend on the lead, we differentiate between atrial and ventricular error variants for the DDDR pacemaker, called $DDDR^A$ and $DDDR^V$ in Table 4.

Table 4. Falsifiable safety constraints related to errors (! = falsifiable), the figures give the run time of the verification

		PA	PV	PSyn	IR	SA	SV	RIA	RIV	RSynIV	RM	UC	OC	PC
Undersensing	VVI	-	0	-	0	-	0	-	0	-	-	!	0	0
	$DDDR^A$	0	0	0	1	0	12	0	0	0	0	!	0	0
	$DDDR^V$	0	0	0	1	0	12	0	0	0	0	!	0	0
Oversensing	VVI	-	0	-	0	-	0	-	0	-	-	0	!	0
	$DDDR^A$	0	0	0	1	0	12	0	0	0	0	0	!	0
	$DDDR^V$	0	0	0	1	0	12	0	0	0	0	0	!	0
Parameter Error	VVI	-	0	-	0	-	5	-	0	-	-	9	0	!
	DDDR	0	0	0	1	0	12	0	1	0	0	!	-	!
Missing Pulse Error	VVI	-	0	-	0	-	0	-	!	-	-	0	0	0
	$DDDR^A$	0	0	0	1	0	12	!	1	1	0	0	0	0
	$DDDR^V$	0	0	!	0	0	12	0	!	!	0	0	0	1
Battery Error	VVI	-	0	-	0	-	0	-	!	-	-	0	0	0
	DDDR	0	0	!	0	0	12	!	!	0	0	0	0	0

5   Conclusion

We presented a model-based, transformational approach to product line design for safety-critical systems that uniformly handles design models, safety analysis, and safety constraints. For safety analysis we extended the STPA approach by Leveson [17] to product lines. By taking the feature-oriented design methodology into account, we are able to identify possibly unwanted feature interaction that may arise from the combination of features as well as from the absence of features in a particular product. For error modeling we employed concepts from AADL in order to have a clear separation between the original design model and the error models. Then we demonstrated the approach within the SCADE framework for the modeling and verification of dependable medical device software and employed VIATRA for transformational product generation.

In the medical device domain products are designed according to the characteristic requirements of individual patients resulting in complex product lines. With our promising approach resulting in a fine-grained safety analysis of software product lines complexity in the verification can be reduced. Furthermore, we offer a seamless tool chain for model-based development. SCADE Suite is approved in practice and provides certified code generation for dependable systems according to several safety standards and, moreover, formal verification by SAT-based model checking.

Our next step will be the fully formal definition of hazards and error models, as well as the development of a more detailed heart model. Furthermore, we plan to apply our approach on a second product line of medical devices, namely analgesia infusions pumps [16].

References

1. Abdulla, P.A., Deneux, J., Stålmarck, G., Ågren, H., Åkerlund, O.: Designing safe, reliable systems using scade. In: Margaria, T., Steffen, B. (eds.) ISoLA 2004. LNCS, vol. 4313, pp. 115–129. Springer, Heidelberg (2006)
2. Apel, S., Kästner, C.: An overview of feature-oriented software development. Journal of Object Technology 8(5), 49–84 (2009)
3. Azanza, M., Batory, D., Díaz, O., Trujillo, S.: Domain-specific composition of model deltas. In: Tratt, L., Gogolla, M. (eds.) ICMT 2010. LNCS, vol. 6142, pp. 16–30. Springer, Heidelberg (2010)
4. Bernstein, Daubert, Fletcher, Hayes, Lüderitz, Reynolds, Schoenfeld, Sutton: The revised NASPE/BPEG generic code for antibradycardia, adaptive-rate, and multisite pacing. Journal of Pacing and Clinical Electrophysiology 25, 260–264 (2002)
5. Classen, A., Heymans, P., Schobbens, P.-Y., Legay, A.: Symbolic model checking of software product lines. In: Intern. Conf. on Software Engineering (ICSE), pp. 321–330 (2011)
6. Esterel Technologies: SCADE Suite KCG 6.1: Safety case report of KCG 6.1.2 (July 2009)
7. Feiler, P., Rugina, A.: Dependability modeling with the architecture analysis & design language (AADL). Tech. rep., Software Engineering Institute, CMU (July 2007)
8. Fischbein, D., Uchitel, S., Brabermann, V.: A foundation for behavioural conformance in software product line architectures. In: ISSTA 2006 Workshop on Role of Software Architecture for Testing and Analysis (ROSATEA), pp. 39–48. ACM (2006)
9. Ortmeier, F., Matthias Güdemann, W.R.: Formal failure models. In: 1st IFAC Workshop on Dependable Control of Discrete Systems, vol. 1, pp. 145–150 (2007)
10. Gray, J.G., Zhang, J., Lin, Y., Roychoudhury, S., Wu, H., Sudarsan, R., Gokhale, A.S., Neema, S., Shi, F., Bapty, T.: Model driven program transformation. In: Intern. Conf. on Generative Programming and Component Engineering (GPCE), pp. 361–378 (2004)

11. Haugen, Møller-Pedersen, Oldevik, Olsen, Svendsen: Adding standardized variability to domain specific languages. In: Intern. Software Product Line Conference, pp. 139–148. IEEE Computer Society (2008)
12. Huhn, M., Bessling, S.: Enhancing product line development by safety requirements and verification. In: Weber, J., Perseil, I. (eds.) FHIES 2012. LNCS, vol. 7789, pp. 37–54. Springer, Heidelberg (2013)
13. IEC: 60812: Analysis techniques for system reliability
14. Jee, E., Lee, I., Sokolsky, O.: Assurance cases in model-driven development of the pacemaker software. In: Margaria, T., Steffen, B. (eds.) ISoLA 2010, Part II. LNCS, vol. 6416, pp. 343–356. Springer, Heidelberg (2010)
15. Jee, Wang, Kim, Lee, Sokolsky, Lee: A safety-assured development approach for real-time software. In: Proceedings of the 2010 IEEE 16th International Conference on Embedded and Real-Time Computing Systems and Applications, pp. 133–142. IEEE Computer Society, Washington, DC (2010), http://dx.doi.org/10.1109/RTCSA.2010.42
16. Larson, B.R.: Integrated clinical environment patient-controlled analgesia infusion pump (January 2012)
17. Leveson, N.G.: Engineering a Safer World: Systems Thinking Applied to Safety (Engineering Systems). The MIT Press (January 2012),
    http://www.worldcat.org/isbn/0262016621
18. Liu, J., Basu, S., Lutz, R.R.: Compositional model checking of software product lines using variation point obligations. Autom. Softw. Eng. 18(1), 39–76 (2011)
19. Liu, J., Dehlinger, J., Lutz, R.R.: Safety analysis of software product lines using state-based modeling. The Journal of Systems and Software 80, 1879–1892 (2007)
20. OptXware Research and Development LLC: The Viatra-I model transformation framework pattern language specification
21. OptXware Research and Development LLC: The Viatra-I model transformation framework users' guide
22. Pahl, G., Beitz, W., Feldhusen, J., Grote, K.H.: Pahl/Beitz Konstruktionslehre: Grundlagen erfolgreicher Produktentwicklung, 7. aufl. edn. Methoden und Anwendung. Springer, Berlin (2006), http://link.springer.com/book/
    10.1007/978-3-540-34061-4/page/1
23. Schaefer, I., Gurov, D., Soleimanifard, S.: Compositional algorithmic verification of software product lines. In: Aichernig, B.K., de Boer, F.S., Bonsangue, M.M. (eds.) Formal Methods for Components and Objects. LNCS, vol. 6957, pp. 184–203. Springer, Heidelberg (2011)
24. Schobbens, P.-Y., Heymans, P., Trigaux, J.-C.: Feature diagrams: A survey and a formal semantics. In: Intern. Conf. on Requirements Engineering (RE), pp. 136–145 (2006)
25. Scientific, B.: PACEMAKER System Specification (January 2007)
26. Thomas, J.: Extending and automating a systems-theoretic hazard analysis for requirements generation and analysis. Tech. rep., SANDIA National Laboratories (July 2012)
27. Tuan, Zheng, Tho: Modeling and verification of safety critical systems: A case study on pacemaker. In: 4th Conf. on Secure Software Integration and Reliability Improvement, pp. 23–32. IEEE (2010)
28. Varró, D., Varró, G., Pataricza, A.: Designing the automatic transformation of visual languages. Science of Computer Programming 44(2), 205–227 (2002)
29. Vesely, W.E., Goldberg, F.F., Roberts, N.H., Haasl, D.F.: Fault Tree Handbook. U.S. Nuclear Regulatory Commission, Washington, DC (1981)

An Investigation of Classification Algorithms for Predicting HIV Drug Resistance without Genotype Resistance Testing

Pascal Brandt[1,2], Deshendran Moodley[1], Anban W. Pillay[1],
Christopher J. Seebregts[1,2], and Tulio de Oliveira[3]

[1] Centre for Artificial Intelligence Research and Health Architecture Laboratory,
University of KwaZulu-Natal, Durban/CSIR Meraka, Pretoria, South Africa
[2] Jembi Health Systems, Cape Town and Durban, South Africa
[3] Africa Centre for Health and Population Studies, Nelson R. Mandela School of
Medicine, University of KwaZulu-Natal, Durban, South Africa

Abstract. The development of drug resistance is a major factor impeding the efficacy of antiretroviral treatment of South Africa's HIV infected population. While genotype resistance testing is the standard method to determine resistance, access to these tests is limited in low-resource settings. In this paper we investigate machine learning techniques for drug resistance prediction from routine treatment and laboratory data to help clinicians select patients for confirmatory genotype testing. The techniques, including binary relevance, HOMER, MLkNN, predictive clustering trees (PCT), RAkEL and ensemble of classifier chains were tested on a dataset of 252 medical records of patients enrolled in an HIV treatment failure clinic in rural KwaZulu-Natal in South Africa. The PCT method performed best with a discriminant power of 1.56 for two drugs, above 1.0 for three others and a mean true positive rate of 0.68. These methods show potential for application where access to genotyping is limited.

Keywords: HIV, treatment failure, machine learning, multi-label classification, clinical decision support.

1 Introduction

South Africa has one of the highest HIV infection rates in the world with more than 5.6 million infected people[1]. Consequently, the country has the largest antiretroviral treatment program in the world with more than one and a half million people on treatment [1]. The recommended treatment for HIV/AIDS (known as highly active antiretroviral therapy (HAART)) is a combination of three drugs from two or more different drug groups. HIV treatment failure occurs when the antiretroviral drugs (ARVs) no longer controls the infection and is due to, amongst other reasons, the development of drug resistance [2].

---

[1] http://www.unaids.org/en/regionscountries/countries/southafrica/

J. Gibbons and W. MacCaull (Eds.): FHIES 2013, LNCS 8315, pp. 236–253, 2014.
© Springer-Verlag Berlin Heidelberg 2014

The standard method to identify resistance to specific drugs is the genotype resistance test (GRT) [3]. The GRT is a biochemical test conducted on a sample of the HIV population in the blood of an infected patient. Resistance algorithms such as Rega [4] or Stanford [3] are used to interpret the results and predict actual resistance from the viral genetic data. While some studies conclude that the cost of including GRT into treatment guidelines might be cost neutral [5], the current South African guidelines do not include GRT for every patient and it is therefore considered a limited resource.

Our aim in this work was to investigate the extent to which six multi-label classification techniques could predict the resistance level without a genotype test. We used data from a comprehensive HIV-1 ART treatment program with access to GRT in South Africa. The performance of the techniques was evaluated by comparing the predictions produced against the results obtained using GRT. The predictions produced by these classification techniques could help care providers to decide whether or not to refer a patient for GRT or to help select an optimal therapy if the regimen is to be changed.

The rest of the paper is organised as follows. In section 2 we describe previous work on factors contributing to HIV drug resistance and the use of machine learning techniques for HIV drug resistance prediction. Section 3 provides a description of the data and the machine learning techniques used in this study. The results are described in section 4 and an analysis is given in section 5. Conclusions are drawn and directions for future work are given in section 6.

2   Previous Work

Studies have shown that poor adherence to treatment regimen is an important factor influencing the development of drug resistance [6,7,8]. Patients who start treatment with a high viral load are more likely to develop resistance [8]. Other factors that influence resistance include exposure to more and greater variation of drugs as well as drug regimens that only partially suppress the virus population [9].

Computerised predictive models have been found to be useful for clinicians in practice and can sometimes even outperform human experts [10,11]. Machine learning techniques such as artificial neural networks, random forests and support vector machines have used genotype data to provide useful predictions about patient outcomes [12,13,14]. Using such methods to select new regimens has also been shown to be viable [15,16,17]. Furthermore, predictions have been shown to be more accurate when clinical data is included in training [15]. However, limited research is available on the efficacy of machine learning techniques for prediction without genotype data. A recent study in this regard is [16]. At a population level, this could potentially help optimise utilization of a scarce resource, such as resistance genotyping.

3   Methods

3.1   Study Data

The training dataset was constructed from anonymised records of adult (age > 16) patients attending the treatment failure management clinic at the Africa Centre in Mtubatuba, KwaZulu-Natal, South Africa[2].

Table 1 summarises the dataset attributes. Patients in the dataset also have a viral isolate associated with their clinical record, which is used to determine the resistance profile of the patient. This resistance profile is then used to construct the label sets associated with each training example. Resistance to a drug is determined using the HIVDB 6.0.5 algorithm [3] and a patient is considered resistant to a drug if the algorithm returns a susceptibility value of ≤ 0.5.

To store patient data, we used RegaDB, an open source patient-centric clinical data management system that stores data related to HIV treatment [18]. The data was stored longitudinally in a relational database. A software utility[3] was developed that uses the RegaDB API to extract patient data in the ARFF[4] format.

3.2   Multi-label Classification

Since each patient may develop resistance to multiple ARVs, multi-label classification is required. Multi-label classification involves associating each input example with multiple labels, rather than a single label [19]. In this study each patient record is associated with a set of 11 binary labels indicating resistance (presence of label) or susceptibility (absence of label) to each ARV drug.

There are three solution groups for solving the problem of multi-label classification. Problem transformation (PT) methods divide the problem into a set of multi-class classification problems and combine the result to form the multi-label prediction. Algorithm adaptation (AA) methods construct specialized algorithms, often by modifying existing multi-class prediction algorithms, to produce a prediction. Ensemble methods (EM) are developed on top of common problem transformation or algorithm adaptation methods [20].

3.3   Stratification

In order for the performance of each cross validation cycle to be representative of the performance if the full dataset was used for training, it is necessary to construct each fold so that the label distribution in the fold is the same as for the complete dataset [21]. In the case of binary classification, the task of stratifying

---

[2] The study and drug resistance analysis of the data was approved by the Biomedical Research Ethics Committee of the University of KwaZulu-Natal (BF052/010) and the Provincial Health Research Committee of the KwaZulu-Natal Department of Health (HRKM176/10).

[3] Source code available at https://github.com/psbrandt/dsm

[4] http://weka.wikispaces.com/ARFF+(book+version)

Table 1. Summary of features used to construct the predictive models

Category	Features	Types	Count
Demographic	Age, Weight, Geographic Location, Ethnicity, Gender, Province, Country of Origin	Numeric, Categorical	7
Clinical	Drug Exposure (Tenofovir, Lopinavir/r, Atazanavir, Zidovudine, Ritonavir, Efavirenz, Abacavir, Nevirapine, Raltegravir, Stavudine, Didanosine, Lamivudine), Recent Blood HB, Recent Blood ALT, Recent Blood Creatinine Clearance, Other Drug Exposure (three features), Tuberculosis Therapy (Prior, During, Post), HTLV-1 Status, HBV Status	Numeric, Categorical	23
Adherence	Treatment Break, Patient Estimated Adherence, Missed, Buddy, Remember, Counseling, Side Effects, Worst Stop, Disclosure, Names, Stop	Categorical	11
Other	Transmission Group, Other Co-morbidities, Partner On Treatment, Exposure to Single Dose NVP, Identified Virological Failure Reason, Traditional Medicine, Alcohol Consumption, TB Treatment Starting Soon, Diarrhea or Vomiting	Categorical	9
Derived	Baseline Viral Load, Time on Failing Regimen, Drug Exposure Count, Pre-Resistance Testing Viral Load, Median Viral Load, Recent CD4 Count Gradient, Post-Treatment CD4 Count, Baseline CD4 Gradient, Pre-Resistance Testing CD4 Count, Mean Viral Load, Pre-Resistance Testing Immunological Failure, Virus Ever Suppressed	Numeric, Categorical	12
Total			**62**

the dataset is simple, since there is only one target label whose distribution must be maintained. However, in multi-label datasets there are multiple distributions that must be maintained.

Since the dataset used in the work is small, the Meka[5] implementation of the iterative stratification algorithm [22] was used to generate 10 folds to be used for cross validation.

3.4   Model Development

Seven multi-label classification models were trained and tested for their ability to predict a known resistance result from demographic and treatment data. The models were selected as a representative sample of those available in the multi-label classification domain [20]. In each case, 10 fold cross validation was done using folds generated by the iterative stratification algorithm described in section 3.3.

Binary Relevance with Support Vector Machine (SVM) base classifier (BR-SVM). The radial basis function kernel was selected because it is able to model non-linear relationships. Model parameters were optimized using the technique in [20,23].

---

[5] http://meka.sourceforge.net/

Binary Relevance with naive Bayes (NB) base classifier (BR-NB). The second experiment conducted replaces the SVM base classifier with a naive Bayes classifier. A naive Bayes classifier models the probability of the class variable using the simplifying assumption that each feature in the feature vector is independent [24].

HOMER. The third experiment used the Hierarchy Of Multi-label classifiERs (HOMER) method [25]. This problem transformation method trains classifiers in a hierarchy on subsets of the labels. The MULAN[6] implementation of this algorithm was used.

MLkNN. The first algorithm adaptation method tested was the Multi-Label k Nearest Neighbours (MLkNN) algorithm [26]. This algorithm, based on the traditional k nearest neighbours method, works by first identifying the k nearest neighbours of an unseen instance and making a prediction based on the labels associated with these neighbours. The MLkNN implementation provided by MULAN was used for this experiment.

Predictive Clustering Trees (PCT). The fifth experiment used the predictive clustering framework algorithm adaptation method [27]. This method builds a clustering tree using top-down induction. The Clus[7] implementation was used.

RAkEL. The first ensemble method tested was RAndom k-labELsets (RAkEL). This method trains ensemble members on small random subsets of labels [28]. The MULAN implementation of the RAkEL algorithm was used and a naive Bayes base classifier was selected.

Ensemble of Classifier Chains (ECC). The MULAN implementation of the ensemble of classifier chains (ECC) method (with a naive Bayes base classifier) was used as the second ensemble method experiment. This method builds on the binary relevance idea by extending the attribute space by adding a binary feature to represent the label relevances of all previous classifiers, thereby forming a classifier chain [29].

3.5   Evaluation Metrics

There are many possible evaluation metrics that can be used to measure the performance of a classifier [30] and an attempt was made select a representative sample of those available. Most metrics are calculated from the confusion matrix generated by a classification or cross validation run. Since the dataset used in this study was highly unbalanced, it was necessary to choose evaluation metrics that are informative in the presence of label imbalance. For this reason, we chose to use true positive rate (TPR, often called sensitivity) and true negative rate (TNR, often called specificity). Along with TPR and TNR, we chose to use Matthew's correlation coefficient, discriminant power and area under the receiver operating characteristic curve (AUC).

---

[6] http://mulan.sourceforge.net/
[7] http://dtai.cs.kuleuven.be/clus/

Matthew's correlation coefficient (MCC) is a correlation coefficient between the observed and predicted classes. Its value is in the range $[-1; 1]$ with 1 indicating perfect prediction, 0 indicating no better than random prediction and -1 indicating total disagreement between prediction and observation [31]. It is defined in equation 1.

$$MCC = \frac{tp \cdot fn - fp \cdot fn}{\sqrt{(tp + fp) \cdot (tp + fn) \cdot (tn + fp) \cdot (tn + fn)}} \qquad (1)$$

where tp is the number of true positives, fn the number of false negatives, tn the number of true negatives and fp the number of false positives from the confusion matrix.

Discriminant power (DP) is a measure that summarizes sensitivity and specificity and is a measure of how well a classifier distinguishes between positive and negative examples [32]. It is defined in equation 2.

$$DP = \frac{\sqrt{3}}{\pi} ln \left(\frac{tp}{fp} \cdot \frac{tn}{fn} \right) \qquad (2)$$

A classifier is a poor discriminant if $DP < 1$, limited if $DP < 2$, fair if $DP < 3$ and good otherwise.

Receiver operating characteristic (ROC) graphs depict relative tradeoffs between benefits (true positives) and costs (false negatives) and are insensitive to changes in class distribution. Area under the receiver operating characteristic curve (AUC) is a single scalar value that represents expected ROC performance [33]. Note that ROC graphs can only be plotted for classifiers that produce a probability estimate and hence no such graphs are plotted for the BR-SVM and PCT methods.

3.6   Validation

In order to ensure valid and robost results, model performance was averaged over the 10 cross validation cycles. Further, the use of stratification during the construction of the folds helps ensure that all training and test cycles are performed using data that is representative of the complete dataset.

4   Results

4.1   Dataset Characteristics

The size of the dataset is 252 patients, with a mean age of 37.49. There are 190 females in the dataset (75.4%). Table 2 shows the number of patients with demonstrated resistance to each number of drugs.

Table 2. Number of patients resistant to each number of drugs

Drugs	0	1	2	3	4	5	6	7	8	9	10	11
Patients	19	0	3	11	5	18	72	5	11	38	45	25
Percent (%)	7.54	0.00	1.19	4.37	1.98	7.14	28.57	1.98	4.37	15.08	17.86	9.92

Table 3. Resistance and susceptibility counts for each drug

	efavirenz	didanosine	emtricitabine	delavirdine	stavudine	nevirapine
Resistant	229 (90.87%)	103 (40.87%)	217 (86.11%)	226 (89.68%)	93 (36.90%)	229 (90.87%)
Susceptible	23 (9.13%)	149 (59.13%)	35 (13.89%)	26 (10.32%)	159 (63.10%)	23 (9.13%)

	tenofovir	etravirine	abacavir	lamivudine	zidovudine
Resistant	61 (24.21%)	196 (77.78%)	123 (48.81%)	217 (86.11%)	77 (30.56%)
Susceptible	191 (75.79%)	56 (22.22%)	129 (51.19%)	35 (13.89%)	175 (69.44%)

The final training dataset consists of 62 features per patient (see table 1). The average feature completeness is 76.84%. 36 of the features (58.06%) are over 90% complete and 24 features (30.71%) are 100% complete. Eight features (12.90%) are over 78% complete. 14 features are between 22% and 78% complete. Four features (6.45%) are less than 10% complete. Completeness here is defined as the number of patients having a value for the specific feature divided by the total number of patients.

It's important to note that in this dataset there are many more patients with resistance than without. As seen in table 2, only 19 (7.54%) showed no resistance. This results in a label imbalance in the training data. Table 3 shows, for each label, how many examples are associated with the label. Since we define label presence as indicating resistance, we can see that resistance heavily dominates that dataset. Tenofovir, zidovudine and stavudine are the only cases where non-resistance dominates over resistance. Didanosine and abacavir are relatively well balanced.

4.2   Model Evaluation

The numeric values for each evaluation metric are given in tables 4–6. Figures 1 - 3 show the ROC curves for the performance of each method that produces a probability estimate to which threshold variation can be applied. The ROC curves are vertically averaged across the 10 folds as put forward in [33]. The AUC along with the standard error is given in the legend for each method in each graph.

Problem Transformation Methods. The BR-SVM method produces blanket positive predictions (which occur when $TPR = 1.0$ and $TNR = 0.0$) for five labels (efavirenz, emtricitabine, delavirdine, nevirapine and lamivudine). These five labels correspond to the five most unbalanced labels in the dataset ($> 86\%$ of examples are resistant). For all other labels except tenofovir the method does not discriminate well, as seen by the low DP values in table 4. Over all, the BR-SVM method performs poorly, with only the performance of predicting tenofovir moderately above the performance of a random classifier based on the MCC value.

When we switched the base classifier to naive Bayes, we saw that BR-NB performed drastically better. There were no blanket positive predictions and the mean DP value increased by over 20%. The mean TPR and TNR values also increased. BR-NB had an MCC value of just over 0.3 for tenofovir, meaning that it is significantly better than a random classifier at predicting, in this case, absence of resistance to this drug. The mean AUC of all the drugs for the BR-NB method was 10% above that of a random classifier (0.5) at 0.6.

HOMER performed slightly worse than the BR-NB method, with the mean of each metric less than BR-NB. The exception was the mean TNR value, which didn't change. HOMER outperforms BR-NB at predicting cases of lamivudine resistance, with a TPR of 0.94. The MCC value for the zidovudine indicates that HOMER performs better than a random classifier for this label. The mean AUC for HOMER is 0.57.

Algorithm Adaptation Methods. MLkNN appears to be the worst performing of all methods. It has the lowest mean value for each statistic and blanket positive predictions for six labels (efavirenz, emtricitabine, delavirdine, nevirapine, etravirine and lamivudine). Further, the mean AUC is 0.49, which indicates worse than random performance. This is confirmed by multiple MCC and DP values less than zero.

The PCT method does not suffer from blanket positive predictions and has the highest mean DP, MCC and TNR values. It has three MCC values above 0.35 and numerous DP values above 1. These values indicate that PCT is substantially better than a random classifier at predicting resistance to efavirenz, delavirdine and nevirapine. PCT performs especially well relative to the other methods for efavirens and nevirapine with a TPR of 0.97 and DP value of 1.56 in both cases. Unlike the other methods, it does not appear to be a good predictor for tenofovir.

Ensemble Methods. The RAkEL method suffers from no blanket positive predictions, but does have MCC and DP values below zero for two drugs, indicating very poor performance in these cases. RAkEL appears at first glance to perform relatively well for lamivudine, with a DP value of 1.06. However, the TNR for this drug is only 0.11, indicating that the method is not good at detecting negative examples. The RAkEL method has an average AUC of 0.58, which puts it between BR-NB and HOMER in terms of this metric.

The ECC method performs worse than random for efavirenz, nevirapine and etravirine, but has relatively high DP values (greater than 1) for emtricitabine, tenofovir and lamivudine. Of the latter three, only tenofovir also shows an MCC value significantly greater than zero (0.38). The average AUC for the ECC method is 0.63 with an AUC value of 0.72 for tenofovir, making it the best performer for this drug and in terms of the ROC analysis in general.

Table 4. Results of the problem transformation methods

	BR-SVM				BR-NB					HOMER				
	TPR	TNR	MCC	DP	TPR	TNR	MCC	DP	AUC	TPR	TNR	MCC	DP	AUC
efavirenz	1.00	0.00	-	-	0.86	0.26	0.10	0.43	0.54	0.89	0.13	0.02	0.09	0.51
didanosine	0.27	0.80	0.08	0.22	0.54	0.62	0.16	0.36	0.62	0.56	0.59	0.15	0.34	0.62
emtricitabine	1.00	0.00	-	-	0.93	0.20	0.15	0.63	0.61	0.94	0.17	0.16	0.70	0.57
delavirdine	1.00	0.00	-	-	0.83	0.23	0.05	0.22	0.56	0.84	0.19	0.02	0.11	0.51
stavudine	0.22	0.85	0.08	0.24	0.38	0.70	0.08	0.18	0.58	0.38	0.81	0.20	0.50	0.60
nevirapine	1.00	0.00	-	-	0.86	0.26	0.10	0.43	0.54	0.89	0.13	0.02	0.09	0.51
tenofovir	0.26	0.94	0.27	0.92	0.43	0.86	0.31	0.85	0.65	0.44	0.84	0.29	0.80	0.66
etravirine	0.99	0.02	0.03	0.31	0.88	0.16	0.05	0.17	0.60	0.52	0.52	0.03	0.08	0.50
abacavir	0.50	0.61	0.12	0.26	0.54	0.64	0.18	0.41	0.63	0.63	0.57	0.19	0.43	0.66
lamivudine	1.00	0.00	-	-	0.93	0.20	0.15	0.63	0.61	0.94	0.17	0.16	0.70	0.57
zidovudine	0.05	0.96	0.03	0.15	0.38	0.79	0.17	0.45	0.63	0.38	0.82	0.22	0.57	0.62
mean	0.66	0.38	0.10	0.35	0.69	0.45	0.14	0.43	0.60	0.67	0.45	0.13	0.40	0.57
std dev	0.40	0.44	0.09	0.28	0.23	0.27	0.07	0.21	0.04	0.23	0.30	0.10	0.28	0.06
best	1.00	0.96	0.27	0.92	0.93	0.86	0.31	0.85	0.65	0.94	0.84	0.29	0.80	0.66

BR-SVM - Binary relevance with support vector machine base classifier, **BR-NB** - Binary relevance with naive Bayes base classifier, **HOMER** - Hierarchy of multi-label classifiers, **TPR** - True positive rate, **TNR** - True negative rate, **MCC** - Matthew's correlation coefficient, **DP** - Discriminative power, **AUC** - Area under the receiver operating characteristic curve

5 Discussion

The multi-label classifiers were evaluated for the ability to predict known resistance to a set of ARVs based only on prior patient biographical and treatment history data excluding the result of a genotype resistance test. Some of the methods were found to be good predictors for specific drugs. For example, PCT predicts resistance to nevirapine with a true positive rate of 0.97.

The mean AUC for the ECC method (0.63) is comparable to the results obtained in the recent study by Revell in [16], which used data from a Southern African dataset on a model trained with a number of international datasets. Revell predicted virological response, while we predicted resistance to specific drugs. Revell achieves a TPR of 0.60 compared to our 0.71 (mean over all drugs) and TNR of 0.62 compared to our 0.38 (mean over all drugs) for ECC. For PCT we have a mean TPR of 0.68 and mean TNR of 0.53, which is comparable to Revell's result. This could imply that if an equally large training set were used in our models, results may improve.

Models that perform well on the highly imbalanced labels (such as BR-NB and PCT) perform less well on the relatively balanced labels (didanosine and abacavir). This supports the idea that no single model should be used to assess resistance to all drugs and the results of multiple models should be combined into an ensemble prediction to produce the best results.

Table 5. Results of the algorithm adaptation methods

	MLkNN					PCT			
	TPR	TNR	MCC	DP	AUC	TPR	TNR	MCC	DP
efavirenz	1.00	0.00	-	-	0.44	0.97	0.35	0.39	1.56
didanosine	0.08	0.83	-0.14	-0.51	0.45	0.47	0.78	0.26	0.62
emtricitabine	1.00	0.00	-	-	0.50	0.94	0.31	0.30	1.09
delavirdine	1.00	0.00	-0.02	-	0.52	0.97	0.31	0.36	1.45
stavudine	0.04	0.97	0.03	0.18	0.48	0.31	0.77	0.09	0.22
nevirapine	1.00	0.00	-	-	0.44	0.97	0.35	0.39	1.56
tenofovir	0.00	0.98	-0.06	-	0.52	0.28	0.87	0.18	0.55
etravirine	1.00	0.00	-	-	0.47	0.91	0.23	0.18	0.60
abacavir	0.39	0.63	0.02	0.04	0.54	0.56	0.70	0.26	0.60
lamivudine	1.00	0.00	-	-	0.50	0.94	0.31	0.30	1.09
zidovudine	0.01	0.99	0.04	0.46	0.53	0.19	0.83	0.04	0.11
mean	0.59	0.40	-0.02	0.04	0.49	0.68	0.53	0.25	0.86
std dev	0.48	0.47	0.07	0.41	0.04	0.32	0.26	0.12	0.52
best	1.00	0.99	0.04	0.46	0.54	0.97	0.87	0.39	1.56

Table 6. Results of the ensemble methods

	RAkEL					ECC				
	TPR	TNR	MCC	DP	AUC	TPR	TNR	MCC	DP	AUC
efavirenz	0.92	0.22	0.13	0.62	0.59	1.00	0.00	-0.02	-	0.68
didanosine	0.52	0.58	0.10	0.23	0.58	0.41	0.73	0.15	0.35	0.64
emtricitabine	0.93	0.20	0.16	0.67	0.60	1.00	0.03	0.09	1.02	0.62
delavirdine	0.96	0.04	0.01	0.05	0.60	1.00	0.04	0.19	-	0.69
stavudine	0.49	0.62	0.11	0.26	0.54	0.25	0.82	0.09	0.24	0.54
nevirapine	0.91	0.22	0.12	0.56	0.60	1.00	0.00	-0.02	-	0.61
tenofovir	0.38	0.88	0.28	0.82	0.66	0.39	0.93	0.38	1.16	0.72
etravirine	0.85	0.11	-0.05	-0.20	0.50	0.97	0.02	-0.02	-0.20	0.56
abacavir	0.42	0.74	0.18	0.42	0.60	0.59	0.70	0.28	0.65	0.68
lamivudine	0.98	0.11	0.19	1.06	0.60	1.00	0.03	0.09	1.02	0.60
zidovudine	0.26	0.82	0.09	0.27	0.55	0.26	0.89	0.19	0.58	0.63
mean	0.69	0.41	0.12	0.43	0.58	0.71	0.38	0.13	0.60	0.63
std dev	0.28	0.32	0.09	0.36	0.04	0.33	0.42	0.13	0.46	0.06
best	0.98	0.88	0.28	1.06	0.66	1.00	0.93	0.38	1.16	0.72

MLkNN - Multi-label k nearest neighbours, **PCT** - Predictive clustering trees, **RAkEL** - Random k-labelsets, **ECC** - Ensemble of classifier chains, **TPR** - True positive rate, **TNR** - True negative rate, **MCC** - Matthew's correlation coefficient, **DP** - Discriminative power, **AUC** - Area under the receiver operating characteristic curve

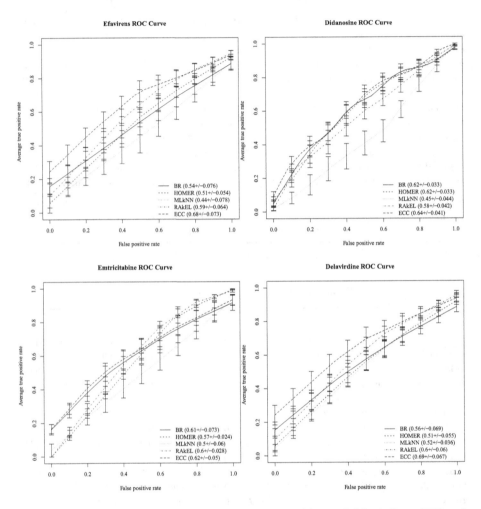

Fig. 1. ROC curves for efavirens, didanosine, emtricitabine and delavirdine. *AUC* and standard error are given for each method in parentheses

ROC - Receiver operating characteristic, **AUC** - Area under ROC curve, **BR** - Binary relevance (with naive Bayes base classifier), **HOMER** - Hierarchy of multi-label classifiers, **MLkNN** - Multi-label k nearest neighbours, **RAkEL** - Random k-labelsets, **ECC** - Ensemble of classifier chains

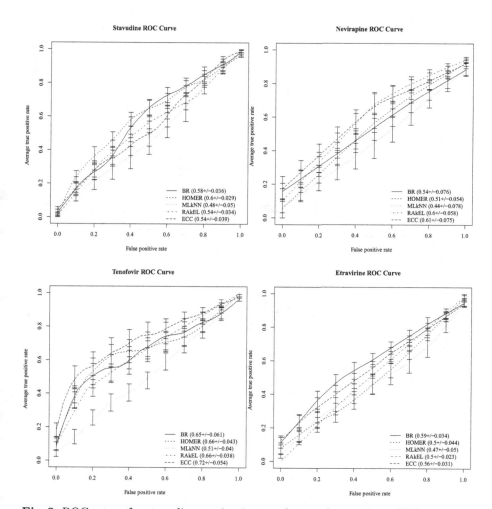

Fig. 2. ROC curves for stavudine, nevirapine tenofovir and etravirine. *AUC* and standard error are given for each method in parentheses

ROC - Receiver operating characteristic, **AUC** - Area under ROC curve, **BR** - Binary relevance (with naive Bayes base classifier), **HOMER** - Hierarchy of multi-label classifiers, **MLkNN** - Multi-label *k* nearest neighbours, **RAkEL** - Random *k*-labelsets, **ECC** - Ensemble of classifier chains

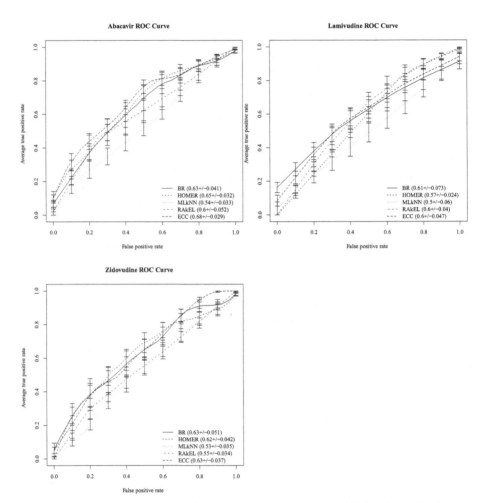

Fig. 3. ROC curves for abacavir, lamivudine and zidovudine. AUC and standard error are given for each method in parentheses

ROC - Receiver operating characteristic, **AUC** - Area under ROC curve, **BR** - Binary relevance (with naive Bayes base classifier), **HOMER** - Hierarchy of multi-label classifiers, **MLkNN** - Multi-label k nearest neighbours, **RAkEL** - Random k-labelsets, **ECC** - Ensemble of classifier chains

Techniques that have high true positive rates often have a relatively low true negative rate, which means that the rate of false positives is high. This could result in an increased number of genotype tests being requested. However, if GRT is not available and/or if the care provider decides that a regimen change is necessary, the false positives can be seen as the algorithms making conservative predictions. It is important to try and retain patients as long as possible on first line treatment regimens since second line therapy costs as much as 2.4 times more than first line therapy and compromises treatment outcomes [5], but if it is decided to switch regimen, conservative prediction results could be used to help design a treatment regimen to which the virus is susceptible.

Algorithms like PCT, BR-NB and ECC have high values for all of the metrics for the drugs that they perform well on. This should give us confidence that the decision support information provided is in fact good and not just the result of a single outlier metric value. Conversely, we should have less confidence in the performance of a technique on a drug if only one of the metrics show good performance, for example, the MLkNN technique has a high TNR value (0.97) for stavudine, but all other metrics indicate very poor performance. Techniques that produce blanket positive predictions provide no information that can be used to support decisions.

The results of this analysis need to be interpreted in light of certain limitations. The most important limitation was the lack of any objective or proxy measures of adherence, such as pharmacy refill data or medication possession ratios, as this information was not available routinely in the program. Adherence is one of the most important determinants of drug resistance and is an essential variable in a predictive dataset. It is also important to consider that certain attributes captured for each patient are self-reported (such as the adherence attributes) and that the reliability of such data may be questionable.

The small number of training examples ($n = 252$) could be partly responsible for the limitations in performance. Another factor that could influence the performance is the presence of features in the dataset that contain incomplete data. Unfortunately, incomplete and inaccurate data are common features of public health ART treatment program data in South Africa and other countries. Patients miss clinic visits for a number of health and socio-economic reasons and it is often the case that laboratory test results are not available when needed by the clinician. Further investigation should be done on the use of feature selection to ensure the optimal subset of features is being used for training and prediction, since irrelevant and redundant features can reduce classification accuracy [34].

Resource-limited public health treatment programs are usually characterised by limited availability of GRT, second line therapy and highly skilled clinicians. In these settings, the predictive power demonstrated by the classifiers may be sufficient to facilitate and improve clinical decision-making. If the primary goal is to optimize the use of GRT, then the method with the highest mean TNR should be selected, which is PCT. If the primary goal is new therapy selection, then

BR-NB should be used, since it has the highest mean TPR. If it is of particular importance to know about the presence of resistance to a specific drug, then the method with the highest TNR for that drug should be selected, since this minimises false positives.

6   Conclusion and Future Work

We have demonstrated that the machine learning techniques examined in this work can be used to a limited degree to predict HIV drug resistance and mostly perform better than a random classifier and in some cases, substantially better. Even though some results show promise there is insufficient evidence to support the conclusion that machine learning prediction models using only clinical, adherence and demographic details, can replace GRT. However, these techniques may be useful in resource-limited public health settings where decisions such as whether to remain on the same therapy, and if not, which new drugs to select, need to be made in the absence of a GRT result or a specialized clinician. While none of the seven methods stands out as a significantly good predictor for resistance to all drugs, some methods perform relatively well on some drugs. For example, PCT is good at identifying resistance to nevirapine. A future area of work could be to construct individual predictive models per drug, using different underlying methods and then combine these results into an ensemble to produce one prediction. The advent of limited resistance testing in the public ART program in South Africa and development of national surveillance data sets [35] will also allow the construction of larger datasets and potentially increase the accuracy of machine learning techniques. The existing techniques will be tested on these larger datasets as they become available. We also plan to extend the analysis and investigate the predictive potential at different stages of treatment failure. Time spent on a failing regimen could lead to accumulation of resistance mutations and this should be taken into consideration when care providers need to decide on a course of action. The software developed could easily be integrated into existing ART programs that use RegaDB and could act as a passive early warning system to alert providers to patients for whom the classifiers predict high levels of resistance.

Acknowledgements. PB received a scholarship for this study from the Health Architecture Laboratory (HeAL) project funded by grants from the Rockefeller Foundation (Establishing a Health Enterprise Architecture Lab, a research laboratory focused on the application of enterprise architecture and health informatics to resource-limited settings, Grant Number: 2010 THS 347) and the International Development Research Centre (IDRC) (Health Enterprise Architecture Laboratory (HeAL), Grant Number: 106452-001). CS, TdO and the Southern African Treatment and Research Network (SATuRN) network were funded by grants from the Delegation of the European Union to South Africa (SANTE 2007 147-790; Drug resistance surveillance and treatment monitoring network for the public sector HIV antiretroviral treatment programme in the Free State) and CDC/PEPFAR via a grant to the Centre for the AIDS Programme of Research in South Africa (CAPRISA) (project title: Health System Strengthening and the HIV Treatment Failure Clinic System (HIV-TFC)). TdO is supported by the Wellcome Trust (grant number 082384/Z/07/Z). The funders had no role in study design, data collection and analysis, decision to publish, or preparation of the manuscript.

References

1. Statistics, S.A.: Statistical release Mid-year population estimates (July 2011), http://www.statssa.gov.za/Publications/statsdownload.asp?PPN=P0302
2. Rossouw, T., Tulio, O., Lessels, R.J.: HIV & TB Drug Resistance & Clinical Management Case Book. South African Medical Research Council Press (2013)
3. Liu, T.F., Shafer, R.W.: Web resources for HIV type 1 genotypic-resistance test interpretation. Clinical Infectious Diseases: An Official Publication of the Infectious Diseases Society of America 42(11), 1608–1618 (2006)
4. Van Laethem, K., De Luca, A., Antinori, A., et al.: A genotypic drug resistance interpretation algorithm that significantly predicts therapy response in HIV-1-infected patients. Antiviral Therapy 7(2), 123–129 (2002)
5. Rosen, S., Long, L., Sanne, I., et al.: The net cost of incorporating resistance testing into HIV/AIDS treatment in South Africa: a Markov model with primary data. Journal of the International AIDS Society 14(1), 24 (2011)
6. Robbins, G.K., Daniels, B., Zheng, H., et al.: Predictors of antiretroviral treatment failure in an urban HIV clinic. Journal of Acquired Immune Deficiency Syndromes 44(1), 30–37 (1999)
7. Parienti, J.J., Massari, V., Descamps, D., et al.: Predictors of virologic failure and resistance in HIV-infected patients treated with nevirapine- or efavirenz-based antiretroviral therapy. Clinical Infectious Diseases: An Official Publication of the Infectious Diseases Society of America 38(9), 1311–1316 (2004)
8. Harrigan, P.R., Hogg, R.S., Dong, W.W.Y., et al.: Predictors of HIV drug-resistance mutations in a large antiretroviral-naive cohort initiating triple antiretroviral therapy. The Journal of Infectious Diseases 191(3), 339–347 (2005)
9. Di Giambenedetto, S., Zazzi, M., Corsi, P., et al.: Evolution and predictors of HIV type-1 drug resistance in patients failing combination antiretroviral therapy in Italy. Antiviral Therapy 14(3), 359–369 (2009)
10. Larder, B., Revell, A., Mican, J.M., et al.: Clinical evaluation of the potential utility of computational modeling as an HIV treatment selection tool by physicians with considerable HIV experience. AIDS Patient Care and STDs 25(1), 29–36 (2011)
11. Zazzi, M., Kaiser, R., Sönnerborg, A., et al.: Prediction of response to antiretroviral therapy by human experts and by the EuResist data-driven expert system (the EVE study). HIV Medicine 12(4), 211–218 (2011)
12. Larder, B., Wang, D., Revell, A., et al.: The development of artificial neural networks to predict virological response to combination HIV therapy. Antiviral Therapy 12(1), 15–24 (2007)

13. Prosperi, M.C.F., Altmann, A., Rosen-Zvi, M., et al.: Investigation of expert rule bases, logistic regression, and non-linear machine learning techniques for predicting response to antiretroviral treatment. Antiviral Therapy 14(3), 433–442 (2009)
14. Altmann, A., Rosen-Zvi, M., Prosperi, M., et al.: Comparison of classifier fusion methods for predicting response to anti HIV-1 therapy. PloS One 3(10), e3470 (2008)
15. Rosen-Zvi, M., Altmann, A., Prosperi, M., et al.: Selecting anti-HIV therapies based on a variety of genomic and clinical factors. Bioinformatics 24(13), 399–406 (2008)
16. Revell, A.D., Wang, D., Wood, R., et al.: Computational models can predict response to HIV therapy without a genotype and may reduce treatment failure in different resource-limited settings. Journal of Antimicrobial Chemotherapy (March 2013)
17. Prosperi, M.C.F., Rosen-Zvi, M., Altmann, A., et al.: Antiretroviral therapy optimisation without genotype resistance testing: a perspective on treatment history based models. PloS One 5(10), e13753 (2010)
18. Libin, P., Beheydt, G., Deforche, K., et al.: RegaDB: Community-driven data management and analysis for infectious diseases. Bioinformatics, 1–5 (April 2013)
19. Tsoumakas, G., Katakis, I., Vlahavas, I.: Mining multi-label data. Data Mining and Knowledge Discovery Handbook, 1–20 (2010)
20. Madjarov, G., Kocev, D., Gjorgjevikj, D., et al.: An extensive experimental comparison of methods for multi-label learning. An Extensive Experimental Comparison of Methods for Multi-label Learning 45, 3084–310 (2012)
21. Kohavi, R.: A Study of Cross-Validation and Bootstrap for Accuracy Estimation and Model Selection. International Joint Conference on Artificial Intelligence 14(12), 1137–1143 (1995)
22. Sechidis, K., Tsoumakas, G., Vlahavas, I.: On the stratification of multi-label data. In: Gunopulos, D., Hofmann, T., Malerba, D., Vazirgiannis, M. (eds.) ECML PKDD 2011, Part III. LNCS, vol. 6913, pp. 145–158. Springer, Heidelberg (2011)
23. Hsu, C.W., Chang, C.C., Lin, C.J.: A Practical Guide to Support Vector Classification. Bioinformatics 1(1), 1–16 (2010)
24. Rish, I.: An empirical study of the naive Bayes classifier. IJCAI 2001 Workshop on Empirical Methods in Artificial Intelligence (2001)
25. Tsoumakas, G.: Effective and efficient multilabel classification in domains with large number of labels. In: Proc. ECML/PKDD 2008 Workshop on Mining Multi-dimensional Data, MMD 2008 (2008)
26. Zhang, M.L., Zhou, Z.H.: ML-KNN: A lazy learning approach to multi-label learning. Pattern Recognition 40(7), 2038–2048 (2007)
27. Blockeel, H., De Raedt, L.: Top-down induction of first-order logical decision trees. Artificial Intelligence 101(1-2), 285–297 (1998)
28. Tsoumakas, G., Vlahavas, I.P.: Random k-labelsets: An ensemble method for multilabel classification. In: Kok, J.N., Koronacki, J., Lopez de Mantaras, R., Matwin, S., Mladenič, D., Skowron, A. (eds.) ECML 2007. LNCS (LNAI), vol. 4701, pp. 406–417. Springer, Heidelberg (2007)
29. Read, J., Pfahringer, B., Holmes, G., et al.: Classifier chains for multi-label classification. Machine Learning 85(3), 333–359 (2011)
30. Sokolova, M., Lapalme, G.: A systematic analysis of performance measures for classification tasks. Information Processing & Management 45(4), 427–437 (2009)
31. Baldi, P., Brunak, S.R., Chauvin, Y., et al.: Assessing the accuracy of prediction algorithms for classification: an overview. Bioinformatics 16(5), 412–424 (2000)

32. Sokolova, M.V., Japkowicz, N., Szpakowicz, S.: Beyond accuracy, F-score and ROC: A family of discriminant measures for performance evaluation. In: Sattar, A., Kang, B.-H. (eds.) AI 2006. LNCS (LNAI), vol. 4304, pp. 1015–1021. Springer, Heidelberg (2006)

33. Fawcett, T.: An introduction to ROC analysis. Pattern Recognition Letters 27(8), 861–874 (2006)

34. Okun, O.: Introduction to Feature and Gene Selection. In: Feature Selection and Ensemble Methods for Bioinformatics: Algorithmic Classification and Implementations, pp. 117–122. IGI Global, Hershey (2011)

35. Conradie, F., Wilson, D., Basson, A., et al.: The 2012 southern African ARV drug resistance testing guidelines by the Southern African HIV Clinicians Society. Southern African Journal of HIV Medicine 13(4), 162–167 (2012)

Characterisation of Knowledge Incorporation into Solution Models for the Meal Planning Problem

Ngonidzashe Zanamwe[1], Kudakwashe Dube[2,*],
Jasmine S. Thomson[3], Fredrick J. Mtenzi[4], and Gilford T. Hapanyengwi[1]

[1] Computer Science Department, Faculty of Science,
University of Zimbabwe
[2] School of Engineering and Advanced Technology,
Massey University, New Zealand
[3] Institute of Food, Nutrition and Human Health,
Massey University, New Zealand
[4] School of Computing, College of Sciences and Health,
Dublin Institute of Technology, Ireland
nzanamwe@science.uz.ac.zw, {k.dube,j.a.thomson}@massey.ac.nz,
fredrick.mtenzi@dit.ie, ghapanyengwi@compcentre.uz.ac.zw
http://www.uz.ac.zw
http://www.massey.ac.nz
http://www.dit.ie

Abstract. This paper is part of work aimed at investigating an approach to knowledge incorporation into solution models of the Meal Planning Problem (MPP) for use in mobile web-based HIV/AIDS nutrition therapy management within the context of developing countries, particularly, in Sub-Saharan Africa. This paper presents a characterisation of the incorporation of knowledge into the models for the MPP. The characterisation is important for assessing the extent to which MPP models can be adapted for use in different clinical problems with different nutrition guideline knowledge and in different regions of the world with differently customised versions of the guidelines. The characterisation was applied to thirty one works in the literature on MPP models. The main outcome of the application of the characterisation was the finding that the existing MPP models do not provide for the incorporation of nutrition guideline knowledge as first class concepts with identifiable and manageable structures, which makes almost impossible the transfer of knowledge from health experts to patients and from one region of the world to another.

Keywords: meal planning, modelling, nutrition guideline, knowledge engineering, algorithms, optimisation problem, evolutionary computing, genetic algorithm, knapsack problem, particle swarm optimisation, constraint satisfaction, linear programming, HIV/AIDS, nutrition therapy.

---

* Corresponding author.

J. Gibbons and W. MacCaull (Eds.): FHIES 2013, LNCS 8315, pp. 254–273, 2014.

1   Introduction

Dissemination and incorporation of Food, Nutrition and Lifestyle Guideline (FNLG) knowledge into the daily life of patients through computing techniques is a challenge whose solution would facilitate knowledge transfer from health experts to patients. FNLGs are evidence-based statements developed from scientific evidence for use in making food and nutrition practice decisions by integrating best available evidence with professional expertise, client values and clinical requirements to improve health outcomes [2]. Solutions to the Meal Planning Problem (MPP) have been widely investigated [10]. However, some of these solutions [5], [31], [47] considered to a lesser extent the context of either patients or diseases. Furthermore, these solutions have not adequately addressed the problem of incorporating FNLG knowledge into MPP models in therapeutic contexts for diseases like HIV/AIDS. Food, Nutrition and Lifestyle Guidelines (FNLGs) refers to food composition data, nutrient reference data, personal data, nutrition guideline knowledge, meal formats and cusine rules. This paper focuses on knowledge incorporation because [39] argues that meal planning tools may be useful only if they are based on comprehensive domain knowledge.

The adoption of mobile applications in Africa is an established and growing trend. Given this background, African countries should exploit mobile applications for improving health outcomes, especially in areas like HIV/AIDS nutrition therapy. In 2012 there were 1937 mobile applications in the care and prevention of HIV/AIDS [28]. However, none provided information on HIV/AIDS nutrition therapy.

This paper presents a characterisation of knowledge incorporation into the MPP models. This characterisation was used in reviewing literature on knowledge incorporation in MPP models. Results of this review suggest that existing MPP models do not provide for the incorporation of FNLG knowledge as first class concepts with identifiable and manageable structures.

The main contribution of this paper is a new characterisation of knowledge incorporation into MPP models. This provides pointers to the next steps in our research project. These steps are i) developing a knowledge intensive, generic and customisable MPP model, ii) developing strategies and software engineering solutions for real uses of the model in HIV/AIDS nutrition therapy and iii) application of the model in the mobile web-based context of developing countries to facilitate knowledge transfer from experts to patients.

The rest of this paper is organized as follows: Section 2 presents the context and motivations of this work and section 3 gives the research problem statement. Theory on modelling the MPP is then presented in section 4. After that, section 5 presents the characterisation of knowledge incorporation into MPP models. This is followed by application of the characterisation to works on meal planning in section 6. Sections 7 and 8 present the summary of findings and implications of results respectively. Section 9 gives the future work and section 10 concludes the paper.

2   The Research Context and Motivations

2.1   The Meal Planning Problem

Meal planning involves designing meals from food ingredients of different nutritional values and volumes. The MPP is the search for a set of meals that satisfy several constraints of nutritional requirements, personal preferences and also meet objectives such as seasonal availability of food items, cost, taste, and method of preparation. A more detailed definition of the MPP is given in [10].

2.2   Food, Nutrition and Lifestyle Guidelines (FNLGs) and HIV/AIDS Nutrition Therapy

FNLGs are important tools for improving outcomes in preventative, curative and therapeutic care [30]. Most African countries have HIV/AIDS FNLGs which exist at several levels [36]. Examples of generic FNLGS include, FANTA and UNICEF/WHO reports [29], [36], national or regional guidelines or initiatives for example, National guidelines for HIV/AIDS and Nutrition in Ethiopia [50], and evidence from scientific literature, and position statements for example, American Dietetic Associations, Nutrition Intervention and Human Immunodeficiency Virus Infection [7]. FNLGs are increasingly being incorporated into computer-based decision-support models [5], [10]. The modelling and incorporation of comprehensive HIV/AIDS FNLGs into mobile applications is a promising vehicle for facilitating the flow of expert knowledge and best practices from experts to individual members of the public.

3   The Research Problem

Existing MPP models do not incorporate highly targeted FNLG knowledge as a first-class concept or structure. This constrains sufficient decoupling within elements of the models and flexibility in the customisation of the knowledge aspects of the models to support knowledge transfer especially in the area of HIV/AIDS nutrition therapy. This work characterises how existing MPP models incorporate FNLGs. The objectives of this research are to i) develop a conceptual framework for characterisation of MPP models and ii) apply the characterisation to existing MPP models.

4   Modelling the Meal Planning Problem

Most MPP studies have used hybrid models which combine computational and mathematical models as in [5], [10], [14]. This section describes the most prevalent models.

4.1 Linear Programming

Works that model the MPP as a Linear Programming (LP) problem include [22], [27]. The MPP can be modelled as a LP problem by starting with a list of food items of various values and volumes and then prepare meals that satisfy objectives and constraints. Some of the constraints include nutritional requirements and personal preferences. Objectives include seasonal availability of food items, cost, taste, just to mention a few.

4.2 Constraint Satisfaction Problem (CSP)

A Constraint Satisfaction Problem is a set of objects whose state satisfy many constraints [51]. Works that model the MPP as a CSP include [1]. The MPP can be modelled as a CSP with hard and soft constraints. Hard constraints are constraints that should be satisfied by every solution whereas soft constraints may or may not be satisfied [38]. Hard constraints include user needs and preferences whereas soft constraints include taste and variety. In a CSP, variables are used for parameters of recipes such as time, cost, energy and protein. Variable domains are based on values in the recipes database and the resulting meal must satisfy all constraints and objectives.

4.3 Knapsack Problem (KP)

A KP assumes that there are n items and each has a value. A knapsack has a maximum capacity it can carry. The objective is to maximise the sum of the values of items in a knapsack so that the sum of the weights must be less than the maximum capacity of a knapsack. Works that model the MPP as a KP include [10], [12], [14], [41]. In mapping a KP to the MPP, a knapsack can represent a meal, a daily meal plan or a weekly meal plan. Firstly, if we assume that a knapsack represents a meal, the task is to pick food items from a set of food items such that constraints and objectives are met. Secondly, if we assume that a knapsack represents a daily meal plan, the task is to pick meals from the previous step such that constraints and objectives are satisfied. Lastly, if we assume that a knapsack represents a weekly meal plan, the task is to pick daily meal plans from a list from the above step in order to achieve an optimal weekly meal plan that satisfy objectives and constraints.

4.4 Genetic Algorithms (GA)

A GA mimics natural evolution by using techniques inspired by the natural processes of inheritance, mutation, selection, and crossover [8]. In a GA, each candidate solution has a set of properties (its chromosomes or genotype) which can be mutated and altered to yield better solutions. Some of the works that model the MPP as a GA include, [5], [10], [11], [41], [48]. In modelling the MPP using a GA, candidate solutions represent meals. These candidate solutions are evolved through application of the operations like, inheritance, mutation, selection, and crossover. The candidate solutions evolve toward meals that meet required constraints and follow FNLGs. The question which always arise is whether or not such meals follow FNLGs for specific diseases?

4.5 Particle Swarm Optimisation (PSO) and Its Quantum Variant (QPSO)

A PSO optimizes a problem by having particles that evolve towards their best form [15], [43]. The QPSO is a variant of the PSO that uses the quantum theory of mechanics to govern the movement of swarm particles [32]. Works that used these MPP models include [21]. In modelling the MPP, particles represent the meals. These meals evolve to better meals in the same way particles evolve to better forms. This evolution process continues until optimal meals satisfying objectives and constraints are obtained.

5   Characterising Knowledge Incorporation into Models for the Meal Planning Problem

5.1 The Typology for Meal Planning Problem Models

There are four types of MPP models namely, nutritional, mathematical, computational and hybrid models. These types of models are shown in Fig. 1. Furthermore, specific models which fall under each type are shown in Fig. 1. For example, GA and Ant Colony Optimisation are computational models. The list of computational models in Fig. 1 is not exhaustive and the same is true of specific models which fall under hybrid model. A nutritional model can be mapped either to a mathematical model like LP or to a computational model like QPSO. Usually, mathematical models often underlie the core conceptualisations of the computational models. This imply that a nutritional model is expressed as mathematical specifications or as computational formalisms. The next sections elaborate on these models.

Nutritional Model of the Meal Planning Problem: This is embodied in the FNLGs and is always domain problem-specific. In this model, a design is required for a temporal schedule of meals such that each meal contains region- or country-specific foods whose combined nutritional value meets a person's nutritional and health requirements as recommended in FNLGs as part of disease-specific nutrition therapy or population grouping-specific feeding scheme. This model is always mapped onto either or both the mathematical and computational models. For this reason, this paper focuses on the mathematical and computational models.

Mathematical Model of the Meal Planning Problem: Is based on some mathematical specifications of domain problem models. LP is the most widely used mathematical model of the MPP.

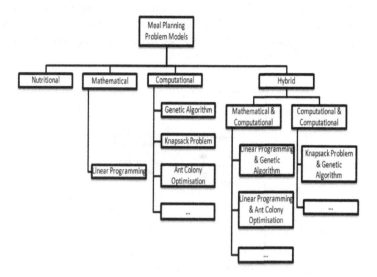

Fig. 1. Types of MPP models

The Computational Model of the Meal Planning Problem: This uses computational formalisms including algorithms. Evolutionary computational models like GA and QPSO have no underlying mathematical model mapping the nutritional model onto them. Therefore, nutritional models map directly onto computational models. In general, computational models of the MPP serve as implementations of the mathematical models.

The Hybrid Model of the Meal Planning Problem: This uses more than one model either i) within the same type, for example, a combination of two computational models like Knapsack Problem and GA, or ii) across the two or more types of models for example, a combination of a mathematical model and a computational model like LP and GA. Both mathematical and computational models may be combined in solving the MPP even though there seems to be no direct mapping relationships between these base models.

5.2 Dimensions of Knowledge Incorporation into the Meal Planning Problem Model

Fig. 2 shows a framework for modelling the MPP. The framework has two dimensions namely the MPP model dimension and the MPP knowledge dimension. In this paper, the MPP model dimension is synonymous with types of MPP models presented in section 5.1. This framework shows that MPP models can be broadly classified as either i) models that are general and more suitable for healthy individuals or ii) models that are specialised and more suitable for patients and specific diseases. Models which are general either incorporate no FNLG knowledge or incorporate non-targeted FNLG knowledge. Models that are specialised either incorporate targeted FNLG knowledge or highly targeted FNLG knowledge. These dimensions are explained below.

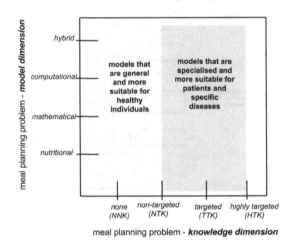

Fig. 2. Framework for the modelling of the meal planning problem - the Meal Planning Problem Model and Knowledge dimensions

Meal Planning Problem Model Dimension: The MPP model dimension includes the nutritional, mathematical, computational and hybrid models described in section 5.1 as types of MPP models.

Meal Planning Problem Knowledge Dimension: The MPP knowledge dimension has four elements: (1) NNK - none or no knowledge which is covered by MPP models that do not incorporate any FNLG knowledge. Solutions from these MPP models are of theoretical value and least useful as they may not be suitable for any group of people; (2) NTK - non-targeted knowledge which is covered by MPP models that incorporate generic and non-targeted FNLG knowledge. Solutions from these MPP models are useful only for healthy individuals; (3) TTK - targeted knowledge which is covered by MPP models that incorporate targeted FNLG knowledge and also incorporate general FNLGs about a specific disease or patient without providing the necessary conceptualisations and structures that are identifiable and manageable as a complete nutrition therapy guideline. Solutions from these MPP models are useful to specific groups of people like patients or sportspersons; and (4) HTK - highly targeted knowledge which is covered by MPP models that incorporate highly targeted FNLG knowledge as first-class concepts and structures. These MPP models are envisaged to make use of systematically developed evidence-based FNLGs that are developed by domain experts. They are envisaged to provide comprehensive conceptualisations and structures that are identifiable and manageable as single units that can be modified and changed, thus making possible the transfer of knowledge from experts to patients.

5.3 Relationships and Implications of the Meal Planning Problem Model and Knowledge Dimensions

The MPP knowledge dimension and the MPP model dimension are related because the MPP models incorporate FNLG knowledge in solving the MPP. For example, a computational model like a GA can incorporate NNK, NTK, TTK or HTK in solving the MPP. The degree of FNLG knowledge incorporated into the MPP model determines the extent to which the meal planning solutions would be useful to people. Also, the degree to which the MPP model supports generic conceptualisation and structuring of the incorporated FNLG knowledge determines the extent to which the MPP model and the knowledge can be customised to specific problem areas and geographic regions of the world.

6 Application of the Characterisation

This section applies the characterisation presented in the above section to existing works on MPP models and also presents outcomes of the application of the characterization. The aim was to determine the extent to which existing works have incorporated FNLG knowledge in MPP models and identify research gaps.

6.1 Methodology

We performed a literature search of papers on MPP models from online sources like Google search engine, ACM and IEEE digital libraries, PubMed and ScienceDirect. This approach was appropriate because it considers and reflects upon international perspectives. Search terms used include: meal planning, meal planning models, MPP, meal planning algorithms, meal planning applications, automatic meal planning. We used advanced search criterion. We searched for the above terms in the title and abstract of each paper. We searched for articles which were published after 2004. After filtering results we remained with 31 relevant papers upon which we applied our characterisation while aiming at: (1) determining the sources of the knowledge; and (2) systematically characterising the knowledge incorporation in models presented in these works.

6.2 Summary of Results

Some of the results of the application of the characterisation are presented in Fig. 3 which shows different types of models used in modelling the MPP.

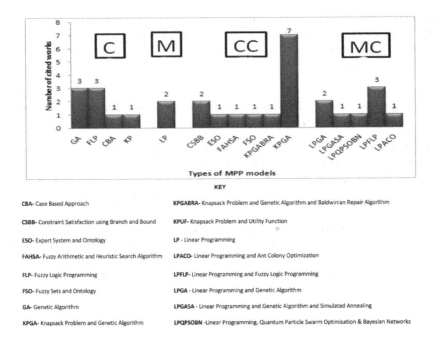

KEY

CBA- Case Based Approach	**KPGABRA-** Knapsack Problem and Genetic Algorithm and Baldwinian Repair Algorithm
CSBB- Constraint Satisfaction using Branch and Bound	**KPUF-** Knapsack Problem and Utility Function
ESO- Expert System and Ontology	**LP -** Linear Programming
FAHSA- Fuzzy Arithmetic and Heuristic Search Algorithm	**LPACO-** Linear Programming and Ant Colony Optimization
FLP- Fuzzy Logic Programming	**LPFLP-** Linear Programming and Fuzzy Logic Programming
FSO- Fuzzy Sets and Ontology	**LPGA -** Linear Programming and Genetic Algorithm
GA- Genetic Algorithm	**LPGASA -** Linear Programming and Genetic Algorithm and Simulated Annealing
KPGA- Knapsack Problem and Genetic Algorithm	**LPQPSOBN -**Linear Programming, Quantum Particle Swarm Optimisation & Bayesian Networks

Fig. 3. Typology of mathematical, computational and hybrid models found in the literature

Models of the Meal Planning Problem: Fig. 3 shows 31 cited works on the MPP. These works can be classified into 16 models. Four of these are computational models marked by a 'C' while one is a mathematical model marked by an 'M' in the figure. Eleven of these are hybrid models. Six of these eleven are a combination of two or more computational models marked by 'CC' and the other five are a combination of a mixture of mathematical and computational models marked by 'MC' in the figure. Each bar in Fig. 3 represents a model. Names of models are shown on the x-axis. For example, the first bar represents a computational model called GA while the eleventh bar represents a hybrid model comprising of a Knapsack Problem and a Genetic Algorithm (KPGA). From Fig. 3, it is clear that KPGA (Knapsack Problem and Genetic Algorithm) is the most prevalent hybrid model since it was used by 7 works. Other fairly prevalent models include GA, LPFLP (Linear Programming and Fuzzy Linear Programming) and FLP (Fuzzy Linear Programming). Each of these 3 models was used by 3 cited works. The remaining models were either used by 2 works (LP, LPGA, CSBB) or by 1 work (LPGASA, LPQPSOBN, ESO, CBA, FAHSA, FSO, KPUF, KPGABRA, LPACO). From Fig. 3, it can be deduced that 21 works used the hybrid model and 10 did not.

Knowledge Dimensions of the Meal Planning Problem Models: Other results from the application of the characterisation model are shown in Fig. 4.

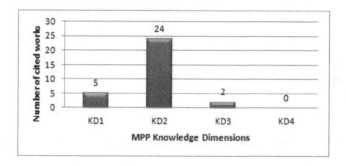

Fig. 4. Meal Planning Problem Knowledge Dimensions

This figure shows the number of cited works which fall under each knowledge dimension. Fig. 4 also shows that 5 cited works fall under KD1. This means that these works did not incorporate any FNLG knowledge in solving the MPP. In addition, 24 works fall under KD2. This means that these works incorporated generic and non-targeted FNLG knowledge in solving the MPP. Furthermore, 2 works fall under KD3. This means that these works incorporated general FNLGs about diseases and patients in solving the MPP. Lastly, no work fall under KD4 meaning that there were no works that incorporated highly targeted FNLG knowledge in solving the MPP. Thus, in total, 26 of these works focus on MPP models that incorporate FNLG knowledge even though it was general.

Knowledge Incorporation in the Meal Planning Problem Models: Fig. 5 is a characterisation of knowledge incorporation into the MPP models found in literature. The column headed type shows the type of model used to solve the MPP. In this column, C stands for computational model; M stands for mathematical model; CC stands for a hybrid model composing of 2 or more computational models and MC stands for a hybrid model comprising of a mixture of mathemactical and computational models. KD stands for knowledge dimension. Fig. 5 also shows that a hybrid model of Knapsack Problem and GA has 2 works which fall under KD1 and 5 works falling under KD2. In addition, the GA and the LP with Fuzzy Logic Programming each has 2 works which fall under KD2 and 1 work under KD1. Similar explanations can be given for the remaining models. Furthermore, most types of models (11 out of 16) are hybrid models of MPP even though none incorporated highly targeted FNLG knowledge. Fig. 5 also shows that 24 out of 31 works fall under KD2. This implies that the highest number of MPP models incorporated general FNLG knowledge. This makes these models less useful to patients. Detailed information on the MPP models and knowledge dimensions is presented in the tables in the appendix section. In these tables a tick means that the cited work falls under that particular knowledge dimension and a cross means the opposite.

Model Dimension/Knowledge Dimension	Type	KD1	KD2	KD3	KD4	Total
Genetic Algorithm	C	1	2	0	0	3
Fuzzy Logic Programming	C	0	2	1	0	3
Case Based Approach	C	0	1	0	0	1
Knapsack Problem	C	0	1	0	0	1
Constraint Satisfaction using Branch and Bound	CC	0	2	0	0	2
Expert System and Ontology	CC	0	1	0	0	1
Fuzzy Arithmetic and Heuristic Search Algorithm	CC	1	0	0	0	1
Fuzzy Sets and ontology	CC	0	1	0	0	1
Knapsack Problem, Genetic Algorithm and Baldwinian Repair Algorithm	CC	0	1	0	0	1
Knapsack Problem and Genetic Algorithm	CC	2	5	0	0	7
Linear Programming	M	0	2	0	0	2
Linear Programming and Genetic Algorithm	MC	0	2	0	0	2
Linear Programming and Genetic Algorithm and Simulated Annealing	MC	0	1	0	0	1
Linear Programming and Quantum Particle Swarm Optimisation with Bayesian Networks	MC	0	1	0	0	1
Linear Programming and Fuzzy Logic Programming	MC	1	2	0	0	3
Linear Programming and Ant Colony Optimization	MC	0	0	1	0	1
Total		5	24	2	0	31

Fig. 5. Characterisation of Knowledge Incorporation into the Meal Planning Problem model for works found in the literature

6.3   Analysis and Discussion of the Results

Our analysis determined the extent to which FNLG knowledge was incorporated in MPP models.

Knowledge Incorporation in Mathematical Models: The diet optimization problem was solved using a LP model by works such as [22] and [27]. Both works used general FNLG knowledge. As such, both models are not very useful to any group of patients. Furthermore, [16] applied Fuzzy Logic in diet therapy for hypertension. The model presented in [16] did not consider constraints like user preferences and cost of meals. In addition to that, this model incorporated general FNLGs instead of highly targeted FNLG knowledge for hypertension.

Knowledge Incorporation in Computational Models: Authors like [5] used a GA to solve the MPP for diabetes. The major weakness of the model presented in [5] is that it considers only a confined number of the factors and model parameters are not easily individualized. Additionally, [5] did not incorporate highly targeted FNLG knowledge in their model. Similarly, [11] used a GA for cardiovascular diseases and used personal medical data combined with general FNLGs for Hungarian lifestyle and cuisine. Both works referenced in this paragraph did not incorporate detailed FNLG knowledge in the models but rather used the FNLG knowledge in testing applications.

Knowledge Incorporation in Hybrid Models: Hybrid models are models that use a combination of two or more models. Hybrid models presented in [10], [14], [41], [12], [42], [42] used a combination of GA and KP. This was a hydrid of two computational models. On the other hand, [47] used a combination of LP, GA and Simulated Annealing. This was a hybrid of a mathematical model with two computational models. Furthermore, 1 study [21] used LP and QPSO. This was a hybrid of a mathematical and a computational model. With respect to the disease or patient context, [10], [12], [21], [41], [42], did not focus on any disease. This means that their models were generic and less useful to any class of patients. However, [47] focused on high blood pressure while [14] focused on life-style related diseases and [24] focused on diabetes. The next section presents a detailed analysis of some of the existing MPP models.

A hybrid MPP model for malnutrition among elderly people is presented in [1]. This is a hybrid of a Constraint Satisfaction Problem and Depth-First Branch and Bound algorithm. In this model, variables for recipe parameters like time, cost, energy and protein were used in the Constriant Satsfaction model. The FNLG knowledge used in [1] cannot be classified as highly targeted FNLG knowledge but as generic knowledge. Further to that, the solution in [1] cannot be used to make meal plans for periods more than a week and only works with small databases of recipes. Furthermore, [1] acknowledges that their model is not time efficient. In addition, a hybrid MPP model for diabetic patients is given in [4]. The model used Fuzzy Arithmetic and Huristic Search algorithm. The main weakness of this model is that it only balances meals individually and not globally. In addition, this model did not focus on incorporating highly targeted FNLGs for diabetic patients but rather on preparing and balancing meals in cases where nutritional requirements are fuzzy.

A hybrid model for optimizing the human diet problem based on price and taste using multi-objective Fuzzy Linear Programming is presented in [6]. This model was for human diet optimisation which means that it cannot be used in specific disease contexts since it did not incorporate FNLG knowledge in the solution to the MPP.

In addition to the above hybrid models, [12] used a model that solves a bi-objective diet problem. One of the weaknesses of this model is that it treats the MPP as a bi-objective rather than a multi-objective problem. Also, the parameters of the model were specified by users instead of by experts. The authors used Dietary Reference Intake and Recommended Dietary Allowance tables established by U.S. Food and Nutrition Board of the National Academy of Sciences. These guidelines are general and as such, the resulting model was only suitable for healthy people. On the contrary, [13] considered the MPP as multi-objective even though the meals prepared using their model did not consist of at least three different kinds of dishes. In [13], a hybrid model composed of the Knapsack Problem and Genetic Algorithm was used. This model did not incorporate any FNLG knowledge in solving the MPP. On the contrary, [17], developed an expert system for diet recommendation using a Case-Based Approach. In this expert system, dietetic information was represented using a ripple down rules tree. The major weakness of their approach is that it cannot be easily adapted to suite a new problem.

Furthermore, [19] looked at diet assessment based on Type-2 Fuzzy Ontology and Fuzzy Markup Language. In [19], an ontology was developed by downloading nutrition facts of various kinds of food from the Internet and convenience stores. These facts were just general FNLGs and as such, the model was less useful to people. In [21], a hybrid model composed of a QPSO algorithm and LP for multi-objective nutritional diet decision making is presented. In this model, only three constraints namely price, disease and quantity restrictions were considered. These are not the only constraints implying that their model is not very useful in real life. Lastly, the authors did not incorporate highly targeted FNLG knowledge into their solution model.

On the contrary, a hydrid model of LP and GA is presented in [48]. This model only considered two objectives namely energy and protein in solving the MPP. Since these are not the only objectives, this model is far from being adequate because it does not incorporate highly targeted FNLG knowledge. Furthermore, their model was for nutrition decision making hence it was more suitable for healthy individuals. In contrast, [44] presents a counselling system for food or menu planning in a restaurant, clinic/hospital, or at home. This system did not incorporate highly targeted FNLG knowledge as evidenced by their suggestion that more nutrition facts must be added in the model. Also, their system was not adaptable to different FNLGs. In solving the MPP, [39] created ontologies to model food composition data, dietary reference values, and cuisine rules. However, their ontologies did not model specific FNLG knowledge for any disease.

Studies cited in the foregoing sections have one thing in common that is, they do not incorporate highly targeted FNLG knowledge as loosely coupled first-class concepts or structures. If a model incorportes FNLG knowledge as a loosely coupled concept, it means the model can incorporate FNLG knowledge from different disease and patient contexts. We are mainly interested in incorporating highly targeted FNLG knowledge in MPP models becuase it is believed that the greater the degree of FNLG knowledge incorporated in a model, the more useful to people the model becomes [39].

Even though no works characterised incorporation of highly targeted knowledge into MPP models, there were efforts to incorporate knowledge in the form user preferences into search and optimisation problem models. The incorporation of preferences [20], [34] and knowledge [18] for coping with computational complexity in methods of solving optimisation problems have been investigated mainly in the context of evolutionary computing approaches. In the literature, investigations have focused mainly on: (1) supporting only one of the two and not both simultaneously; and (2) knowledge that can only be gathered from results of intermediate steps [46] in the search for a solution while not providing for domain knowledge that cannot be cast into the class of user preferences, such as FNLG guideline knowledge in the case of the MPP.

7   Summary of Findings

Our results seem to suggest that, (1) most studies (21) used hybrid models and some of these models incorporate FNLG knowledge of some sort. (2) In some works that used hybrid models, the knowledge incorporated was not targeted to any specific disease or patient context. (3) In cases where, disease or patient contexts were considered, the models did not incorporate highly targeted domain specific knowledge in the form of specific FNLGs in their entirety as first class concepts and structures. (4) No study was done to solve the MPP for HIV/AIDS patients yet HIV/AIDS is a significant health problem in sub-Saharan Africa.

8   Implications of the Findings

Since there are no solutions to the MPP that incorporate highly targeted FNLG knowledge, especially in the area of HIV/AIDS nutrition therapy, this is a research gap that should be filled by developing a MPP model that leads to a solution that incorporates highly targeted FNLG knowledge about HIV/AIDS. Once national and international FNLG knowledge is incorporated into the solution in a loosely coupled and manageable way, it becomes easy to transfer knowledge from health experts to patients. A loosely coupled model has elements which do not depend on one another and it can accommodate different FNLG knowledge. This solution to the MPP will help dieticians, nutritionists, caregivers and even People Living With HIV and Aids (PLWHA) to make fast and improved decisions about nutrition which will improve health outcomes of PLWHA.

The implication for mobile applications for HIV/AIDS nutrition therapy in developing countries is that meal planning applications will facilitate transfer of knowledge from experts to patients. Fig. 6 presents an architecture that facilitates this knowledge transfer. This is achieved by incorporating FNLG knowledge in MPP models and then developing mobile applications based on the MPP models. In addition to that, PLWHA will easily, quickly and cost effectively access information about nutrition via mobile devices thereby improving their health.

9   Future Work

Today it remains less unknown how highly targeted FNLG knowledge can be incorporated into MPP models in a loosly coupled, flexible and customisable way. This makes the model flexible and easy to customise so that it can be used with different FNLGs. Further on-going work on our doctoral research project being undertaken at the University of Zimbabwe in collaboration with researchers at Massey University, New Zealand, and the Dublin Institute of Technology, Ireland aims at investigating a generic model for the MPP, which can result in easy facilitation of transference of FNLG knowledge from health experts to patients. The next steps in this research are:

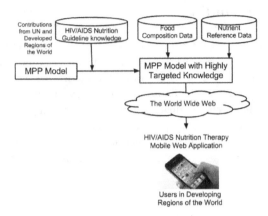

Fig. 6. The mobile web-based application conceptual scenario for HIV/AIDS nutrition therapy

1. Developing specific techniques for FNLG knowledge incorporation into computational formalisms and algorithms used by MPP models;
2. Developing a knowledge intensive, generic and customisable model of the MPP
3. Developing strategies and software engineering solutions for real uses of the model in HIV/AIDS nutrition therapy and
4. Application of the model in the mobile web-based context of developing countries to facilitate knowledge transfer.

10   Summary

This work focused on characterising the incorporation of FNLG knowledge into existing MPP models. The paper presented a characterisation of the MPP models which was subsequently applied to 31 works on MPP models found in literature. Our results seem to suggest that most of these works used the nutrition model, at least, in its basic form as well as either or both of the computational and mathematical models. It was also established that most works used the hybrid model and some models incorporated FNLG knowledge. However, in most works that incorporated FNLG knowledge, the knowledge was not targeted to any specific disease or patient context. In cases where, disease or patient contexts were considered, the models did not incorporate highly targeted knowledge in the form of full FNLGs as first-class concepts and structures that can be managed to allow problem-specific and regional customisation. No study has addressed this gap nor has any study solved the MPP for PLWHA, which is a significant health problem in Sub-Saharan Africa.

Acknowledgments. Ngonidzashe Zanamwe gratefully acknowledges the University of Zimbabwe who are sponsoring his research work.

References

1. Aberg, J.: Dealing with Malnutrition: A Meal Planning System for Elderly. In: AAAI Spring Symposium on Argumentation for Consumers of Health Care, American Association for Artificial Intelligence (2006)
2. American Dietetic Association. HIV/AIDS evidence-based nutrition practice guideline. Chicago (IL): American Dietetic Association. Technical Report (2010)
3. Bonissone, P.P., Subbu, R., Eklund, N., Kiehl, T.R.: Evolutionary Algorithms + Domain Knowledge = Real-World Evolutionary Computation. IEEE Transactions on Evolutionary Computation 10, 256–280 (2006)
4. Buisson, J.C.: Nutri-Educ, a nutrition software application for balancing meals, using fuzzy arithmetic and heuristic search algorithms. Artificial Intelligence in Medicine 42, 213–227 (2008),
http://www.intl.elsevierhealth.com/journals/aiim
5. Bulka, J., Izworski, A., Koleszynska, J., Lis, J., Wochlik, I.: Automatic meal planning using artificial intelligence algorithms in computer aided diabetes therapy. In: Proceedings of the 4th International Conference on Autonomous Robots and Agents, Wellington, New Zealand, February 10-12 (2009)
6. Eghbali, H., Eghbali, M.A., Kamyad, A.V.: Optimizing Human Diet Problem Based on Price and Taste Using Multi-Objective Fuzzy Linear Programming Approach. IJOCTA 2(2), 139–151 (2012)
7. Fields-Gardner, C., Campa, A.: Position of the American Dietetic Association: Nutrition Intervention and Human Immunodeficiency Virus Infection. J. Am. Diet. Assoc. 110, 1105–1119 (2010)
8. Fraser, A., Burnell, D.: Computer Models in Genetics. McGraw-Hill, New York (1970) ISBN 0-07-021904-4
9. Fratczak, Z., Muntean, G., Collins, K.: Electronic Monitoring of Nutritional Components for a Healthy Diet. In: Digital Convergence in a Knowledge Society: The 7th Information Technology and Telecommunication Conference IT and T, pp. 91–97 (2007)
10. Gaal, B.: Multi-level genetic algorithms and expert system for health promotion. PhD Thesis (2009)
11. Gaal, B., Vassnyi, I., Kozmann, G.: A Novel Artificial Intelligence Method for Weekly Dietary Menu Planning. Methods Inf. Med. 44, 655–664 (2005)
12. Kahraman, A., Seven, H.A.: Healthy Daily Meal Planner. In: Genetic and Evolutionary Computation Conference (GECCO) 2005, Wshington, D.C. USA, June 25-29 (2005)
13. Kaldirim, E., Kose, Z.: Application Of A Multi-Objective Genetic Algorithm To The Modified Diet Problem. In: Genetic and Evolutionary Computation Conference (GECCO) 2006, Seattle, WA, USA, July 8-12 (2006)
14. Kashima, T., Matsumoto, S., Ishii, H.: Evaluation of Menu Planning Capability Based on Multidimensional 0-1 Knapsack Problem of Nutritional Management System. IAENG International Journal of Applied Mathematics 39, IJAM_39_04 (2009)
15. Kennedy, J., Eberhart, R.: Particle Swarm Optimization. In: Proceedings of IEEE International Conference on Neural Networks, IV, pp. 1942–1948 (1995)
16. Kljusuri, J.G., Rumora, I., Kurtanjek, Z.: Application of Fuzzy Logic in Diet Therapy - Advantages of Application, Fuzzy Logic - Emerging Technologies and Applications. In: Dadios, E. (ed.), InTech (2012)
17. Kovasznai, G.: Developing an Expert System for Diet Recommendation. In: 6th IEEE International Symposium on Applied Computational Intelligence and Informatics, Timioara, Romania, May 19-21 (2011)

18. Landa-Becerra, R., Santana-Quintero, L.V., Coello, C.A.: Knowledge Incorporation in Multi-objective Evolutionary Algorithms. In: Ghosh, A., Dehuri, S., Ghosh, S. (eds.) Multi-Objective Evolutionary Algorithms for Knowledge Discovery from Databases. SCI, vol. 98, pp. 23–46. Springer, Heidelberg (2008)

19. Lee, C.S., Wang, M.H., Acampora, G., Hsu, C.Y.: Diet Assessment Based on Type-2 Fuzzy Ontology and Fuzzy Markup Language. International Journal of Intelligent Systems 25, 1187–1216 (2010)

20. Li, Z., Liu, H.L.: Preference-Based Evolutionary Multi-objective Optimization. In: Eighth International Conference on Computational Intelligence and Security (CIS), pp. 71–76 (2012)

21. Lv, Y.: Combined Quantum Particle Swarm Optimization Algorithm for Multi-objective Nutritional Diet Decision Making. IEEE 978, 4244–4520 (2009)

22. Maillot, M., Vieux, F., Amiot, M.J., Darmon, N.: Individual diet modelling translates nutrient recommendations into realistic and individual-specific food choices. American Journal of Clinical Nutrition 91, 421–430 (2010)

23. Mák, E., Pintér, B., Gaál, B., Vassányi, I., Kozmann, G., Németh, I.: A Formal Domain Model for Dietary and Physical Activity Counseling. In: Setchi, R., Jordanov, I., Howlett, R.J., Jain, L.C. (eds.) KES 2010, Part I. LNCS, vol. 6276, pp. 607–616. Springer, Heidelberg (2010)

24. Manat, M., Deraman, S.K., Noor, N.M.M., Rokhayati, Y.: Diet Problem and Nutrient Requirement using Fuzzy Linear programming Approach. Asian Journal of Applied Sciences 5, 52–59 (2012)

25. Mamat, M., Zulkifli, N.F., Deraman, S.K., Noor, N.M.M.: Fuzzy Linear Programming Approach in Balance Diet Planning for Eating Disorder and Disease-related Lifestyle. Applied Mathematical Sciences 6, 5109–5118 (2012)

26. Mamat, M., Rokhayati, Y., Noor, N.M.M., Mohd, I.: Optimizing Human Diet Problem with Fuzzy Price Using Fuzzy Linear Programming Approach. Pakistan Journal of Nutrition 10, 594–598 (2011)

27. Masset, G., Monsivais, P., Maillot, M., Darmon, N., Drewnowski, A.: Diet Optimization Methods Can Help Translate Dietary Guidelines into a Cancer Prevention Food Plan. Journal of Nutrition 139, 1541–1548 (2009)

28. Muessig, K.E., Pike, E.C., LeGrand, S., Hightow-Weidman, L.B.: Mobile Phone Applications for the Care and Prevention of HIV and Other Sexually Transmitted Diseases: A Review. Journal of Medical Internet Research 15 (2013)

29. Neuman, I., Mebratu, S.: Eastern and Southern Africa Regional Meeting on Nutrition and HIV/AIDS. Meeting report. UNICEF ESARO, Nairobi Kenya (2008)

30. National Food and Nutrition Commission (NFNC).: Nutrition Guidelines for Care and Support of People Living with HIV and AIDS. Technical Report, Republic of Zambia Ministry of Health (2011)

31. Noor, N.M., Saman, M.Y.M., Zulkifli, N., Deraman, S.K., Mamat, M.: Nutritional Requirements to Prevent Chronic Diseases using Linear Programming and Fuzzy Multi-Objective Linear Programming. In: ICCIT, pp. 565–570 (2012)

32. Pant, M., Thangaraj, R., Abraham, A.: A new quantum behaved particle swarm optimization. In: Keijzer, M. (ed.) Proceedings of the 10th Annual Conference on Genetic and Evolutionary Computation (GECCO 2008), pp. 87–94. ACM, New York (2008)

33. Pei, Z., Liu, Z.: Nutritional Diet Decision Using Multi-objective Difference Evolutionary Algorithm. In: IEEE International Conference on Computational Intelligence and Natural Computing (2009)

34. Rachmawati, L., Srinivasan, D.: Incorporation of imprecise goal vectors into evolutionary multi-objective optimization. In: IEEE Congress on Evolutionary Computation, pp. 1–8. IEEE (2010)

35. Rachmawati, L., Srinivasan, D.: Preference Incorporation in Multi-objective Evolutionary Algorithms: A Survey. In: IEEE Congress on Evolutionary Computation, pp. 962–968. IEEE (2006)

36. Regional Centre for Quality of Health Care (RCQHC):Handbook: Developing and Applying National Guidelines on Nutrition and HIV/AIDS. Technical Report, US-AID and UNICEF, Kampala, Uganda (2003)

37. Rusin, M.: Zaitseva. E.: Hierarchical Heterogeneous Ant Colony Optimization. In: Proceedings of the Federated Conference on Computer Science and Information Systems, pp. 197–203. IEEE (2012)

38. Schiex, T.: Possibilistic Constraint Satisfaction Problems or "How to handle soft constraints?". In: Proceedings of the Eighth Conference on Uncertainty in Artificial Intelligence (UAI 1992), pp. 268–275 (2013)

39. Seljak, B.K.: Computer-Based Dietary Menu Planning: How to Support It by Complex Knowledge? In: Setchi, R., Jordanov, I., Howlett, R.J., Jain, L.C. (eds.) KES 2010, Part I. LNCS, vol. 6276, pp. 587–596. Springer, Heidelberg (2010)

40. Seljak, B.K.: Dietary Menu Planning Using an Evolutionary Method. Electrotechnical Review 74, 285–290 (2007)

41. Seljak, B.K.: Computer-Based Dietary Menu Planning. In: Proceedings of the 7th WSEAS International Conference on Evolutionary Computing, Cavtat, Croatia, June 12-14, pp. 39–44 (2006)

42. Seljak, B.K.: Evolutionary Balancing of Healthy Meals. Informatica 28, 359–364 (2004)

43. Shi, Y., Eberhart, R.C.: A modified particle swarm optimizer. In: Proceedings of IEEE International Conference on Evolutionary Computation, pp. 69–73 (1998)

44. Snae, C.: Bruckner. M.: FOODS: A Food-Oriented Ontology-Driven System. In: Second IEEE International Conference on Digital Ecosystems and Technologies (2008)

45. Sundmark, N.: Design and implementation of a constraint satisfaction algorithm for meal planning. MSc. Thesis, Linkpings Universitet (2005)

46. Wagner, T., Trautmann, H.: Integration of Preferences in Hypervolume-Based Multi-Objective Evolutionary Algorithms by Means of Desirability Functions. Special Issue: Preference-based Multiobjective Evolutionary Algorithms, IEEE Transactions on Evolutionary Computation 14, 688–701 (2010)

47. Wang, G., Sun, Y.: An Improved Multi-objective evolutionary Algorithm for hypertension nutritional diet Problems IT in Medicine Education. In: IEEE International Symposium, vol. 1, pp. 312–315 (2009)

48. Wang, G., Bai, L.: Game Model Based Co-evolutionary Algorithm and Its Application for Multiobjective Nutrition Decision Making Optimization Problems. In: Wang, Y., Cheung, Y.-m., Liu, H. (eds.) CIS 2006. LNCS (LNAI), vol. 4456, pp. 177–183. Springer, Heidelberg (2007)

49. Yang, S., Wang, M., Jiao, L.: A quantum particle swarm optimization. In: Congress on Evolutionary Computation, vol. 1, pp. 320–324 (2004)

50. The Federal Democratic Republic of Ethiopia Ministry of Health. National Guidelines for HIV/AIDS and Nutrition in Ethiopia (2008)

51. Tsang, E.: Foundations of Constraint Satisfaction. Academic Press (1993)

Appendix: *The Characterisation of Knowledge incorporation into solution models for the Meal Planning Problem in the literature*

Cited Work	Target Disease/ Population	MPP Models	KD1 (NNK)	KD2 (NTK)	KD3 (TTK)	KD4 (HTK)
[1] Aberg (2006)	Malnutrition Among Elderly People	1. Constraint Satisfaction 2. Depth-First Branch And Bound Algorithm	×	√	×	×
[7] Gaál et al(2005)	Cardio-Vascular Diseases in Hungary.	1. Genetic Algorithm	×	√	×	×
[10] Gaal (2009)	Health Promotion,	1. Knapsack Problem 2. Genetic Algorithm	×	√	×	×
[42] Seljak (2004)	No Specific Disease	Fractional Knapsack 2. Genetic Algorithms	×	√	×	×
[14] Kashima et al(2009)	Lifestyle-Related Diseases in Japan	1. Knapsack Problem 2. Genetic Algorithm	×	√	×	×
[13] Kahraman et al(2005)	For Healthy People	1. Knapsack Problem 2. Genetic Algorithm	√	×	×	×
[41] Seljak (2006)	For Healthy People	1. Knapsack Problem 2. Genetic Algorithm 3. Baldwinian Repair Algorithm	×	√	×	×
[5] Bulka et al(2009)	Diabetes	1. Genetic Algorithms	×	√	×	×
[26] Manat et al(2011)	Diabetes and Cardiovascular Diseases in Malaysia.	1. Linear Programming 2. Fuzzy Objective Coefficient Using Linear Membership Function.	√	×	×	×
[37] Rusin et al(2012)	Diabetes	1. Linear Programming; 2. Ant Colony Optimization	×	×	√	×
[21] Lv (2009)	Health Promotion	1. Linear Programming 2. Quantum Particle Swarm Optimization 3. Bayesian Networks	×	√	×	×
[48] Wang And Bai (2007)	Nutrition Decision Making	1. Linear Programming 2. Nash Genetic Algorithm	×	√	×	×
[47] Wang & Sun (2009)	Hypertension for China	1. Linear Programming 2. Genetic Algorithm 3. Simulated Annealing	×	√	×	×
[31] Noor et al(2012)	Balanced Diet and Chronic Diseases in Malaysia	1. Linear Programming 2. Fuzzy Multi-Objective Linear Programming	×	√	×	×
[6] Eghbali (2012)	Human Diet	1. Formulated As Linear Multi-Objective Fuzzy Programming Problem 3. Fuzzy Programming	×	√	×	×
[13] Kaldirim & Köse (2006)	Health Promotion	1. Knapsack Problem; 2. Genetic Algorithm (NSGA-II)	√	×	×	×
[44] Snae & Bruckner (2008)	Health Promotion for Bangkok, in Thailand	1. Expert System Using Some Ontology	×	√	×	×

Appendix: *The Characterisation of Knowledge incorporation into solution models for the Meal Planning Problem in the literature*

Cited Work	Target Disease/ Population	MPP Models	KD1 (NNK)	KD2 (NTK)	KD3 (TTK)	KD4 (HTK)
[33] Pei & Liu (2009)	Nutritional Diet Decision Making for Asians.	1. Difference Evolutionary (Improved Version of GA)	√	×	×	×
[23] M´ak, et al(2010)	Nutrition and Lifestyle Counselling	1. Linear Programming 2. Multi-Level Genetic Algorithm	×	√	×	×
[3] Buisson(2008)	Diabetic Patients	1. Fuzzy Arithmetic And 2. Heuristic Search Algorithms	√	×	×	×
[17] Kov´asznai(2011)	Diet Recommendation	1. Case-Based Approach and Developed An Expert System	×	√	×	×
[39] Seljak (2010)	For People Without Specific Dietary Requirements In Republic Of Slovenia	1. Multidimensional Knapsack Problem (MDKP) 2. NSGA-II (Elitist Non-Dominated Sorting Genetic Algorithm)	×	√	×	×
[45] Sundmark (2005	Malnutrition Amongst the Elderly	1. Constraint Satisfaction Problem 2. Depth First Branch And Bound 3. Item-Based Collaborative Filtering For User Preferences.	×	√	×	×
[19] Lee et al(2010)	Diet Assessment in Taiwan	1. Type-2 Fuzzy Sets (*T2fss*) 2. Type-2 Fuzzy Ontology	×	√	×	×
[16] Kljusurić et al(2012)	"DASH Diet" (Dietary Approaches to Stop Hypertension)	1. Fuzzy Logic Modelling	×	×	√	×
[25] Mamat et al(2012a)	Obesity in Malaysia,	1. Fuzzy Linear Programming	×	√	×	×
[24] Manat et al(2012b)	For Eating Disorder And Disease-Related Lifestyle to Prevent Chronic Diseases	1. Fuzzy Linear Programming	×	√	×	×
[9] Fratcazak Et al(2007)	Obesity , Irish, Incorporated General Information About The Nutrients In The Utility Function	1. Knapsack Problem 2. Utility Function	×	√	×	×
[40] Seljak (2007)	Diet-Planning,	1. Knapsack Problem (MDKP) 2. Elitist Non-Dominated Sorting Genetic Algorithm (NSGA-II)	×	√	×	×
[22] Maillot et al(2010)	Nutrient-Based Recommendations For Each Individual In A French Adult Population	1. Linear Programming	×	√	×	×

A Quantitative Analysis of the Performance and Scalability of De-identification Tools for Medical Data

Zhiming Liu, Nafees Qamar, and Jie Qian

United Nations University
International Institute for Software Technology
Macau SAR China
{lzm,nqamar,qj}@iist.unu.edu

Abstract. Recent developments in data de-identification technologies offer sophisticated solutions to protect medical data when, especially the data is to be provided for secondary purposes such as clinical or biomedical research. So as to determine to what degree an approach– along with its tool– is usable and effective, this paper takes into consideration a number of *de-identification* tools that aim at reducing the *re-identification* risk for the published medical data, yet preserving its statistical meanings. We therefore evaluate the residual risk of re-identification by conducting an experimental evaluation of the most stable research-based tools, as applied to our Electronic Health Records (EHRs) database, to assess which tool exhibits better performance with different quasi-identifiers. Our evaluation criteria are quantitative as opposed to other descriptive and qualitative assessments. We notice that on comparing individual disclosure risk and information loss of each published data, the μ-Argus tool performs better. Also, the generalization method is considerably better than the suppression method in terms of reducing risk and avoiding information loss. We also find that sdcMicro has the best scalability among its counterparts, as has been observed experimentally on a virtual data consisted of 33 variables and 10,000 records.

1 Introduction

Interoperable electronic health records are one of the current trends characterizing and empowering the most recent Health Information Systems (HISs). With the advent of EHR standardizations, for instance, HL7 and *open*EHR [8], sharable EHR systems are now at the edge of practice. Notably, huge amount of patients' EHRs is being stored, processed, and transmitted across several healthcare platforms and among clinical researchers for online diagnosis services and other clinical research. Alternatively, the secondary use of de-identified data could be for instance in health system planning, public health surveillance, and generation of de-identified data for system testing [6]. However, if EHRs are directly made available to the public (i.e., without applying a de-identification technique), occurrences of serious data confidentiality issues are very likely to

J. Gibbons and W. MacCaull (Eds.): FHIES 2013, LNCS 8315, pp. 274–289, 2014.

occur. In reality, hospitals have confidential agreements with patients, which strictly forbid them not to disclose any identifiable information on individuals. Further to that, laws such as HIPAA [5] explicitly state the confidentiality protection on health information, where any sharable EHR system must legally comply with.

De-identification is defined [5] as a technology to remove the identifiable information such as name, and SSN from the published dataset so that the medical data may not be re-identified, even if it is being offered for a secondary use. Specifically, it is meant to deal with data privacy challenges by protecting the data under a maximum tolerable disclosure risk while still preserving the data of an acceptable quality.

One naive approach on confidentiality protection of patient's data is to remove any identifiable information (i.e., patient's name, SSN, etc.) of an EHR. However, adversary can still re-identify a patient by inferring from external information. A research [17] indicates that 87 percent of the population of U.S. can be distinguished by sex, date of birth and zip code. Such a combination of attributes, which can uniquely identify an individual, is defined as quasi-identifiers. More specifically, we can define quasi-identifiers as the background information about one or more people in the dataset. If an adversary has knowledge of these quasi-identifiers, it makes it possible to recognizing an individual and taking the advantage of his clinical data. On the other hand, we can find out most of these quasi-identifiers have statistical meanings in clinical researches. Thus, there exists a paradox between reducing the likelihood of disclosure risk and retaining the data quality. For instance, if any information of patient's residence were excluded from the EHR, it would disable related clinical partners to catch the spread of a disease. Conversely, releasing data including total information of patient's residence, sex and date of birth would bring a higher disclosure risk.

In recent years, several typical privacy criteria (i.e., k-anonymity [19], l-diversity [13], and t-closeness [11]) and anonymization methods (e.g., generalization, suppression, etc.) have been proposed. A detailed description on the formal definition of anonymity can be found in [16]. Based on these endeavors, a number of research-based de-identification tools (i.e., CAT, μ-Argus, and sdcMicro) now exist that offer data anonymization services to avoiding with the disclosure risks of patients' original data and other legal pitfalls. Each tool has its sample demonstration and even some of these have been applied on real datasets [21]. Nonetheless, these methods and tools lack in providing a sufficient evidence of their adoptability as well as usability. Thus, an experimental evaluation is dearly needed that could provide a systemic and directly usable analyses of these tools. The study should also allow choosing the most appropriate tool for de-identifying healthcare data such that any healthcare organization could know the efficacy of a tool before opting for it. To the extent of our knowledge, our conducted study is the first work that finds answers to such questions by examining the characteristics of a de-identification tool with respect to its ability to minimizing data closure risks and avoiding the distortion of results which is as much important as the de-identification process itself.

We propose an experiment on our EHR database to evaluate the performance and effectiveness of each de-identification tool. Then we find the most suitable tool for releasing EHRs by judging its capability of minimizing data disclosure risk and the distortion of de-identified data. To ensure meaningful quantitative analyses, we successfully borrowed a dataset from a local dialysis center in Macau SAR China, consisting of 1000 electronic health records. This moderate-size dataset could provide necessary quasi-identifiers for finding the possibilities of linking back an entry to the original patient even after applying a de-identification tool. Some contemporary and partly similar works include [6] and [9] that also evaluate such tools. However, most of these efforts target the technical details of the internal functioning and anonymization processes and methods such as [6], instead of providing insights on the usability and effectiveness of tools against re-identifiability of a published medical dataset. Another study [7] also summarizes some anonymization techniques. It discusses operations, metric and optimality principles of recent anonymization algorithms, and shows weakness of these algorithms through examples of different attack models. However, it does not provide a comparison of these techniques by means of quantitative analyses, or a criterion to follow, in order to find a best anonymization solution for a certain type of data.

Organization: In Section 2, we briefly introduce the experimented tools. Section 3 analyses the EHR database and then lists the potential quasi-identifiers. Section 4 introduces the design of experiment. Section 5 presents the results of our experiments. We also discuss the limitations of this study in Section 6. Section 7 draws some important conclusions and lists future directions.

2   State-of-the-Art Tools for Data De-identification

A number of research groups [14][20][22] are actively developing their de-identification tools, aiming to enabling their users to have more confidence in publicly-published dataset. They have adopted different approaches that reflect their particular interests and expertise. However, all these tools include a similar anonymization process in which a privacy criterion can be iteratively approximated. In this paper we include the following most stable tools.

CAT (Cornell Anonymization Kit). [22] is developed by a database group at Cornell University. This tool anonymizes data using generalization, which is proposed by [1] as a method that specifically replaces values of quasi-identifiers into value ranges. This tool also provides graphical user interface, which eases users' operations like adjusting parameters of a privacy criterion or checking current disclosure risk. Users can apply anonymization process iteratively until they obtain a satisfactory result. To ensure privacy criterion, users have to delete unsafe data manually. Therefore, there is no optimal principle implemented in this tool. In terms of usability, this tool presents contingency tables and density graphs between original and anonymous data, which implicitly offers users an

Table 1. Featuring the three de-identification tools

Tools	Input Data	Privacy Criterion	Anonymization Approach	Data Evaluation
CAT	Meta and microdata	l-diversity, t-closeness	Generalization	Comparison, Risk analysis
μ-Argus	Meta and microdata	k-anonymity	Global recoding, Local Suppression, etc.	Risk analysis
sdcMicro	Database	k-anonymity	Global recoding, Local Suppression, etc.	Comparison, Risk analysis

intuitive way to learn the information loss that caused during a de-identification process.

μ-Argus. [14] is part of the CASC project http://neon.vb.cbs.nl/casc/, which is partly sponsored by the European Union. μ-Argus is an acronym for Anti-Re-identification General Utility System. This tool is based on a view of safety and unsafety of microdata that is used at Statistics Netherlands, which means the rules it applies to protect data comes from practice rather than the precise form of rules. Besides handling the specific requirements of Statistics Netherlands, this tool also implements general methods for producing safe data. In particular, it supports de-identification approaches such as global recoding, local suppression, top and bottom coding, the Post RAndomisation Method (PARM), aggregation, swapping, synthetic data and record linkage, which enable a variety of selections to enhancing data security against some foreseeable re-identification risks. Users are allowed to apply their strategies through a graphical user interface and make adjustments upon an observation of the re-identifiable risk of the results. Privacy criterion is guaranteed by an automatic mechanism, in which unsafe variables in record are removed.

sdcMicro. [20] is developed by Statistics Austria based on R as a highly extensive system for statistical computing. Since R is an open platform, it offers a facility for designing and writing functions for particular research purposes. Like μ-Argus, this tool implements several anonymization methods considering different types of variables. Users are able to try out several settings of global recording method iteratively, while have a detailed look at each step of the anonymization. Since anonymization process is applied via scripts, all the steps can easily be reproduced. In addition, this tool provides functions for the measurement of disclosure risk and the data utility for numerical data.

Table 1 illustrates a preliminary summary of the similarities and differences of these tools, allowing an security specialist to have a better intuition of the techniques behind their automations.

3   Electronic Health Records of Patients

From an ongoing collaborative work with the Kiang Wu Hospital Dialysis Center Macau SAR China, we have implemented a software system for capitalizing on its electronic health records. Our acquired test database consists of 1000 EHR samples in which a total of 183 variables have been recorded.

De-identifying such a moderate-size dataset is considerably challenging since the de-identified data would always have a chance of re-identification attack, if published. Suppose that while responding to an organization's request asking for a published dataset on patients' infectious disease histories, the corresponding quasi-identifiers (already known by an intruder) can indirectly cause a disclosure of patient's information. An adversary could determine one of the quasi-identifiers referenced to a female born on 12/04/64, sent to Kiang Wu Hospital Dialysis Center last Friday, and living in Taipa (Macau) is exactly his neighbor. Then he could find out that his neighbor has an infectious disease history of HCV (i.e., an acronym for Hepatitis C). Even though the likelihood of such a scenario is relatively difficult but yet possible with or without using the automated re-identification attacks. For VVIP personalities such a leakage can bring about far more catastrophic results than for general public records.

Preliminaries: Here, we consider a subset of the combination of the following variables in the database: Gender, Date of Birth, Place of Birth, Province of Residence, and Zip Code as a set of quasi-identifiers. From now on we use the following abbreviations:

QID = quasi-identifier, ZC = zip code, DoB = date of birth,
YoB = year of birth, DoR = district of residence, PoB = place of birth

Given a quasi-identifier, a set of records which have the same values of this quasi-identifier is defined as an anonymity set; the number of distinct values of this quasi-identifier in the database indicates the number of anonymity sets; the number of patients who share a specific value of this quasi-identifier represents the anonymity set size k. Here, anonymity is the state of being not identifiable within a set of subjects, the anonymity set. We choose quartiles as a means of indicating the value distribution of the anonymity set size for each quasi-identifier.

Table 2 shows the statistical characteristics of anonymity set size k for various quasi-identifiers. The second column indicates the number of anonymity sets in our database for a given quasi-identifier. Generally, during the de-identification process, the larger the number of distinct anonymity sets, the less information distortion on the published dataset because the anonymity set tends to be smaller in that case and removing one affects only little on the overall dataset. The min and max values denote the size of smallest and size of largest anonymity set.

According to Table 2, it is clear that some quasi-identifiers lead to particularly high disclosure risks, because more than half of their anonymity sets are smaller than 2, which means a large portion of patients can be unambiguously identifiable by that quasi-identifier. For instance, for {ZC+DoB}, we can find that 'k=1' is

Table 2. Anonymity set size k for various quasi-identifiers

Quasi-identifiers	Numbers of sets	Min.	1st Qu.	Median	3rd Qu.	Max
ZC	38	9	20	25	31	51
ZC+gender	76	2	10	13	16	30
ZC+DoB	997	1	1	1	1	2
ZC+YoB	659	1	1	1	2	5
ZC+PoB	280	1	1	1	2	37
ZC+gender+YoB	804	1	1	1	1	4
ZC+gender+PoB	341	1	1	1	2	22
gender+DoB	998	1	1	1	1	2
gender+YoB	70	5	10	13	19	38
gender+DoR	14	55	62	72	77	91
gender+PoB	44	2	5	7	9	369
gender+DoR+PoB	191	1	1	2	2	67
gender+PoB+YoB	336	1	1	1	2	31
gender+DoR+YoB	398	1	1	2	3	11
gender+DoR+PoB+YoB	638	1	1	1	2	9

up to the 3rd quartile, which means at least 75 percents of the patients are unambiguously identifiable by zip code and date of birth. Also, some quasi-identifiers are weaker because their smallest anonymity set is more than 5, such as {ZC}, {gender+DoR} and {gender+YoB}. Overall, it turns out that quasi-identifier that contains date of birth, place of birth and year of birth are most identifiable.

We also found that the size of anonymity sets for which quasi-identifiers contain 'place of birth' has a significant increase between the third quartile and max value. It means that a relatively large group of patients converge to one characteristic. This is because most of the patients of Kiang Wu Hospital Dialysis Center are Macau citizens. Consequently, patients who were born elsewhere are of sparse distribution and more likely to be unambiguously identifiable by their {gender+PoB} or {ZC+PoB}. Table 2 also clearly shows that year of birth, a reduction of date of birth, increases the de-identifiability: the median anonymity set size for {gender+YoB} is 13, whereas for {gender+DoB} is only 1.

Table 3 shows the actual number of patients that belongs to those anonymity sets, for example, for {ZC+DoB}, only two patients can be found in anonymity sets that have $k \leq 5$. The larger the value in the columns '$k=1$' and '$k \leq 5$', the larger the portion of the patients that is covered by anonymity sets of small sizes, and the stronger the quasi-identifier identify patients. The number indicates that {ZC+DoB} is the strongest quasi-identifier, because almost all patients have $k=1$. However, zip code alone is a weaker quasi-identifier, because none of patients is in the first two columns.

Similarly, {gender+DoB} is a very strong quasi-identifier mainly because date of birth poses a significant privacy risk for nearly all the patients in our database. In this experiment, we replaced date of birth to year of birth before the experiment.

The numbers for {ZC+gender+YoB} indicates that 63.7 percent of the patients can be unambiguously identified by this quasi-identifier.
For {gender+DoR+PoB+YoB}, it shows that nearly half of the patients can be unambiguously identified.

Table 3. Number of EHR data per anonymity set size, for various quasi-identifiers

Quasi-identifiers	$k=1$	$k \leq 5$	$k \leq 10$	$k \leq 50$
ZC	0	0	9	949
ZC+gender	0	2	179	1000
ZC+DoB	994	1000	1000	1000
ZC+YoB	418	1000	1000	1000
ZC+PoB	199	294	309	1000
ZC+gender+YoB	637	1000	1000	1000
ZC+gender+PoB	237	333	664	1000
gender+DoB	994	1000	1000	1000
gender+YoB	0	10	188	1000
gender+DoR	0	0	0	0
gender+PoB	0	57	242	294
gender+DoR+PoB	90	294	304	542
gender+PoB+YoB	240	354	575	1000
gender+DoR+YoB	134	864	989	1000
gender+DoR+PoB+YoB	435	958	1000	1000

4   The Assessment Criteria

In order to assess the performance and effectiveness of the listed de-identification tools with our EHR database, we design our experiment of the following four main aspects.

1. Selection of Quasi-identifiers. Judging from Table 3, we found {ZC+gender +YoB} (denoted as QID^1) and {gender+DoR+PoB+YoB} (denoted as QID^2) are the most representative quasi-identifiers for this database (note that we excluded the quasi-identifiers that contained date of birth).

2. Selection of Privacy Criteria. Our comparison on the tools is independent on the parameter of selected privacy criteria. Specifically, the factors we think that affect the performance of a tool are its optimization algorithms and approaches. To ease our comparison, we provided k-anonymity for this dataset. In this experiment, we set the parameter k to 2, which means the minimum value of anonymity set size that is safe for QID^1 and QID^2.

3. Dimensions of Comparison. Three dimensions of comparison are identified. The first dimension is the individual disclosure risk of the published datasets regarding the above quasi-identifiers. An accurate measure in terms of the individual risk on a quasi-identifier was defined as the following formula [10].

$$\xi = \frac{1}{n} \sum_{k=1}^{K} f_k r_k \qquad (1)$$

For a quasi-identifier, f_k denotes the size of $k - th$ anonymity set of the database; r_k denotes the probability of re-identification of a $k - th$ anonymity set; K depends on which k-anonymity to be preserved (for 2-anonymity K=2); n denotes the total number of the records. A higher number indicates that the published database undergoes a higher probability of disclosing patient's privacy. Generally, individual disclosure risk is related to the threshold value. Suppose that a threshold r^* has been set on the individual risk (see formula (1)), unsafe records are those for which $r_k \leq r^*$. When threshold value is set to 0.5, it ensures the dataset to achieve 2-anonymity. Similarly, when it is 0.2, it requires the dataset to achieve 5-anonymity.

The second dimension is the information loss for the published datasets. A strict evaluation of information loss must be based on a comparison between original dataset and published dataset. A metric called *Prec* has been proposed by Sweeny [18]. For each quasi-identifier, *Prec* counts the ratio of the practical height applied to the total height of the generalization hierarchy. Consequently, the more the variables are generalized, the higher the information loss. However, *Prec* has been criticized not considering the size of the generalized cells. Also, it does not account for the information loss caused by suppression method. Another commonly used metric is DM* [3], which addresses on the weakness of *Prec*. But it has also been criticized by [12] because it does not give intuitive results when the distributions of the variables are non-uniform. Therefore, these two metrics are not suitable for this experiment.

As described in Section 3, for a quasi-identifier QID, the distribution of its anonymity set size (denoted as F (QID)) should be equivalent to the distribution of the values of variables in QID. If some of these values are modified in the anonymization process, it will have an impact on F (QID). Such an impact depends on the frequency of the modified values in total values. Therefore, it is feasible to calculate the information loss of anonymization by comparing F (QID) of original data and published data. Looking into Table 2, it is clear that the anonymity set size of {gender+PoB} (denoted as QID^3) and {gender+DoR+PoB} (denoted as QID^4) has a significant increase between the third and forth quartile than other quasi-identifiers. In other words, the individual disclosure risk has a significant decrease in the third and fourth quartile because the larger the anonymity set size, the safer the published data is. To simplify the results, we measure the information loss in terms of the slope of anonymity set size for each QID^3 and QID^4 in the third and fourth quartile.

The information loss for a quasi-identifier is:

$$\lambda = \frac{\frac{\partial R'}{\partial Num'}}{\frac{\partial R}{\partial Num}} = \frac{\frac{k(n+1)' - k(n)'}{Sum'}}{\frac{k(n+1) - k(n)}{Sum}} \tag{2}$$

Where $k(n)$ represents the anonymity set size at the n-th quartile of the original dataset, its primed version $k(n)'$ is the result of the published data; Sum represents the number of distinct anonymity sets in the dataset, its primed version Sum' is the number after de-identification. The above formula usually yields a positive value. A higher number suggests a higher information loss of the original dataset.

The third dimension is the scalability of these tools. A virtual dataset consisted of 33 variables and 10,000 records are used as a test case, which includes 4 numeric variables, 3 categorical ones, and the rest are plain-text. We construct this synthetic dataset by enlarging the sample dataset of μ-argus from 4,000 to 10,000 records, of which the additional 6,000 records are copies that randomly selected from the original dataset. Using this relatively large database, we evaluate the ability of these tools to deal with large data sets.

4. Principal Methods Used for De-identification. Although different methods for acquiring k-anonymity criterion have been implemented in these tools, we present here a broad classification depending on the main techniques used to de-identify quasi-identifiers. Specifically, we classify anonymization methods in two categories as follows: Generalization and Suppression, as proposed in [2]. Other methods, which randomly replace the values of quasi-identifiers (e.g., adding noise), distort the individual data in ways that often result in incorrect clinical inferences. As these methods tend to have a low acceptance among clinical researchers, we decided not to apply them to the EHR database.

Generalization: provides a feasible solution to achieving k-anonymity by transforming the values in a variable to the optimized value ranges referencing to the user-defined hierarchies. Particularly, global recording means that generalization is performed on the quasi-identifiers across all of the records, which ensures all the records have the same recoding for each variable.

Suppression: means the removal of values from data. There are three general approaches to suppression: case-wise deletion, quasi-identifier removal, and local cell suppression, where CAT applies the first approach; μ-argus and the sdcMicro applied the third approach. For the same affected number of records, casewise deletion always has a higher degree of distortion on the dataset than local cell suppression. In most case, suppression leads to less information loss than generalization because the former affects single records whereas the latter affects all the records in the dataset. However, the negative effect of missing values should be considered.

5   Experimental Results

Before starting our experiment, we indexed our EHR database into microdata and metadata. For instance, we mapped 7 identifiable variables in PatientRecord table to categorical variables, 1 to numerical variables, 9 to string variables and removed 18 variables that were either illegal to release (i.e., patient's name, SSN) or irrelevant to research purpose (i.e., time stamp, barcode). We also truncated the value of date of birth variable into year of birth.

We started by anonymizing our dataset using μ-Argus. First, we specified the combination of variables to be inspected as QID^1 and QID^2 with the threshold set to 1 (maximum value of anonymity set size k, which is considered unsafe). It should be noted that the individual risk model was restricted in μ-Argus because there was an overlap between the quasi-identifiers. Then the tool counted the number of the unsafe records that are unambiguously identifiable for each combination of variables. By following its user's manual, the first anonymization method we applied was global recoding. Specifically, 22 different values in place of birth variable were equivalently generalized to 8 categories; 35 different values in year of birth variable were generalized to 12 categories; the last digit of zip code was removed. As shown in figure 1, the number of unsafe records decreased from 637 to 0 and 435 to 252, respectively for QID^1 and QID^2. It is clear that global recoding significantly decreases the risk of re-identification on QID^1. However, for QID^2, 252 out of 1000 patients remain to be unambiguously identifiable.

After dealing with categorical variables, we found that micro aggregation method was not practical, because the minimum frequency of the numeric variable is far above the minimum requirement for safe anonymity set size. Then we applied local suppression method to protect the remaining unsafe records. This led to 75 values in gender variables and 121 values in place of birth variables suppressed from the dataset.

In what follows we used sdcMicro. Due to the character encoding issue on ODBC, we collated our dataset from Traditional Chinese to UTF-8, which resulted in character loss on some of the values in place of birth and district of residence variables. Then we used freqCalc function in sdcMicro to calculate the number of unsafe records for QID^2. The result shows that 411 records could be unambiguously identified by QID^2, contrast to 435 in Table 3, which indicates an inaccuracy deviation of 5.5% on QID^2.

Similarly, we first applied the sdcMicro function globalRecode to the dataset. It turns out year of birth variable generalized to the same 12 categories, which reduced the number of unsafe records to 244 and 254, respectively for QID^1 and QID^2.

Then the function localSupp could be used to apply local suppression method. Using the threshold value of 0.5 (to achieve 2-anonymity as mentioned in Section IV), localSupp was first applied to QID^1. This led to a suppression of 244 values in zip code variable and 20 values in year of birth variable. Again, calculating the number of unsafe records for this quasi-identifier, we found that the published dataset reached 4-anonymity and the maximum value of individual risk decreased to 0.143. For QID^2, we notice that most of the unsafe records has a

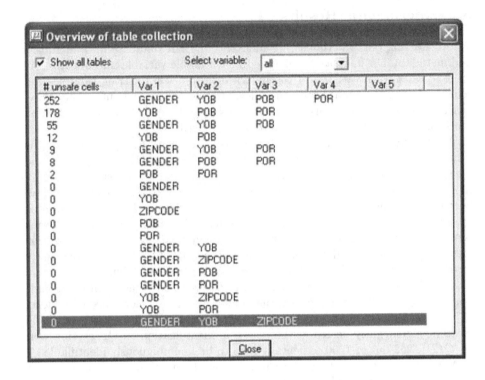

Fig. 1. An overview of unsafe records for various quasi-identifiers

re-identification risk over 0.89. With the threshold value to 0.89, suppression of 254 values in place of birth variable were done. We observed only 3 records with anonymity set size $k=1$. Then suppression (threshold value = 0.5) was applied, 3 values in district of residence variable were suppressed.

The left side of figure 2 shows the distribution of individual risk of the original dataset for QID^2, while the right side shows the result of the published dataset. It is clear that the maximum value of individual risk decreased from 1.0 to 0.5. After three suppressions were done, for each quasi-identifier, the dataset satisfied 2-anonymity.

The third tool is CAT. As the tool restricts one quasi-identifier per anonymization process, we specified two quasi-identifiers respectively. Since CAT doesn't provide k-anonymity directly, we choose t-closeness criteria instead. We first provided t-closeness criteria on the QID^1 with a threshold value t to 0.5, which means the maximum value of individual disclosure risk is 0.5. This led to generalization method applied to year of birth and zip code variables. Specifically, every ten values in zip code variable were generalized into one category, which addressed the same effect on the published dataset as a truncation of the last digit of this variable; every two values in year of birth variable were generalized into one category.

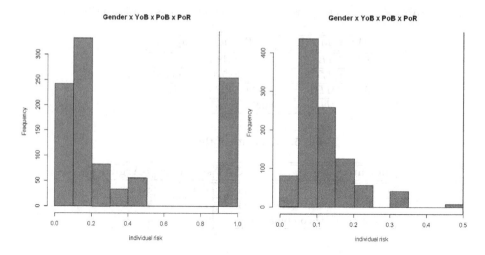

Fig. 2. The individual risk of the dataset for QID^2

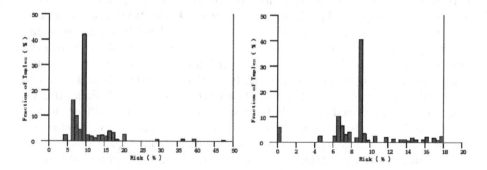

Fig. 3. The individual risk of the dataset for QID^1

As the left side of figure 3 shows, the current maximum value of individual disclosure risk is 0.5. After deleting 58 records, the maximum value decreased to 0.18. Looking into the right side of figure 3, which presents the distribution of individual disclosure risk of QID^1 on the published dataset, we found that less than 20 percent of the records have the risk above 0.1 and 2-anonymity was reached.

We then provided the t-closeness criteria with a threshold value t set to 0.978 on QID^2. This led to generalization method applied on year of birth variable, place of residence variable and place of birth variable. In particular, the values in place of residence variable were mapped into one category. The values in year of birth variable were equivalently mapped to 12 categories. The values in place of birth variable were equivalently mapped to 5 categories. After removing 57 records, the maximum value of individual risk decreased to 0.15.

Table 4. Two dimensions of comparison for various quasi-identifiers

Maximum level	CAT	sdcMicro	μ-Argus
ξ for QID^1	0.149	0.143	0
ξ for QID^2	0.402	0.500	0.384
λ for QID^3	3.600	2.028	1.682
λ for QID^4	86.631	3.261	1.783

Table 5. Scalability of three tools

Indicators	CAT	sdcMicro	μ-Argus
pass testcase	Yes	Yes	Yes
maximum vars in QID	4	33	5
maximum QID combination	1	6	5

For each quasi-identifier, these de-identification tools were able to publish the EHR dataset that satisfy 2-anonymity. We then analyzed the published datasets in terms of two aspects: 1) individual disclosure risk and 2) information loss.

Here we calculate the individual disclosure risk ξ of all published dataset using formula (1). Table 4 indicates that μ-Argus has produced safer dataset than the others, because it could protect patient's privacy under the lowest maximum individual risk for both quasi-identifiers. In particular, all records in the dataset produced by μ-Argus satisfy 2-anonymity for QID^1 as ξ equals 0. Following, we evaluated each published dataset in terms of their information loss λ (see formula (2)). Since CAT generalized all the values in the place of residence variable into one category, it led to a significant information distortion on QID^4. In contrast to CAT and sdcMicro, μ-Argus takes the lowest information loss for both quasi-identifiers to reach 2-anonymity.

Finally, we apply a virtual dataset of 10,000 records on these tools so as to evaluate their scalability. To compare the scalability of each tool, we first check whether it can load the test case. Then we examine the maximum variables in a quasi-identifier as well as the combination of quasi-identifiers. When evaluating maximum combination, we set the number of variables in a quasi-identifiers to the least maximum variables. Here, this experiment is carried out by a personal computer running the Windows 7 operating system.

As Table 5 shows, all three tools are capable of handling test case. For CAT, it can only handle one quasi-identifier at a time, which limits its scalability a lot. For μ-Argus, it has a limitation of its acceptance of variables of quasi-identifier. When exceeding its maximum, it fails with an error message which reports that the program ran out of memory (Note that this error is caused by the tool itself since memory resource is still adequate.) Since sdcMicro is able to handle 33 variables as a quasi-identifier and 6 combinations, we cannot observe its limitation using test case. Judging from Table 5, we conclude that sdcMicro has the best scalability among three tools.

6   Discussion on Results

Numerical methods are proposed to anonymize quasi-identifiers in order to avoid disclosing individual's sensitive information. However, not all these de-identifications methods such as masking were implemented in the discussed de-identification tools. Therefore, we are unable to report on the effectiveness of those methods on our EHR database. One of the constraints that our experiment has is the exclusion of a commercially available tool, i.e., The Privacy Analytics Risk Assessment Tool (PARAT) (http://www.privacyanalytics. ca/privacy-analytics-inc-releases-version-26-of-parat/, which is the only commercial product available so far. However, it has been reported that [4]) PARAT performs better than the algorithm implemented in CAT. Furthermore, PARAT, with its risk estimator, is able to produce more accurate de-identification results than the one incorporated in μ–Argus.

The results in this paper not only show the performance of the de-identification tools, but it also indicates the differences among tools based on the adopted algorithms to optimize the generalization steps. For instance, 254 values in place of birth variable were suppressed in sdcMicro, while all the values were generalized to 8 categories in μ-Argus. As μ-Argus generalized more variables than sdcMicro, it benefits from less records being suppressed and, thus, the statistical meanings of these variables can be preserved. This also shows a specialty of our controlled experiment that shows that the generalization method causes a lower information loss than suppression when the latter takes certain percent of the total records. Consequently, as applied to our EHR database, generalization method is more suitable than the suppression method.

For the purpose of comparison, we consider k-anonymity as the only privacy criteria that may lead to attribute disclosure problem on patient's clinical data. More considerably, no de-identification approach is being applied to clinical variables (i.e., infectious disease, blood type in PatientRecord table) leading an attacker to discover a patient's clinical information merely on finding a small variation in those clinical variables. Such an anticipated problem will also be resolved in the future development of our de-identification component for the ongoing EHR project. Likewise, identifying and implementing access control rules for external stakeholders accessing particular de-identified medical data is a complex task. Therefore, an appropriate access control and corresponding validation mechanism [15] must be placed to ensure better protection of any medical data to be offered for a secondary purpose.

7   Conclusion and Future Directions

This paper presented a rigorous assessment of the state-of-the-art de-identification tools that are available to researchers to publish datasets using anonymization techniques. The tools that have been evaluated, are CAT (Cornell Anonymization Kit), μ-Argus, and sdcMicro. We also discussed the significant features of each tool, their underlying anonymization methods, and the privacy criteria adopted.

Following, we analyzed the EHR database in terms of two categories: anonymity set size k and number of EHR data per anonymity set size for 15 quasi-identifiers. Our one of the important findings included that quasi-identifiers that contain place of birth and year of birth variables were the most identifiable. We selected two quasi-identifiers to be observed and anonymized. We also included two formulas, based on which the published dataset of each tool could be examined with respect to two dimensions: individual disclosure risk and information loss. For each tool, we outlined the anonymization process and provide 2-anonymity. Finally, we calculated the information loss and individual risk of each published dataset. As μ-Argus produced the safest records and caused the lowest information loss among these tools, it makes it more appropriate de-identification tool for anonymizing our EHR database. However, the study revealed that sdcMicro has the best scalability among three tools.

In this paper we evaluated the research-based de-identification tools dealing with structured data only. Before applying any of the de-identification tools, it is however important to know specific user requirements for de-identifying medical data. One of the future research directions includes investigating the de-identifications tools for unstructured data (e.g., clinical notes, reports, summaries, etc.), that we consider particularly relevant and usable for de-identifying legacy healthcare databases to avoid and mitigate data compromises.

Acknowledgments. This work has been supported by the project SAFEHR funded by Macao Science and Technology Development Fund. We are also grateful to the Kiang Wu Hospital Dialysis Center Macau SAR China, for their continuous support.

References

[1] di Vimercati, S.D., Foresti, S., Livraga, G., Samarati, P.: rotecting privacy in data release. In: 11th International School on Foundations of Security Analysis and Design, pp. 1–34 (2011)

[2] Emam, K.E.: Methods for the de-identification of electronic health records for genomic research. Genome Medicine 3(4), 25 (2011)

[3] Emam, K.E., Dankar, F.K., Issa, R., Jonker, E., Amyot, D., Cogo, E., Corriveau, J.-P., Walker, M., Chowdhury, S., Vaillancourt, R., Roffey, T., Bottomley, J.: Research paper: A globally optimal k-anonymity method for the de-identification of health data. J. Am. Med. Inform. Assoc. (JAMIA) 16(5), 670–682 (2009)

[4] Emam, K.E., Dankar, F.K., Issa, R., Jonker, E., Amyot, D., Cogo, E., Corriveau, J.-P., Walker, M., Chowdhury, S., Vaillancourt, R., Roffey, T., Bottomley, J.: Research paper: A globally optimal k-anonymity method for the de-identification of health data. JAMIA 16(5), 670–682 (2009)

[5] Fitzgerald, T.: Building management commitment through security councils. Information Systems Security 14(2), 27–36 (2005)

[6] Fraser, R., Willison, D.: Tools for de-identification of personal health information (September 2009), http://www.infoway-inforoute.ca/index.php/.../624-tools-for-de-identification-of-personal-health-information

[7] Fung, B.C.M., Wang, K., Chen, R., Yu, P.S.: Privacy-preserving data publishing: A survey of recent developments. ACM Comput. Surv. 42(4) (2010)

[8] Garde, S., Hovenga, E.J.S., Buck, J., Knaup, P.: Ubiquitous information for ubiquitous computing: Expressing clinical data sets with openehr archetypes. In: MIE, pp. 215–220 (2006)

[9] Gupta, D., Saul, M., Gilbertson, J.: Evaluation of a deidentification (de-id) software engine to share pathology reports and clinical documents for research. American Journal of Clinical Pathology, 176–186 (2004)

[10] Hundepool, A., Domingo-Ferrer, J., Franconi, L., Giessing, S., Lenz, R., Longhurst, J., Nordholt, E.S., Seri, G., Wolf, P.-P.D.: Handbook on statistical disclosure control (December 2006)

[11] Li, N., Li, T., Venkatasubramanian, S.: t-closeness: Privacy beyond k-anonymity and l-diversity. In: 23rd International Conference on Data Engineering (ICDE 2007), pp. 106–115 (2007)

[12] Li, T., Li, N.: Optimal k-anonymity with flexible generalization schemes through bottom-up searching. In: IEEE International Conference on Data Mining Workshops (ICDMW 2006), pp. 518–523 (2006)

[13] Machanavajjhala, A., Gehrke, J., Kifer, D., Venkitasubramaniam, M.: l-diversity: Privacy beyond k-anonymity. In: 23rd International Conference on Data Engineering (ICDE 2006), p. 24 (2006)

[14] Netherlands, S.: u-argus user's manual, http://neon.vb.cbs.nl/casc/Software/MuManual4.2.pdf

[15] Qamar, N., Faber, J., Ledru, Y., Liu, Z.: Automated reviewing of healthcare security policies. In: 2nd International Symposium on Foundations of Health Information Engineering and Systems (FHIES), pp. 176–193 (2012)

[16] Samarati, P., Sweeney, L.: Generalizing data to provide anonymity when disclosing information (abstract). In: PODS, p. 188 (1998)

[17] Sweeney, L.: Simple demographics often identify people uniquely. Pittsburgh: Carnegie Mellon University, Data Privacy Working Paper 3, 50–59 (2000)

[18] Sweeney, L.: Computational disclosure control - a primer on data privacy protection. Technical report, Massachusetts Institute of Technology (2001)

[19] Sweeney, L.: k-anonymity: A model for protecting privacy. International Journal of Uncertainty, Fuzziness and Knowledge-Based Systems 10(5), 557–570 (2002)

[20] Templ, M.: Statistical disclosure control for microdata using the r-package sdcmicro. Transactions on Data Privacy 1(2), 67–85 (2008)

[21] Templ, M., Meindl, B.: The anonymisation of the cvts2 and income tax dataset. an approach using r-package sdcmicro (2007)

[22] Xiao, X., Wang, G., Gehrke, J.: Interactive anonymization of sensitive data. In: Proceedings of the ACM SIGMOD International Conference on Management of Data (SIGMOD 2009), pp. 1051–1054 (2009)

Author Index